# Applying Quality of Life Research

## Best Practices

**Series editor**
Helena Alves, Department of Management and Economics, University of Beira
Interior, Covilhã, Portugal

This book series focuses on best practices in specialty areas of Quality of Life research, including among others potentially: community development, quality of work life, marketing, healthcare and public sector management.

In today's world, governments, organizations and individuals alike are paying increasingly more attention to how their activities impact on quality of life at the regional, national and global levels. Whether as a way to tackle global resource shortages, changing environmental circumstances, political conditions, competition, technology or otherwise, the far-reaching impact of decisions made in these and other areas can have a significant impact on populations regardless of their level of development. Many lessons have been learned; yet many are still to be realized. Across a number of volumes on diverse themes, this book series will address key issues that are of significant importance to decision makers and participants across all sectors. The series will be invaluable to anyone with an interest in applying quality of life knowledge in contemporary society.

More information about this series at http://www.springer.com/series/8364

Margareta Friman • Dick Ettema • Lars E. Olsson
Editors

# Quality of Life and Daily Travel

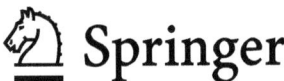 Springer

*Editors*
Margareta Friman
CTF Service Research Center,
Department of Social and
Psychological Studies
Karlstad University
Karlstad, Sweden

Dick Ettema
Department of Human Geography
and Spatial Planning
Utrecht University
Utrecht, The Netherlands

Lars E. Olsson
CTF Service Research Center,
Department of Social and
Psychological Studies
Karlstad University
Karlstad, Sweden

ISSN 2213-994X      ISSN 2213-9958   (electronic)
Applying Quality of Life Research
ISBN 978-3-030-09537-6      ISBN 978-3-319-76623-2   (eBook)
https://doi.org/10.1007/978-3-319-76623-2

Printed on acid-free paper

This Springer imprint is published by the registered company Springer International Publishing AG part of Springer Nature.
The registered company address is: Gewerbestrasse 11, 6330 Cham, Switzerland

# Preface

The purpose of this book *Quality of Life and Daily Travel* is to introduce and demonstrate the importance of daily travel in people's daily life. In doing so, we bring together distinguished researchers from a variety of academic backgrounds to provide conceptualizations and applications, presented as case studies, of what today is known to have relevance for daily travel and quality of life. The overall goal is to provide a broad understanding of the links between life satisfaction, well-being, and travel; the importance of commuting; and different evaluations and measures to assess the experience of commuting and quality of life.

This book should be of interest to specialists, including researchers as well as politicians and journalists, who have a professional need for knowledge on how travel can affect people's daily life. In addition, we hope that the book will attract practitioners such as transport planners, transport marketers, public transport authorities, and environmental professionals.

We thank all chapter authors and their coauthors for their contributions. They have fulfilled or exceeded our expectations leading to, as we think, an excellent coverage of most of the relevant research findings on travel behavior.

Karlstad, Sweden Margareta Friman
Utrecht, The Netherlands Dick Ettema
Karlstad, Sweden Lars E. Olsson
December 22, 2017

# About the Editors

**Margareta Friman** graduated in 2000 with a Ph.D. from the University of Gothenburg (Göteborg, Sweden). After having held positions as Assistant and Associate Professor at Karlstad University (Sweden), she was in 2010 appointed as Professor of Psychology at Karlstad University. For the last 10 years, she has been the director of the Service and Market Oriented Transport (SAMOT) Research Group at Karlstad University. In 2014, she received the Håkan Frisinger Foundation for Transportation Research Award by the Volvo Research and Educational Foundations. Today, Margareta Friman is conducting research in consumer psychology, environmental psychology, and transportation psychology at the Service Research Center (CTF), Karlstad University.

**Dick Ettema** graduated from Eindhoven University of Technology with a Ph.D. in Architecture, Building, and Planning. After working both in academia and consulting, he is now professor of Urban Accessibility and Social Inclusion in the Department of Human Geography and Spatial Planning in Utrecht University. His research focuses on how accessibility of cities and urban regions changes as a result of demographic, economic, societal and technological developments, and how this affects citizens' daily activity and travel patterns, social inclusion and well-being. Dick is editor of the *Journal of Transport and Land Use*, board member of the World Society for Transport and Land Use Research and director of the Urban Futures research program in Utrecht University.

**Lars E. Olsson** graduated from Göteborg University with a Ph.D. in Psychology of decision making. After a position as researcher at the Center for Consumer Research at the School of Business, Economics, and Law in Gothenburg, he was in 2009 recruited to the Service and Market Oriented Transport (SAMOT) Research Group. He is now Associate Professor of Psychology at Karlstad University. Lars E. Olsson has done research in the areas of sustainability, environmental behavior, consumer experiences, travel behavior, and well-being. His articles have been published in international journals in psychology, environmental studies, economics, and transportation.

# Contents

# Contributors

**Maya Abou-Zeid** American University of Beirut, Beirut, Lebanon

**Moshe Ben-Akiva** Massachusetts Institute of Technology, Cambridge, MA, USA

**Amit Birenboim** Utrecht University, Utrecht, The Netherlands

**Martijn Burger** Erasmus Happiness Economics Research Organization (EHERO), Erasmus University Rotterdam, Rotterdam, The Netherlands

**Melanie Crane** The University of Sydney, Sydney, Australia

**Graham Currie** Monash University, Clayton, VIC, Australia

**Jonas De Vos** Geography Department, Ghent University, Ghent, Belgium

**Alexa Delbosc** Monash University, Clayton, VIC, Australia

**Ahmed El-Geneidy** McGill University, Montreal, Canada

**Dick Ettema** Department of Human Geography and Spatial Planning, Utrecht University, Utrecht, The Netherlands

**Lesley Fordham** McGill University, Montreal, Canada

**Margareta Friman** CTF Service Research Center, Department of Social and Psychological Studies, Karlstad University, Karlstad, Sweden

**Tommy Gärling** University of Gothenburg, Göteborg, Sweden

Karlstad University, Karlstad, Sweden

**Charles R. Jonassaint** University of Pittsburgh, Pittsburgh, PA, USA

**Ronny Kutadinata** The University of Melbourne, Melbourne, VIC, Australia

**Sascha Lancée** Erasmus Happiness Economics Research Organization (EHERO), Erasmus University Rotterdam, Rotterdam, The Netherlands

**Fotis K. Liotopoulos** SBOING.net, Thessaloniki, Greece

**Patricia L. Mokhtarian** Georgia Institute of Technology, Atlanta, GA, USA

**Charles Musselwhite** Swansea University, Swansea, UK

**Zahra Navidi** The University of Melbourne, Melbourne, VIC, Australia

**Enrico M. Novelli** University of Pittsburgh, Pittsburgh, PA, USA

**Lars E. Olsson** CTF Service Research Center, Department of Social and Psychological Studies, Karlstad University, Karlstad, Sweden

**Ram M. Pendyala** Arizona State University, Tempe, AZ, USA

**Nicholas Petrunoff** The University of Sydney, Sydney, Australia

**Chris Rissel** The University of Sydney, Sydney, Australia

**Yusak O. Susilo** KTH Royal Institute of Technology, Stockholm, Sweden

**Dea van Lierop** McGill University, Montreal, Canada

**Ruut Veenhoven** Erasmus Happiness Economics Research Organization (EHERO), Erasmus University Rotterdam, Rotterdam, The Netherlands

Opentia Research Program, North-West University, Potchefstroom, South Africa

**Isabel Viegas de Lima** Massachusetts Institute of Technology, Cambridge, MA, USA

**E. Owen D. Waygood** Laval University, Quebec City, Canada

**Stephan Winter** The University of Melbourne, Melbourne, VIC, Australia

**A. Yair Grinberger** Heidelberg University, Heidelberg, Germany

**Fang Zhao** Singapore-MIT Alliance for Research and Technology, Singapore, Singapore

# Part I
# Introduction

# Chapter 1
# Quality of Life and Daily Travel: An Introduction

**Lars E. Olsson, Margareta Friman, and Dick Ettema**

**Abstract** In this chapter, we provide an introduction to the topic and a brief overview of *Quality of Life and Daily Travel*. A short background of why it is relevant to study travel and wellbeing, along with definitions and concepts related to quality of life research – such as objective and subjective outcomes, and hedonic and eudaimonic outcomes – will be followed by an overview of the chapters of the book arranged in three parts: theoretical perspectives and conceptualizations, case studies, and future directions. The aim of this book, *Quality of Life and Daily Travel*, is to compile current knowledge into one edited volume, where several areas of research are integrated – including traffic and transport psychology, transport planning and engineering, transport geography, transport economics, consumer services, and wellbeing research – in order to discuss the various facets of the links between travel and wellbeing. The importance of mobility, accessibility, experiences and emotions for the wellbeing of people will be highlighted.

**Keywords** Daily travel · Quality in life · Life satisfaction · Hedonic wellbeing · Eudaimonic wellbeing · Happiness · Subjective wellbeing

## 1.1 Introduction

In one of his Ted Talks, the late Professor Hans Rosling told a story of an extremely poor Sub-Saharan farmer and his family who saved money for a long time to finally be able to afford a bicycle. This new travel mode revolutionized their lives. His wife wouldn't have to carry water on foot the five miles from the well, they would be able

L. E. Olsson (✉) · M. Friman
CTF Service Research Center, Department of Social and Psychological Studies, Karlstad University, Karlstad, Sweden
e-mail: lars.e.olsson@kau.se; margareta.friman@kau.se

D. Ettema
Department of Human Geography and Spatial Planning, Utrecht University, Utrecht, The Netherlands
e-mail: D.F.Ettema@uu.nl

© Springer International Publishing AG, part of Springer Nature 2018
M. Friman et al. (eds.), *Quality of Life and Daily Travel*, Applying Quality of Life Research, https://doi.org/10.1007/978-3-319-76623-2_1

to start growing more crops in fields further away from home, he would be able to carry more produce to sell at the market, which would also take much less time to travel to, giving him more time for other chores. Things started to get better for the family, they gained a substantial increase in their life quality thanks to their new daily travel opportunities. The relationship between travel and wellbeing is rather obvious in this story. But, as will be shown in this book, the relationship between travel and quality of life is also apparent for people in more developed societies; not only through travel being a means of reaching important daily activities, but also as an important activity in itself.

The pursuit of wellbeing has interested researchers in many disciplines for decades, which can be seen in the starting up of several journals dedicated to this issue, e.g. the Journal of Happiness Studies, Applied Research in Quality of Life and Social Indicators Research. In transport research, no outlet has yet specifically been devoted to wellbeing, although some journals have published a number of articles on the topic over the past 8 years. The aim of this book *Quality of Life and Daily Travel* is to compile current knowledge into one edited volume, where several areas of research are integrated – including traffic and transport psychology, transport planning and engineering, transport geography, transport economics, consumer services, and wellbeing research – in order to discuss the various facets of the links between travel and wellbeing.

In the book, objective and subjective outcomes, as well as hedonic and eudaimonic outcomes will be discussed. It will highlight the importance of mobility, accessibility, and experiences for the wellbeing of people. Conceptualizations and applications of mobility in an ageing society, mode use, leisure trips, social exclusion, travel satisfaction and emotions will all be discussed by researchers from a variety of academic backgrounds. Case studies of what is known today to be relevant to daily travel and quality of life will be presented. In this introductory chapter, we provide a brief overview of *Quality of Life and Daily Travel*. In this introduction (Part I), a short background of why it is relevant to study travel and wellbeing, along with definitions and concepts related to quality of life research, will be followed by an overview of the chapters of the book arranged in three parts: theoretical perspectives and conceptualizations (Part II), case studies (Part III), and future directions (Part IV).

## 1.2 Background

Compared to 30 years ago, we travel more and further to take part in our daily activities, e.g. work, healthcare, social and leisure activities, and shopping. Work commutes have alone increased in length by 30%, to an average of 17 km, and today we spend on average about 40–80 min per day just on those trips (Frändberg and Vilhelmson 2011; Olsson et al. 2013). Children also travel further today to get to the schools of their choice, and to do other preferred activities (Andersson et al. 2012). In addition, the elderly population is growing and is projected to get even older over the next 30 years, approaching 2.1 billion in 2050 (UN 2015), while still being active and in need of transportation. To meet this demand, and create policies for future sustainable transport systems without reducing the life quality of people, a better understanding is needed of the relationship between daily travel and wellbeing (Ettema et al. 2014).

'Quality of life' (QoL) is often used as an umbrella term variously defined in dictionaries as: "The standard of health, comfort, and happiness experienced by an individual or groups" (Oxford Dictionaries), "The happiness, independence and freedom available to an individual" (Merriam-Webster Dictionary), or "The full range of factors that influence what people value in living, beyond the purely material aspects" (Eurostat 2015). The roots of QoL can be traced back to ancient Greek philosophy (McMahon 2008; Veenhoven 2016) argues, however, that a unified definition of the concept has never been agreed upon. This may include objective components such as health or wealth, or subjective components such as life satisfaction. Subjective components may furthermore be presented as hedonic or eudaimonic, where the hedonic defines wellbeing in terms of pleasure and pain, and the eudaimonic in terms of meaning, personal functioning, and personal growth (Deci and Ryan 2001). It has, however, been shown that measures of hedonic and eudaimonic wellbeing are moderately correlated, indicating both overlapping and distinct features, and that an understanding of wellbeing may thus be enhanced by measuring it in differentiated ways (Compton et al. 1996). There is also growing interest in the concept of health-related QoL (HRQoL), where both the objective and subjective dimensions of health-related experiences are taken into account when measuring health. Several scholars have applied the same line of reasoning to quality of life in general, arguing that combinations of measures would better measure and depict changes in life quality (Dolan et al. 2011). It has, for instance, been proposed that, in order to correctly assess and design policy, standard metrics of wealth and economic progress are valuable but should be complemented with wellbeing measures in order to better portray changes in life quality (Adler and Seligman 2016). Although most agree that no single measure would exhaustively capture the QoL of an individual or a society, the subjective factors of QoL have gained increased attention during recent decades.

Since 1972, the Himalayan Kingdom of Bhutan has been using measures of Gross National Happiness as a guide to policy design. It took almost 40 years for other national governments and international institutions to follow in their footsteps. In 2011, the United Nations adopted a resolution encouraging its member states "to pursue the elaboration of additional measures that better capture the importance of the pursuit of happiness and wellbeing in development with a view to guiding their public policies" (UN General Assembly Resolution A/65/309). The OECD has developed the Better Life Index to advocate for wellbeing in its 34 member states. In their guidelines, it is furthermore stated that, among other things, subjective wellbeing should be measured, which is defined as: "Good mental states, including all of the various evaluations, positive and negative, that people make of their lives and the affective reactions of people to their experiences" (OECD 2013).

For decades, happiness, subjective wellbeing, and life satisfaction have been the focus of economics research (e.g. Dolan et al. 2008), psychology (e.g. Diener et al. 1999), and sociology (e.g. Veenhoven 1984), with several reliable subjective measures having been developed to capture these (Diener et al. 1985; Dolan et al. 2011; Pavot 2008). Data from international panels has been collected over a number of years (e.g. Helliwell et al. 2012 [The Happiness Report]), and some nations have recently started to implement their own measures, e.g. in the UK, Japan, and Australia, in an attempt to comply with guidelines given by the UN.

There is an increasing interest in understanding how domain-specific contexts, e.g. consumption, improved schools, and public facilities, relate to the perceived quality of life (Diener and Seligman 2004). Studies looking at different life-domains and wellbeing in general have indeed found support for the relative importance of specific domains (Schimmack and Oishi 2005). Shimmack (2008) argues that domain satisfaction and life satisfaction are highly correlated even after controlling for shared method effects and the common influences of personality traits. He also stresses that this relationship is more due to the bottom-up influences of domain satisfaction on life satisfaction than the reverse. Thus, changes in domain satisfaction are likely to produce changes in life satisfaction. Travel has been argued to be one domain of relevance to general wellbeing (Ettema et al. 2010). This claim has indeed gained attention over the past decade, followed by publications of conceptual models and empirical research on the topic. This can be seen in scientific articles on mobility, accessibility, and transportation research looking into subjective, hedonic, and eudaimonic wellbeing and happiness, and their relationship with daily travel (e.g. Delbosc and Currie 2011; De Vos et al. 2013; Ettema et al. 2010, 2016).

The activity-based approach used in travel behavior research (Axhausen and Gärling 1992; Jones Dix et al. 1983) argues that travel is valued as it provides possibilities of engaging in important daily activities. It has been demonstrated that these daily activities are important for our wellbeing (Lyubomirsky et al. 2005; Jakobssson-Bergstad et al. 2011; Deci and Ryan 2008). For instance, Pychyl and Little (1998) measured individuals' wellbeing and activities whereby individuals engage and find positive correlations between personal and social meaning relating to their activities and life satisfaction, but also that stress associated with these activities adds to their negative emotional wellbeing. Similar findings have been reported by Oishi et al. (1999), who showed the positive influence on daily satisfaction of engaging in rewarding social activities. It has also been proposed that activities trigger positive or negative affect, e.g. feeling good, happy or stressed, and that activities help people to recognize their potential and to progress toward personal goals and growth (Deci and Ryan 2008; Waterman et al. 2008). From this, it follows that, if changes in a transport system affect individuals' opportunities for engaging in certain activities, this may influence their wellbeing. Due to urban sprawl, activities (destinations) are being spread more widely, leading to travel taking more time and playing a greater role in people's daily lives, which could potentially affect their wellbeing. Some scholars argue, furthermore, that travel should not only be seen as a means to an end (an opportunity to engage in activities), but also as an important activity in itself (Mokhtarian and Salomon 2001; Mokhtarian et al. 2001), an activity that can be experienced as positive or negative. In a conceptual model presented by Ettema et al. (2010), it is suggested that improvements to travel options, e.g. greater reliability and shorter travel and waiting times, will result in less stressful experiences, more rapid progress toward goals, and thus an increased level of subjective wellbeing. These findings have been supported empirically with respect to both life satisfaction and emotional wellbeing (Jakobsson-Bergstad et al. 2011; Olsson et al. 2013; Friman et al. 2017a, b). However, some researchers are calling for more research before such conclusions are drawn (see, for instance, Mokhtarian and Pendyala, Chap. 2 of this book).

We concur with previous research on quality of life, i.e. that it is a multifaceted concept that no single measure would exhaustively capture. With respect to travel and QoL, we specifically agree with Nordbakke and Schwanen (2014) when they urge that future work on wellbeing and mobility should consider the objective, subjective, hedonic, and eudaimonic dimensions, and be aware of the multiple ways in which wellbeing and its linkages with mobility may be context-dependent. The final section of this introduction will highlight the above-mentioned aspects in greater detail by giving a brief overview of the chapters included in the book, divided into three sections: i.e. theoretical conceptualizations (Part II), empirical case studies (Part III), and future directions (Part IV).

## 1.3   Contributions in the Book

### 1.3.1   Conceptualizations

Part II of the book consists of three chapters with theoretical perspectives and conceptualizations of different aspects of travel-related QoL. In Chap. 2, Patricia L. Mokhtarian and Ram M. Pendyala discuss the quality of life associated with a person's daily travel. Their chapter provides several useful insights into the conceptual differences between various short-term measures concerning transportation-domain-specific subjective wellbeing. Travel satisfaction is found to be directly influenced by five components of travel, in addition to socio-economic/demographic traits, attitudes, and trip-/travel-related characteristics. The authors provide the reader with an illustrative example by analyzing data from the American Time Use Survey. One of their conclusions is that travel does not necessarily generate moods that are all that different from those associated with other activities. After reviewing previous studies, the authors conclude that more research is needed to understand the extent to which travel satisfaction really affects, or is affected by, subjective wellbeing. Mokhtarian and Pendyala emphasize that timeframe, focus, the exclusion/inclusion of activities, the importance of other life domains, the five components of travel, and causal directions are all important aspects to be considered in future studies.

In Chap. 3, on conceptualizations, Tommy Gärling argues that previous research on travel satisfaction has largely failed to study both the feelings evoked by travel and, more specifically, how the residual effects of such feelings influence the experience of activities subsequent to travel. This chapter describes and discusses how travel-related feelings have been conceptualized and measured retrospectively.

Theoretical constructs developed in basic emotion research are presented and used as the basis for how travel-related feelings should be conceptualized and measured, emphasized by equations forming the logical arguments of a number of parameters of importance. Specifically, a theoretical model presented by Gärling states that evaluations of events evoke emotional responses, that emotional responses to events are stronger and more transient than mood, and that the influence of emotional responses on mood depends on the mood at the time the influence occurred. Numerical experiments quantitatively show how discrete events and continuous factors influence positive and negative mood during and immediately after travel. It is concluded that measurements of mood may be less susceptible to any biased self-reports that may be present in traditional travel satisfaction measures.

In the final piece on conceptualizations (Chap. 4), Alexa Delbosc and Graham Currie present, based on a thorough literature review, a conceptual framework of the relationship between mobility, accessibility, social exclusion, and wellbeing. They argue for the importance of taking both eudaimonic and hedonic outcomes into account in order to fully understand the relationship between travel and wellbeing. They reflect on where research has taken us today, identifying research gaps and where future research needs to focus. A discussion is presented regarding the difference between mobility and accessibility, and how this distinction is conceptualized in the literature on transport and wellbeing. They conclude that, to date, many hypothesized links between transport, accessibility, mobility, subjective wellbeing, and social exclusion remain relatively unexplored, providing fertile ground for future research.

### 1.3.2  Case-Study Applications

Part III of the book consists of ten chapters containing specific case studies. In Chap. 5, Sascha Lancée, Martijn Burger, and Ruut Veenhoven concentrate on commuting and happiness. They ask which ways feel best for which kinds of people? In order to answer this question, they review previous research and establish that it has mainly focused on the average effect of commuting. By collecting data using the Day Reconstruction Method, and creating travel profiles, they can show that there are considerable differences in happiness between different segments when commuting. In their chapter, they present optimal ways of commuting, considering happiness levels for different kinds of people, and it is concluded that there is no single way of commuting that is perfect for everybody. Based on this case from the Netherlands, they discuss and suggest an agenda for further research.

In Chap. 6, Viegas de Lima et al. develop a dynamic Ordinal Logit Model based on smartphone Future Mobility Sensing data from Australia, discussing estimation results in the context of Hedonic Theory. In their chapter, they indicate how different activity types (work, education, personal, discretionary, travel, staying at home, and other) affect individuals' experienced happiness. The results show that educational activities, followed by work and travel, are the most disliked, while discretionary activities, such as social activities, meals, and recreation, lead to more positive feelings of happiness. The model is then used to test for the presence of an intra-activity Hedonic Treadmill Effect, and it is found that people do remember their activities as being more neutral during later reports of happiness. This followed by a discussion about when, and for what reason, experiences and happiness should be measured.

In Chap. 7, Yusak O. Susilo and Fotis K. Liotopoulos present a case regarding how to measure door-to-door journey travel satisfaction using a cell phone application. They summarize lessons learned from designing, deploying, and analyzing the results of door-to-door, multi-modal, travel satisfaction in eight different European cities. The authors compare the results produced by the application with results that can be obtained by other methods. This is an interesting case that gives us in-depth knowledge of cell phone applications' advantages and disadvantages. One conclusion is that, although the application is attractive both from the respondents' and the surveyors' perspectives, the technical development process faces many weaknesses and difficulties.

In Chap. 8, Jonas De Vos looks into how travel satisfaction, defined as the mood during trips and the evaluation of these trips, can be affected by trip characteristics. By analyzing leisure trips in the city of Ghent (Belgium), the effect on travel satisfaction of trip characteristics, travel-related attitudes, and residential location is examined. Based on the results, it is argued that it is possible for satisfactory trips using a certain travel mode to increase the likelihood of choosing that mode again for future trips of the same kind, whether indirectly or through changes in attitude. It is furthermore argued that repetitive positively- or negatively-perceived trips might also affect longer-term wellbeing, e.g. life satisfaction, both directly and indirectly through the performance of, and satisfaction with, activities at destinations. De Vos highlights the fact that there might be a reverse causality between travel and life satisfaction, whereby people's life satisfaction is able to influence how satisfied they are with short-term activity episodes, e.g. satisfaction with leisure trips and activities.

In Chap. 9, Lesley Fordham, Dea van Lierop, and Ahmed El-Geneidy write about the impact of commuting on overall life satisfaction. This study is based on the results of the McGill Commuter Survey, a university-wide travel survey in which students, staff, and faculty describe their commuting experiences to McGill University, located in Montreal, Canada. Using a Factor-Cluster Analysis, it is shown that there is a positive linear relationship between trip satisfaction and overall life satisfaction. Cyclists and pedestrians have the highest trip satisfaction, being impacted most by their commute and reporting the highest overall life satisfaction. Modal outliers, those exhibiting lower trip satisfaction relative to other users of the same mode, report that satisfaction with their commute does not greatly influence their life satisfaction, also claiming to have access to and use fewer modes. Based on the results, the authors propose that building well-connected multi-modal networks, which incorporate active transportation, will improve the travel experience of all commuters (including current modal outliers) and, accordingly, overall life satisfaction.

In Chap. 10, Nick Petrunoff, Melanie Crane, and Chris Rissel present a case study of the relationship between quality of life, in the form of stress, and daily commutes to work by car and using active modes. While the authors acknowledge that the importance of travel satisfaction is increasingly being used as a measure of transport-related wellbeing, they argue that more emphasis should be specifically placed on stress as an important measure for further consideration as regards how we value travel and appraise transport options. The main study, which had the objective of evaluating the effects of the 3-year workplace travel plan on active travel to work, concluded that a workplace travel plan that only included strategies aimed at encouraging active travel to work achieved significant increases in active travel. More importantly, those commuting by active modes reported less stress than car commuters did. The authors conclude that too narrow a focus on transport satisfaction, when informing policy, is a limitation that disregards the larger benefits of active travel for quality of life.

In Chap. 11, Owen D. Waygood present an overview of how transport affects children's health and wellbeing. He summarizes previous research, showing that transport affects children's health and wellbeing in a multitude of ways through access to activities, through the mode used, and through the external impacts of others' transport choices. Child wellbeing includes impacts on children's physical, psychological, cognitive, social, and economic domains. The case, from Quebec City, shows that active and independent travel is positively associated with many measures of wellbeing. Also, the built environment cannot be ignored when it comes to securing children's wellbeing. When traveling, certain environments support incidental interactions, in turn being shown, in this case, to have a positive influence on children's wellbeing.

In Chap. 12, Amit Birenboim, Yair Grinberger, Enrico M. Novelli, and Charles R. Jonassaint present a case study of the potential for employing smartphone location tracking to investigate the association between deteriorating mobility during daily activities and the wellbeing of individuals with chronic disease. The locations of 36 patients suffering from sickle cell disease, a genetic disorder that affects the production of hemoglobin, were tracked continuously every 2 min using their smartphones to allow the calculation of movement parameters, e.g. walking and driving distances and speed. The results showed that the association between daily mobility parameters and physical and mental wellbeing (i.e. depression, pain level) were as expected, but mostly non-significant. There is some discussion that, while this could be attributed to the small sample of the study, it might also be the case that other indicators better representing the tempo-spatial context of human behavior should be considered in the future. In line with findings presented by Susilo and Liotopoulos (Chap. 7), they emphasize the potential limitations of mobile tracking devices.

In Chap. 13, Charles Musselwaith locates the need for mobility among the elderly in three principal motivational domains: i.e. utility (mobility as a need to get from A to B), psychosocial (mobility in relation to independence, identity, and roles), and aesthetic needs (mobility for its own sake), in a hierarchical structure. He presents case studies of the life with the car, and without the car of elderly people using public transport, of elderly people as pedestrians, and of elderly people receiving lifts from friends and family. Musselwaith also studies a group of elderly drivers who identify the extent to which the three levels of need (utility, psychosocial, and aesthetic) are met. The results of this qualitative case show that driving a car meets all three levels of mobility need. It is furthermore shown that transport provision without the car neglects psychosocial needs for mobility, and only sporadically meets aesthetic needs.

## 1.3.3   Future Directions

Part IV, the final section of the book, includes a concluding Chap. 14 by Margareta Friman, Lars E. Olsson, and Dick Ettema in which ideas and directions for future research are provided. Various interventions, as a means of counteracting mispredictions by the individual traveler and breaking travel habits, are discussed and illustrated. The authors elaborate upon what is known about individuals' predictions and their accompanying thoughts about possible consequences regarding wellbeing when performing a travel mode change. It is argued that one overall goal of every transport policy should be providing sustainable travel, accompanied by sustained or increased wellbeing. Friman, Olsson, and Ettema come to the conclusion that, while there is a vast amount of research on judgment and decision making, there is still a need for knowledge of how to aid people's judgments as regards switching to sustainable alternatives. Specifically, researchers are urged to unveil how to prevent a loss of, or support a gain in, wellbeing when switching to sustainable travel.

**Acknowledgements**   Financial support provided to Margareta Friman and Lars E Olsson for their work on this chapter was obtained through grant #43210-1 from the Swedish Energy Agency.

# References

Adler, A., & Seligman, M. E. P. (2016). Using wellbeing for public policy: Theory, measurement, and recommendations. *International Journal of Wellbeing, 6*(1), 1–35. https://doi.org/10.5502/ijw.v6i1.1.

Andersson, E., Malmberg, B., & Östh, J. (2012). Travel-to-school distances in Sweden 2000–2006: changing school geography with equality implications. *Journal of Transport Geography, 23,* 35–43.

Axhausen, K., & Gärling, T. (1992). Activity-based approaches to travel analysis: Conceptual frameworks, models, and research problems. *Transport Reviews, 12,* 323–341.

Compton, W. C., Smith, M. L., Cornish, K. A., & Qualls, D. L. (1996). Factor structure of mental health measures. *Journal of Personality and Social Psychology, 71*(2), 406.

Deci, E. L., & Ryan, R. M. (2008). Hedonia, eudaimonia, and well-being: An introduction. *Journal of Happiness Studies, 9,* 1–11.

De Vos, J., Schwanen, T., Van Acker, V., & Witlox, F. (2013). Travel and subjective well-being: A focus on findings, methods and future research needs. *Transport Reviews, 33*, 421–442.

Delbosc, A., & Currie, G. (2011). The spatial context of transport disadvantage, social exclusion and well-being. *Journal of Transport Geography, 19*(6), 1130–1137.

Diener, E., & Seligman, M. E. P. (2004). Beyond money: Toward an economy of well-being. *Psychological Science in the Public Interest, 5*(1), 1–31.

Diener, E., Emmons, R. A., Larsen, R. J., & Griffin, S. (1985). The satisfaction with life scale. *Journal of Personality Assessment, 49*(1), 71–75.

Diener, E., Suh, E. M., Lucas, R. E., & Smith, H. L. (1999). Subjective well-being: Three decades of progress. *Psychological Bulletin, 125*(2), 276–302.

Dolan, P., Peasgood, T., & White, M. (2008). Do we really know what makes us happy: A review of the economic literature on the factors associated with subjective well-being. *Journal of Economic Psychology, 29*, 94–122.

Dolan, P., Layard, R., & Metcalfe, R. (2011). *Measuring subjective well-being for public policy.* London: Office for National Statistics.

Ettema, D., Gärling, T., Olsson, L. E., & Friman, M. (2010). Out-of-home activities, daily travel, and subjective well-being. *Transportation Research Part A, 44*, 723–732.

Ettema, D., Friman, M., & Gärling, T. (2014). Overview of handbook on sustainable travel. In T. Gärling, D. Ettema, & M. Friman (Eds.), *Handbook of sustainable travel.* Dordrecht: Springer.

Ettema, D., Friman, M., Gärling, T., & Olsson, L. E. (2016). Travel mode use, travel mode shift and subjective well-being: Overview of theories, empirical findings and policy implications. In D. Wang & S. He (Eds.), *Mobility, sociability and wellbeing of urban living.* Berlin: Springer.

Eurostat. (2015). *Quality of life: Facts and views* (p. 2015). Luxembourg: Publications Office of the European Union.

Frändberg, L., & Vilhelmson, B. (2011). More or less travel: Personal mobility trends in the Swedish population focusing gender and cohort. *Journal of Transport Geography, 19*(6), 1235–1244.

Friman, M., Olsson, L. E., Ettema, D., & Gärling, T. (2017a). How does travel affect emotional well-being and life satisfaction? *Transport Research Part A: Policy and Practice, 106*, 170–180.

Friman, M., Olsson, L. E., Ståhl, M., Ettema, D., & Gärling, T. (2017b). Travel and residual emotional well-being. *Transportation Research Part F: Transport Psychology and Behaviour, 49*, 159–176.

Helliwell, J., Layard, R., & Sachs, J. (Eds.). (2012). *World happiness report.* New York: The Earth Institute, Columbia University.

Jakobsson Bergstad, C., Gamble, A., Hagman, O., Polk, M., Gärling, T., Ettema, D., Friman, M., & Olsson, L. E. (2011). Influences of affect associated with routine out-of-home activities on subjective well-being. *Applied Research in Quality of Life, 7*, 49–62.

Jones, P. M., Dix, M. C., Clarke, I., & Heggie, I. G. (1983). *Understanding travel behaviour.* Aldershot: Gower.

Lyubomirsky, S., Sheldon, K. M., & Schkade, D. (2005). Pursuing happiness: The architecture of sustainable change. *Review of General Psychology, 9*, 111–131.

McMahon, D. M. (2008). The pursuit of happiness in history. In M. Eid & R. J. Larsen (Eds.), *The science of subjective well-being* (pp. 80–93). New York: Guildford Press.

Mokhtarian, P. L., & Salomon, I. (2001). How derived is the demand for travel? Some conceptual and measurement considerations. *Transportation Research Part A: Policy and Practice, 35*, 695–719.

Mokhtarian, P. L., Salomon, I., & Redmond, L. S. (2001). Understanding the demand for travel: It's not purely 'derived'. *Innovation: The European Journal of Social Science Research, 14*(4), 355–380.

Nordbakke, S., & Schwanen, T. (2014). Well-being and mobility: A theoretical framework and literature review focusing on older people. *Mobilities, 9*(1), 104–129. https://doi.org/10.1080/17450101.2013.784542.

OECD. (2013). *OECD guidelines on measuring subjective well-being*. Paris: OECD Publishing. https://doi.org/10.1787/9789264191655-en.

Oishi, S., Diener, E. F., Lucas, R. E., & Suh, E. M. (1999). Cross-cultural variations in predictors of life satisfaction: Perspectives from needs and values. *Personality and Social Psychology Bulletin, 25*, 980–990.

Olsson, L. E., Gärling, T., Ettema, D., Friman, M., & Fujii, S. (2013). Happiness and satisfaction with work commute. *Social Indicators Research, 111*, 255–263.

Pavot, W. (2008). The assessment of subjective well-being. In M. Eid & R. J. Larsen (Eds.), *The science of subjective well-being* (pp. 124–167). New York: Guilford Press.

Pychyl, T. A., & Little, B. R. (1998). Dimensional specificity in the prediction of subjective well-being: personal projects in pursuit of the Phd. *Social Indicators Research, 45*, 423–473.

Ryan, R. M., & Deci, E. L. (2001). On happiness and human potentials: A review of research on hedonic and eudaimonic well-being. *Annual Review of Psychology, 52*(1), 141–166.

Schimmack, U. (2008). The structure of subjective well-being. In M. Eid & R. J. Larsen (Eds.), *The science of subjective well-being* (pp. 97–123). New York: Guilford Press.

Schimmack, U., & Oishi, S. (2005). The influence of chronically and temporarily accessible information on life satisfaction judgments. *Journal of Personality and Social Psychology, 89*(3), 395–406.

UN General Assembly Resolution A/65/309. *Happiness: Towards a holistic approach to development*. Retrieved from http://www5.cao.go.jp/keizai2/koufukudo/shiryou/5shiryou/s-1.pdf

United Nations (UN). (2015). *World population ageing*. New York: United Nations.

Veenhoven, R. (1984). *Conditions of happiness*. Dordrecht: D. Reidel.

Veenhoven, R. (2016). Happiness: History of the concept. In J. Wright (Ed.), *International encyclopedia of social and behavioral sciences* (pp. 521–525). Oxford: Elsevier.

Waterman, A. S., Schwartz, S. J., & Conti, R. (2008). The implications of two conceptions of happiness (hedonic enjoyment and eudaimonia) for the understanding of intrinsic motivation. *Journal of Happiness Studies, 9*, 41–79.

# Part II
# Conceptualizations

# Chapter 2
# Travel Satisfaction and Well-Being

Patricia L. Mokhtarian and Ram M. Pendyala

**Abstract** One approach to assessing the quality of life associated with a person's daily travel is to obtain a summary judgment of that individual's satisfaction with travel. Such a judgment could be considered a measure of the transportation-domain-specific subjective well-being (SWB). A number of such summary measures have been developed, including happiness, liking, pleasantness, a subjective valuation of the time spent traveling, and two different Satisfaction with Travel Scales (STS). In this chapter, we discuss some of the conceptual differences among these various measures, and review some key empirical results associated with them. In particular, we conceive of travel satisfaction as being directly influenced by five components of travel, as well as by socio-economic/demographic (SED) traits, attitudes, and trip-/travel-related characteristics. The chapter includes an analysis of data drawn from the well-being module of the 2013 American Time Use Survey (ATUS), to offer preliminary insights into how people feel about their travel episodes, differences in travel-related emotions across socio-economic groups, and how travel compares with other activities in terms of engendering feelings of well-being. We follow with a discussion of the relationship of travel satisfaction to overall well-being, and conclude with some brief reflections on the role of this research domain in our rapidly changing transportation milieu.

**Keywords** Activities while traveling · American Time Use Survey (ATUS) · Positive utility of travel · Quality of life · Satisfaction with travel · Service quality · Subjective well-being · Travel experience

P. L. Mokhtarian (✉)
Georgia Institute of Technology, Atlanta, GA, USA
e-mail: patmokh@gatech.edu

R. M. Pendyala
Arizona State University, Tempe, AZ, USA
e-mail: ram.pendyala@asu.edu

© Springer International Publishing AG, part of Springer Nature 2018
M. Friman et al. (eds.), *Quality of Life and Daily Travel*, Applying Quality of Life Research, https://doi.org/10.1007/978-3-319-76623-2_2

## 2.1  Introduction

Research suggests that travel experiences have consequential implications for well-being, with the effects being quite context-dependent. Travel for tourism purposes generally results in health and wellness benefits (Chen and Petrick 2013), while long distance (international) travel or commuting is often associated with feelings of stress (Waterhouse et al. 2004; Novaco and Gonzalez 2009). One approach to assessing the quality of one's travel is to obtain a summary judgment of one's satisfaction with travel; such a judgment could be considered a measure of the transportation-domain-specific subjective well-being or SWB (it could also be considered a measure of "remembered utility", which is a type of "experienced utility"; see Ettema et al. 2010; De Vos et al. 2016). A number of such summary measures have been proposed in the literature. In this chapter, we review and comment on a broad selection of those measures. To keep the scope manageable, we focus on measures that accommodate positive evaluations of travel,[1] and not those that only address negative aspects of travel, such as stress (Evans et al. 2002) or disgruntlement (Stradling et al. 2007).

In the remainder of this chapter, Sect. 2.2 reviews a number of travel satisfaction metrics, from conceptual as well as empirical standpoints. Section 2.3 presents a descriptive analysis of well-being-related emotions associated with travel and activity episodes in the well-being module of the 2013 American Time Use Survey (ATUS) data. Section 2.4 sketches some highlights from research on the influence of travel satisfaction on well-being (WB). Finally, Sect. 2.5 offers some concluding comments.

## 2.2  A Review of Travel Satisfaction Measures and Their Causes

### 2.2.1  An Overview of Conceptualizations of Travel Satisfaction

The travel satisfaction measures identified for this chapter can be loosely classified into three groups (for convenience, the bibliography is organized around these three groups, together with a fourth category to account for references not falling into one of these categories; some categories include some entries that are useful references but not mentioned in the text due to space limitations). First, there is a long history of

---

[1]This admittedly arbitrary choice for narrowing the scope is motivated by the positive orientation of the very concept of well-being (although of course one's well-being can also be adverse, just as a "satisfaction" scale can register a dissatisfied traveler), and by the desire to offer a partial counter-weight to the still-prevalent tendency, especially in engineering and economic fields, to view travel as entirely a disutility to be minimized.

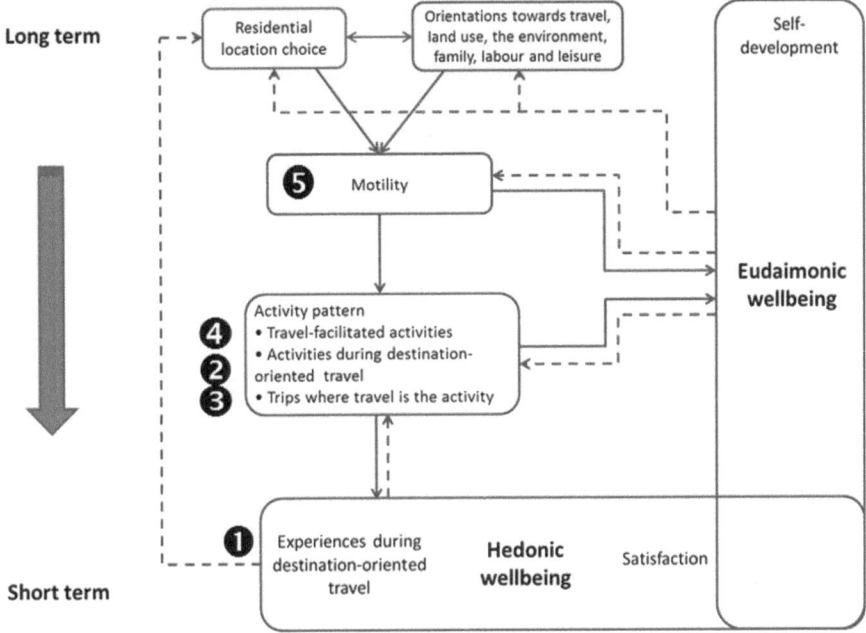

**Fig. 2.1** Five avenues of influence on travel satisfaction. The numbers have been added, to correspond to the discussion in Sect. 2.2.1 (Adapted from De Vos et al. 2013)

consumer-oriented industries measuring the satisfaction of their customers with the goal of identifying ways to improve their products and services. Among such industries, transportation service providers (notably transit operators) have devised a number of *service quality measures* over the years. Second and more recently, the *subjective well-being* literature has given rise to several scales intended to capture WB in the transportation domain. The third group contains a variety of *other summary measures* associated with an affective and/or cognitive evaluation of one's own travel. The boundaries between these groups are unavoidably blurry. For example, Olsson et al. (2012) applied a measure associated with the second group (the Satisfaction with Travel Scale) in a service quality evaluation (first group) context; we placed it in Group 2. Eiro and Martinez (2014) modeled satisfaction with one's current "mobility chain" involving multiple modes, but because they highlighted the public transit mode and positioned their research in the service quality context, we placed it in Group 1. Several studies linked their research to subjective well-being, but since their measurements of travel satisfaction were idiosyncratic or unusual, we placed them in Group 3.

A useful framework within which to place the travel satisfaction construct is offered by De Vos et al. (2013); see Fig. 2.1. Note first that De Vos et al. propose this framework to explain the influence of travel in general on overall SWB; we are suggesting that it can also be used to identify specific avenues of influence on travel satisfaction in particular. Note second that De Vos et al. appear to view travel satisfaction as primarily a short-term measure associated with hedonic well-being (HWB), but seem to allow for the possibility that it can be associated with eudaimonic well-being (EWB) also, and accordingly that it can apply in a longer-term sense. As a general principle, with respect to time frame, the measures of travel satisfaction discussed here can pertain to a specific recent trip, to a specific type (e.g., mode or purpose) of travel without a time referent, or to one's travel overall.

The figure suggests five specific components of, or avenues of influence on, travel satisfaction. We briefly define each of the components, roughly in order from shorter term to longer term (for reviews of the literature on each one, see De Vos et al. 2013; Mokhtarian 2017):

1. **Experiences during travel:** We distinguish this from the next component by suggesting that "experiences" are events or feelings that *passively happen* to the traveler, whereas "activities" refers to things *done by* the traveler. When the experience is a direct consequence of the activity, the boundary between the two may become indistinct, but some experiences, whether positive (a beautiful sunset) or negative (loud or aggressive strangers), occur involuntarily. Although not often considered in this way, the definition of this component could be broadened to include mode-performance and other trip-based attributes, naturally including traits such as comfort and safety, and less naturally but still somewhat logically including traits such as travel time, distance, and cost; presence of companions; and so on.

2. *Activities conducted while traveling:* Activities undertaken by the traveler can increase satisfaction with the trip (or [type of] travel), whether by enhancing the pleasure of a trip that was already enjoyable (taking photos of the passing scenery), diminishing the impact of negatives about the trip (listening to music to block out nuisances or to keep boredom or impatience at bay), or allowing the travel time to be used productively. Conversely, activities while traveling may decrease satisfaction, by diminishing the pleasure of an otherwise enjoyable trip (having to work instead of chatting with a companion) or magnifying the impact of negatives about the trip (increasing stress) (Shaw et al. 2018).

3. *Travel AS the activity:* Although perhaps not the dominant motivation for travel, it is sometimes undertaken for its own sake (for reasons such as curiosity, escape, the need to move/exercise, physical/mental therapy, mastery or exhibition of a skill, display of status, and so on; see, for example, Mokhtarian and Salomon 2001; Ory and Mokhtarian 2005). The resulting "autotelic" travel is often of a recreational nature (jogging, skiing, sailing, hiking, hang-gliding), but may also "masquerade" as ordinary daily travel (such as going out to eat primarily to "get out of the house" rather than to eat out per se). If the fulfillment of the motivation for traveling is successful, it can be expected to contribute positively to satisfaction, but experiences/activities while traveling may detract from satisfaction.

4. *Engagement in out-of-home activities:* This is the traditional reason assumed for traveling—the ability to conduct desired, but spatially-dispersed, activities (generally at fixed locations, as opposed to while traveling). From this perspective, the research interest may often lie in how the travel supports the activity rather than

the contribution of the activity at the destination (and/or origin) of the trip to travel satisfaction. Nevertheless, when travel satisfaction *is* the research focus, it is certainly possible for the activities at either end of the trip to affect how the trip itself is perceived.

5. *Motility:* This is defined as the potential, or ability, to travel, regardless of whether that potential is realized (enacted) or not (Kaufmann et al. 2004). A number of studies, often of the elderly, have confirmed that satisfaction is derived simply from *having the option* to travel.

Of course, the respective contribution that each of these five components makes to travel satisfaction is certain to vary by trip type, time scale, context, and other variables.

Beyond these five components, a number of other covariates with travel satisfaction have been identified, including socio-economic/demographic (SED) traits and attitudes, built environment attributes, and trip-/travel-context characteristics. As we present each category of satisfaction measures in the following subsections, we will sketch some key results associated with influences on those measures.

## 2.2.2  Service Quality Measures

Eiro and Martinez (2014) briefly review several scales designed to measure customer satisfaction with transportation service—predominantly public transit service. These scales include:

- the Service Quality Method (Parasuraman et al. 1985), and its refinements—the ServPerf index (Cronin and Taylor 1994) and Normed Quality Model (Teas 1993);
- the Customer Satisfaction Index (CSI; Hill et al. 2003) and its variant, the Heterogeneous Customer Satisfaction Index (HCSI; Eboli and Mazzulla 2009); and
- the Service Quality Index (SQI; Hensher and Prioni 2002).

Various modeling approaches have been used in this area, including linear, discrete choice, and structural equations models. Representative results include findings that satisfaction tends to be greater with more positive perceptions of mode performance, fewer transfers, a greater ability to do "extra tasks" on board, and being lower-income or less-educated (Eiro and Martinez 2014).

## 2.2.3  Subjective Well-Being-Based Measures

In view of the theme of this book, the group of travel satisfaction measures with the largest number of studies examined in this review is the group based on the subjective well-being (SWB) concept. Although we do not claim to have performed an exhaustive review, our intentional search of the literature identified at least 20 such studies appearing in the 15 years between 2002 and 2017, with the peak appearing to occur in 2013 (6) and 2014 (5).

Bergstad et al. (2011) introduced a Satisfaction with Travel Scale (STS), consisting of the average of five items, each rated on 7-point scales. To expand the incorporation of affective components, Ettema et al. (2011) devised a different STS, based on nine semantic-differential items rated on 7-point scales. Responses to these nine items are either summed across all scales to produce an overall rating, or summed separately across subscales to produce ratings of affect and cognitive evaluation. The latter scale has especially gained considerable attention, with a number of subsequent studies either adopting it or proposing modifications to it (De Vos et al. 2015).

Studies in this group often measure satisfaction for a broader set of modes than do those in the service quality-based group. The object of the satisfaction measure may be "daily travel" (Bergstad et al. 2011), the most recent leisure trip (De Vos et al. 2015), the commute trip (St-Louis et al. 2014; Ye and Titheridge 2017), the most recent tourist trip (Sirgy et al. 2010), and so on. A common theme (at least for the studies of local travel) among the findings is that users of active modes (walking and biking) tend to be most satisfied, while bus users tend to be least satisfied and car drivers fall somewhere in between (Gatersleben and Uzzell 2007; Ye and Titheridge 2017; Smith 2017; De Vos et al. 2016; St-Louis et al. 2014). Susilo and Cats (2014) report on a study noteworthy for involving more than 500 respondents across eight European cities. They found, ironically, that greater use of a given mode was associated with lower satisfaction with it. At least two studies have investigated the influence of the built environment on travel satisfaction, with mixed findings. Cao and Ettema (2014) found a significant impact of the built environment on satisfaction with daily travel, even after controlling for travel and location preferences, while Ye and Titheridge (2017) found that the influence of the built environment on commute satisfaction was completely mediated by its influence on commute characteristics.

### 2.2.4 Other Summary Judgments

A number of other studies have been conducted involving single or multiple measures representing summary judgments about one's travel. Again, the time scale involved can range from an individual trip to travel in general. We briefly describe the measures we have identified, and a few results:

- **Predicted satisfaction:** Whereas most or all of the other measures discussed in this chapter are based on reactions to actual current or past trips, some studies have asked respondents to predict how satisfied they think they would be with particular types of trips (notably public transit trips). For example, Pedersen et al.

(2011) obtained such predictions from 62 car users in Sweden, who then used public transportation for 1 month and reported *experienced satisfaction* during that period, as well as *remembered satisfaction* afterwards. Results showed no significant differences between predicted and remembered overall satisfaction, but significantly higher experienced satisfaction—suggesting a recall bias on the part of the study participants.

- *Liking:* Ory and Mokhtarian (2005) analyzed 1358 San Francisco Bay Area commuters who were asked to report how much they liked traveling in each of 13 categories (overall for short- and long-distance travel, plus for specific modes and purposes), on a 5-point ordinal scale ranging from "strongly dislike" to "strongly like". For all but three of those variables, the share of "likers" outweighed the "dislikers"; even the least popular type of travel, commuting, was liked or strongly liked by more than a fifth of the sample. Linear regression models explaining those 13 travel liking variables showed the relative importance of personality and attitudes, compared to objective travel amounts and SED traits.
- *Happiness:* In a novel methodological approach, Duarte et al. (2010) used cartoons to capture expected happiness as an explanatory variable in models of the choice between car and metro rail. For the most part, the happiness variables were extremely significant in the models, although it must be admitted that the goodness-of-fit appeared to be slightly better in a model not including those variables.

  For a mode-switching experiment in Switzerland in which habitual car commuters were given a free transit pass and "required" to commute by transit for at least 2 days in a given week, Abou-Zeid et al. (2012) also referred to their measure as capturing happiness. In their case, the measure was obtained by asking respondents to rate their satisfaction with their car commute (before and after treatment), on a 5-point ordinal scale from very dissatisfied to very satisfied. They found that satisfaction with car increased after the treatment (perhaps due to a shift in reference point), but the difference from the pre-treatment measure diminished to negligibility over time (suggesting a hedonic treadmill effect, or a return to a natural "set point"; Brickman et al. 1978).
- *Enjoyment:* Páez and Whalen (2010) compared the ideal (IT) and actual (AT) commute times of 1251 students at McMaster University in Hamilton, Canada, to create a measure they referred to as "enjoyment of commuting". Specifically, they defined the measure as

  R= (IT − AT)/AT, which, when expressed as a percentage, represents "the percentage increase or decrease needed in actual travel time (AT) to meet the ideal commute time (IT)" (p. 543). Among other results, they found greater enjoyment among those using active modes (walking or bicycling) to commute, those who intrinsically valued the commute, and those who were able to use their commute time productively.
- *Subjective valuation of travel time:* In addition to asking about satisfaction with the current journey, the National [Rail] Passenger Survey of Great Britain asked the respondent to choose whether "I made very worthwhile use of my time on this train today"; "I made some use of my time on this train today"; or "My time spent

on this train is wasted time" (Susilo et al. 2012; Lyons et al. 2016). Overall, more than half of the 19,715 respondents to the 2010 survey (54%) reported making some use of the time, and a substantial minority (30%) indicated making very worthwhile use of their time. Among other variables, these shares varied by trip purpose, ticket class, level of preparation (in terms of items brought by the traveler), sufficiency of seating, and age.

These studies have stimulated the inclusion of similar questions in surveys elsewhere. For example, Circella et al. (in progress) report on a survey of 2571 Northern California commuters, who were asked, "In terms of its *value to you*, how would you rate the time you spent on this recent commute?" (emphasis original), with responses obtained on a 5-point ordinal scale anchored by "mostly wasted time" and "mostly useful time". About half (49%) of the sample perceived their travel time as being somewhat or mostly useful, and only 20% saw it as being somewhat or mostly wasted. In another study (Frei et al. 2015), "riding the CTA is a better use of time/money than driving" was the most-often reported reason for choosing transit over driving or carpooling, offered by 59% of a sample of 336 train riders in Chicago.

• *Pleasantness and fatigue:* The 2007–2008 French National Travel Survey asked about the pleasantness and fatigue (both mental and physical) associated with a random sample of the trips made by its nationally representative sample of some 13,000 respondents (Mokhtarian et al. 2015). Only about 8% perceived the trip to be tiring (some of which still considered it pleasant), while fewer than 4% saw it as unpleasant and 46% considered it pleasant (with the remaining 51% rating it as neither of the two). These evaluations differed by socioeconomic traits and trip characteristics in mostly expected and congruent ways, but in several cases the same variable acted oppositely on pleasantness compared to its impact on fatigue—pointing to the need to account for both dimensions in fully assessing a trip's contribution to well-being.

• *Satisfaction with travel amounts:* Most studies of travel satisfaction focus on the *quality* of one's travel. However, satisfaction with one's *quantity* of travel is also important. Using the previously-cited sample of San Francisco Bay Area commuters, Choo et al. (2005) analyzed responses to questions about how much respondents wanted to travel compared to their current amounts, measured on a 5-point ordinal scale from "much less" to "much more" for ten mode-, purpose-, and distance-based categories of travel. Majorities of respondents were satisfied with their current amounts of travel for most categories, with exceptions being commuting (50% wanted to do it less or much less); and long-distance travel overall, for entertainment, and by airplane (with about 56%, 61%, and 59% wanting to do it more or much more, respectively). The authors classified the influences on these measures into categories such as complementarity, substitution, competing preferences, saturation, relative deprivation, and insatiability.

Etezady et al. (2017) asked an abbreviated form of this question in a 2016 survey of 1965 millennial and Generation X commuters and non-commuters in California as a whole. Specifically, respondents rated their satisfaction with their current travel amount (overall), on a 5-point ordinal scale ranging from extremely dissatisfied to extremely satisfied. About 70% of the sample was satisfied or extremely so, with little difference between commuters and non-commuters.

## 2.2.5   A Discussion of Semantic and Conceptual Issues

The preceding subsections have illustrated the diversity of ways in which concepts associated with travel satisfaction have been operationalized. The associated empirical results have exhibited a number of common themes, such as the relative satisfaction with active transport and dissatisfaction with buses. We believe it would be inadvisable, however, to indiscriminately lump all of the previously-defined measures into a single category and assume that they all measure the same thing.

Consider the *travel liking* construct, for example. At least as operationalized to date, this variable is less about one's travel experience for a particular trip, and more about one's general attitude toward travel in a certain category (although that attitude is presumably based on a body of past experiences). A *liking for* travel is not the same as *satisfaction with* travel—one can imagine being *satisfied* with an unwanted but necessary experience such as going to the dentist (it went as well as could be expected, or it wasn't as painful as was feared, or it was unavoidably painful but I had been told what to expect and I was satisfied that the dentist was competent and the staff were cheerful, doing everything possible to make me comfortable) while not particularly *liking* it.

Similarly, *liking* is not quite *happiness* either. The distinctions may be difficult to articulate, and can depend a great deal on how each construct is operationalized. But as a generalization based on the current travel-oriented literature, perhaps it could be said that *liking* has a somewhat forward-looking, anticipatory, and general sense to it, whereas *happiness* can have more of a present-looking, momentary, and specific connotation. For example, an individual may *like* a certain category of travel in general, and anticipate enjoying a trip in that category, but may end up *unhappy* when actually taking (and then remembering) that trip, due to idiosyncratic experiences associated with it.

Along the same lines, we have already seen that the same trip could be both *pleasant* and *fatiguing*, indicating that *fatiguing* and *unpleasant* are not at all synonymous. Similarly, experiencing a trip as (passively) *pleasant* is not the same as (actively) *liking* it, and saying that a trip *made me happy* seems like a stronger statement than saying it was *pleasant*, while saying it was *satisfactory* seems weaker. For that matter, saying it was *satisfactory* seems weaker than saying it was *satisfying*, which even more sharply illustrates the importance of semantic nuance. Similarly, "I am *happy* with my commute" (in which "happy" actually *does* function as a rough synonym to "satisfied") seems weaker than "my commute makes me *happy*".

In some cases, a given study will use multiple terms interchangeably. For example, as mentioned in Sect. 2.2.4, Abou-Zeid et al. (2012) referred to a *satisfaction* measure as capturing *happiness*, whereas we would again suggest that a trip to the dentist could engender the former but not necessarily the latter. Similarly, Páez and Whalen (2010, emphases added) called their $R = (IT - AT)/AT$ measure the *"enjoyment* of commuting", and implicitly equate it to *satisfaction* (p. 538 and throughout), but then add (p. 538), "or more accurately, a *desire to spend more time* commuting". We suggest that the latter designation is truer to the mathematics of the formula used, since we would expect commuters on *both* sides of $R = 0$ (the point at which the ideal has been achieved) to be dissatisfied, whereas R, the variable actually being measured, increases monotonically with $IT - AT$.

In short, there is considerable semantic ambiguity in the definition and application of the various travel satisfaction-related constructs we have identified. We suggest that future research could benefit from (1) an awareness of semantic differences as possible reasons for disparities in results across studies; (2) a purposeful choice among alternative metrics; and (3) a circumspection in language, i.e., a caution about constructs that may not truly be interchangeable. Of course, this is more easily said than done, and the present authors do not claim to be faultless in this respect.

## 2.3   Analysis of Episode-Specific Emotional Measures of Well-Being

Based on the discussion thus far, it is clear that the field is increasingly attempting to associate travel-related satisfaction with feelings of subjective well-being (SWB), recognizing that the extent to which individuals are satisfied with their travel experiences plays a potentially significant role in shaping their assessment of their overall well-being—and by extension, quality of life. As noted in the previous section, travel-related satisfaction may be measured and interpreted in a number of different ways. This section focuses on an analysis of momentary feelings of subjective well-being, which may be treated as akin to moods (affective balance) that people feel during travel (or any activity) episodes. Such momentary emotional feelings are likely to be related to, but are certainly not synonymous with, the degree of satisfaction that a person may derive from the activity or travel experience itself. On the one hand, we have probably all experienced being in a good mood for some completely unrelated reason, despite being in the midst of what would otherwise be an unpleasant trip or activity, and conversely been in a bad mood despite being in pleasant surroundings. On the other hand, the activity itself can invoke "mixed emotions"; for example, a vigorous run may induce feelings of tiredness and pain, but the activity may be extremely satisfying and actually enhance wellness and quality of life. Thus, we view these momentary feelings of well-being as very short-term measures of SWB, but the fact that they are measured in the context of specific episodes within well-defined time intervals means that, across large samples, we can expect them to provide some insights into the satisfaction associated with a given activity/travel type.

Accordingly, we present an investigation of momentary feelings of well-being associated with travel and activity episodes, as reported by respondents to the 2013 well-being module of the American Time Use Survey (ATUS) data set collected by the United States Bureau of Labor Statistics (BLS).[2] Respondents were asked to rate three random episodes from their time use diary on six different emotional measures using a seven-point scale (0–6). The six measures are: happiness, meaningfulness, sadness, stressfulness, tiredness, and painfulness. This data set allows an assessment of the momentary feelings of well-being that are associated with different travel episodes, and how they in turn compare with emotions associated with *other* activity episodes.

Table 2.1 presents average emotional ratings for travel episodes by mode of travel. Statistics are provided for a number of different socio-economic and demographic groups. A larger score implies a stronger feeling of a respective emotion. An exhaustive discussion of the statistics reported in the table is beyond the scope of this chapter, but a few patterns and trends are noteworthy. Younger individuals (18 to 34-year-old individuals are largely millennials in this data set) generally report lower levels of happiness for travel episodes by all means of transportation, except for public transit. This is consistent with the notion that millennials are generally more travel averse, but are more embracing of public transit than prior generations. This age group also finds travel episodes to be less meaningful, suggesting that this generation may be deriving meaningfulness from other pursuits and types of interactions. On the other hand, this does not necessarily translate to higher degrees of negative emotions for this age group; in other words, they don't necessarily find travel more painful or stressful than older age groups, but they don't necessarily derive the same level of happiness or meaningfulness from travel episodes either.

The difference in the make-up of trips between employed and unemployed individuals largely explains the differences in emotion measures between these two groups. A substantial fraction of travel for employed individuals is commute-related; on the other hand, unemployed individuals report travel for an array of purely non-work related purposes, including personal enrichment activities such as education, volunteering, caring for non-household members, and religious and spiritual activities. As many who are not employed also belong to the 55+ year age group, both of these segments depict higher average scores on the painfulness measure—this may be attributed to the higher prevalence of medical/dental episodes within their portfolio of activities.

Individuals in lower-income households report higher levels of happiness and meaningfulness for travel episodes, on average, when compared to individuals in higher-income households. They also report higher levels of emotion for the negative moods as well. In other words, individuals in lower-income households appear

---

[2]Similar data were analyzed by Morris and Guerra (2015), but (1) our analysis uses the 2013 sample whereas theirs uses the 2010 sample, and (2) our analysis focuses on presenting descriptive statistics, segmented by particular variables of interest, while theirs focuses on modeling the summary variable of affect balance.

**Table 2.1** Average emotional ratings for travel episodes by mode (2013 American Time Use Survey)

| Emotion | Travel by mode | 18–34 years | 35–54 years | 55+ years | Male | Female | Employed | Not employed | ≤$20K income[a] | >$75K income[a] | Weekday | Weekend | Sample size |
|---|---|---|---|---|---|---|---|---|---|---|---|---|---|
| Sample Size | | 1661 | 2564 | 2040 | 2941 | 3324 | 4417 | 1848 | 873 | 688 | 3195 | 3070 | 6265 |
| Happiness | Car driver | 4.34 | 4.34 | 4.63 | 4.34 | 4.53 | 4.40 | 4.54 | 4.45 | 4.28 | 4.32 | 4.56 | 4817 |
| | Car passenger | 4.62 | 4.75 | 4.96 | 4.61 | 4.85 | 4.77 | 4.80 | 4.80 | 4.76 | 4.69 | 4.83 | 986 |
| | Public transit | 4.20 | 3.79 | 4.22 | 3.97 | 4.12 | 3.83 | 4.53 | 4.21 | 3.45 | 3.93 | 4.28 | 139 |
| | Non-motorized | 4.36 | 4.50 | 4.48 | 4.34 | 4.56 | 4.35 | 4.58 | 4.33 | 4.26 | 4.32 | 4.56 | 286 |
| Meaningfulness | Car driver | 3.67 | 4.01 | 4.34 | 3.95 | 4.12 | 3.95 | 4.27 | 4.27 | 3.63 | 3.95 | 4.13 | 4784 |
| | Car passenger | 3.99 | 4.46 | 4.76 | 4.34 | 4.45 | 4.37 | 4.48 | 4.54 | 4.27 | 4.56 | 4.35 | 978 |
| | Public transit | 3.04 | 3.81 | 4.68 | 3.52 | 4.04 | 3.25 | 5.05 | 3.71 | 2.30 | 3.88 | 3.68 | 138 |
| | Non-motorized | 3.76 | 4.31 | 4.21 | 3.89 | 4.27 | 3.95 | 4.23 | 4.24 | 3.95 | 4.02 | 4.10 | 285 |
| Sadness | Car driver | 0.44 | 0.54 | 0.52 | 0.50 | 0.52 | 0.50 | 0.56 | 0.69 | 0.38 | 0.52 | 0.50 | 4829 |
| | Car passenger | 0.40 | 0.50 | 0.63 | 0.52 | 0.51 | 0.39 | 0.65 | 0.43 | 0.44 | 0.62 | 0.46 | 988 |
| | Public transit | 0.76 | 1.06 | 0.98 | 0.92 | 0.95 | 0.93 | 0.96 | 1.00 | 1.00 | 1.00 | 0.81 | 141 |
| | Non-motorized | 0.72 | 0.71 | 0.49 | 0.73 | 0.58 | 0.68 | 0.63 | 1.12 | 0.64 | 0.70 | 0.63 | 288 |
| Stressfulness | Car driver | 1.42 | 1.43 | 1.00 | 1.18 | 1.40 | 1.32 | 1.19 | 1.40 | 1.40 | 1.44 | 1.12 | 4832 |
| | Car passenger | 1.15 | 1.23 | 1.03 | 1.07 | 1.16 | 1.05 | 1.23 | 1.09 | 1.04 | 1.40 | 0.99 | 990 |
| | Public transit | 1.69 | 1.89 | 1.12 | 1.53 | 1.63 | 1.66 | 1.44 | 2.00 | 1.80 | 1.69 | 1.38 | 141 |
| | Non-motorized | 1.49 | 1.38 | 1.00 | 1.43 | 1.20 | 1.36 | 1.29 | 1.88 | 1.31 | 1.36 | 1.30 | 288 |

| | | | | | | | | | | | | |
|---|---|---|---|---|---|---|---|---|---|---|---|---|
| Tiredness | Car driver | 2.30 | 2.06 | 1.61 | 1.82 | 2.14 | 2.09 | 1.64 | 2.28 | 1.88 | 2.11 | 1.83 | 4831 |
| | Car passenger | 2.45 | 2.25 | 1.97 | 1.99 | 2.29 | 2.42 | 1.96 | 2.55 | 2.55 | 2.36 | 2.12 | 987 |
| | Public transit | 2.84 | 2.92 | 1.63 | 2.16 | 2.77 | 2.78 | 1.91 | 2.86 | 2.25 | 2.48 | 2.55 | 141 |
| | Non-motorized | 2.29 | 2.19 | 1.70 | 2.15 | 2.06 | 2.18 | 2.01 | 2.29 | 2.08 | 2.24 | 1.97 | 288 |
| Painfulness | Car driver | 0.53 | 0.77 | 0.79 | 0.70 | 0.74 | 0.64 | 0.95 | 0.74 | 0.43 | 0.74 | 0.69 | 4832 |
| | Car passenger | 0.56 | 0.89 | 1.27 | 0.93 | 0.93 | 0.69 | 1.20 | 0.77 | 0.72 | 1.16 | 0.80 | 992 |
| | Public transit | 0.40 | 0.92 | 1.49 | 0.87 | 0.96 | 0.65 | 1.50 | 0.86 | 0.65 | 0.97 | 0.83 | 139 |
| | Non-motorized | 0.59 | 0.83 | 1.46 | 0.93 | 0.83 | 0.58 | 1.38 | 0.74 | 0.56 | 0.98 | 0.79 | 288 |

Note: Scores are averages based on a scale of 0–6 with a higher score implying a greater degree of the emotion
[a]Computed only on valid cases with no missing income information

to experience a greater range in their feelings of well-being, both in positive and in negative ways, than those in higher-income households. Individuals in lower-income households report greater levels of pain, stress, and tiredness than their higher-income counterparts; this is, at least in part, explained by the fact that individuals in lower-income households are more likely to use alternative (non-car-driver) modes of transport. The use of such modes may entail greater levels of physical exertion and stress on the part of the individual. As expected, weekend travel episodes offer greater levels of happiness and lower levels of the negative emotions, largely owing to the greater prevalence of discretionary leisure activities on those days of the week (but are not necessarily all that more meaningful; weekday travel, which exhibits a high degree of work- and school-related travel, offers levels of meaningfulness similar to those of weekend travel except in the case of car-driver travel episodes—presumably because of the arduousness of commuting as a driver).

Comparison across modes suggests that the car passenger mode generally engenders greater feelings of happiness than other modes of transportation. Consistent with research cited in Sect. 2.2.3, public transit is found to provide the lowest ratings on the positive emotions and some of the highest ratings on the negative emotions. In other words, except for a few instances, travel by public transit is seen as less pleasant than travel by other modes of transportation. From a happiness standpoint, traveling as a car passenger depicts the highest scores, suggesting that being free of the guidance and navigation task and in the company of others while traveling engenders stronger feelings of happiness than traveling by other modes. This may at least partially explain the success of new mobility-on-demand services that may be hailed using mobile app platforms. The same is largely true for the meaningfulness emotion. Similarly, car passengers report the lowest levels of sadness. On the other hand, they do report slightly higher levels on the pain scale; this may reflect a selection effect, in that people in pain may be less able to drive themselves, walk/bike, or even take transit. Non-motorized travel is associated with lowest levels of tiredness, suggesting that leisurely strolls are seen as relaxing. Across all four negative emotions, however, tiredness is rated the highest regardless of mode, suggesting that people do experience some level of fatigue as they expend energy (physical and mental) in accomplishing travel episodes. The lowest average scores are associated with the sadness and painfulness measures, suggesting that individuals feel these emotions only to a small degree in the context of travel.

Table 2.2 presents the happiness rating for activity episodes by type and location of activity (outside home or inside home). In the interest of brevity, average emotional ratings are not presented for every one of the six mood indicators for all activity types. Also, detailed activity purposes coded in the lexicon of the American Time Use Survey were aggregated into fewer categories for purposes of this analysis. The categorization adopted in this chapter is as follows:

- *Personal and Household Maintenance:* Personal care, professional and personal care services, caring for and helping household members, household activities, household services, government services, and civic obligations
- *Eat Meal:* Eating and drinking

**Table 2.2** Average happiness scores by activity type (2013 American Time Use Survey)

| Activity category | Location | 18–34 years | 35–54 years | 55+ years | Male | Female | Employed | Not employed | ≤$20K income[a] | >$75K income[a] | Weekday | Weekend | Sample size |
|---|---|---|---|---|---|---|---|---|---|---|---|---|---|
| Personal and household maintenance | Out-of-home | 4.42 | 4.38 | 4.43 | 4.39 | 4.42 | 4.42 | 4.38 | 4.54 | 4.31 | 4.35 | 4.47 | 858 |
| | In-home | 4.47 | 4.26 | 4.26 | 4.26 | 4.32 | 4.28 | 4.33 | 4.28 | 4.19 | 4.30 | 4.31 | 6093 |
| | Sample size | 1519 | 2773 | 2659 | 2333 | 4618 | 3898 | 3053 | 794 | 617 | 3508 | 3443 | 6951 |
| Eat meal | Out-of-home | 4.62 | 4.64 | 4.94 | 4.58 | 4.89 | 4.63 | 5.08 | 4.82 | 4.54 | 4.58 | 4.90 | 1205 |
| | In-home | 4.65 | 4.54 | 4.48 | 4.46 | 4.60 | 4.61 | 4.45 | 4.56 | 4.64 | 4.46 | 4.60 | 3260 |
| | Sample size | 982 | 1625 | 1858 | 2146 | 2319 | 2646 | 1819 | 555 | 418 | 2178 | 2287 | 4465 |
| Social/recreational | Out-of-home | 4.72 | 4.73 | 5.05 | 4.75 | 4.92 | 4.72 | 5.07 | 4.82 | 4.65 | 4.71 | 4.93 | 1581 |
| | In-home | 4.47 | 4.31 | 4.34 | 4.27 | 4.43 | 4.42 | 4.28 | 4.44 | 4.36 | 4.28 | 4.42 | 5205 |
| | Sample size | 1378 | 2248 | 3160 | 3304 | 3482 | 3564 | 3222 | 751 | 531 | 3135 | 3651 | 6786 |
| Shopping | Out-of-home | 4.16 | 4.11 | 4.43 | 4.20 | 4.26 | 4.19 | 4.33 | 4.23 | 4.32 | 4.22 | 4.25 | 1086 |
| | In-home | 4.43 | 3.47 | 4.63 | 4.07 | 3.93 | 3.94 | 4.08 | 4.14 | 2.67 | 4.14 | 3.96 | 30 |
| | Sample size | 249 | 483 | 384 | 462 | 654 | 755 | 361 | 148 | 108 | 464 | 652 | 1116 |
| Work and work-related | Out-of-home | 3.84 | 3.99 | 4.28 | 3.93 | 4.11 | 4.01 | n/a | 4.27 | 3.91 | 4.02 | 3.98 | 1530 |
| | In-home | 3.49 | 3.71 | 3.92 | 3.83 | 3.58 | 3.75 | n/a | 3.70 | 3.65 | 3.83 | 3.59 | 366 |
| | Sample size | 509 | 966 | 421 | 1082 | 814 | 1848 | n/a | 305 | 301 | 1399 | 497 | 1896 |
| Travel | Out-of-home | 4.39 | 4.39 | 4.67 | 4.36 | 4.60 | 4.43 | 4.61 | 4.51 | 4.30 | 4.36 | 4.62 | 6446 |
| | Sample size | 1718 | 2631 | 2097 | 3011 | 3435 | 4533 | 1913 | 895 | 710 | 3289 | 3157 | 6446 |

(continued)

**Table 2.2** (continued)

| Activity category | Location | 18–34 years | 35–54 years | 55+ years | Male | Female | Employed | Not employed | ≤$20K income[a] | >$75K income[a] | Weekday | Weekend | Sample size |
|---|---|---|---|---|---|---|---|---|---|---|---|---|---|
| Personal enrichment | Out-of-home | 4.41 | 4.83 | 5.08 | 4.69 | 4.93 | 4.75 | 4.95 | 4.97 | 4.56 | 4.54 | 5.00 | 645 |
|  | In-home | 3.81 | 4.71 | 5.18 | 4.48 | 4.78 | 4.55 | 4.80 | 4.08 | 4.67 | 4.77 | 4.60 | 343 |
|  | Sample size | 249 | 316 | 423 | 389 | 599 | 550 | 438 | 153 | 76 | 391 | 597 | 988 |
| Other | Out-of-home | 4.41 | 4.74 | 4.70 | 4.48 | 4.73 | 4.60 | 4.66 | 4.81 | 4.67 | 4.34 | 4.91 | 177 |
|  | In-home | 4.33 | 4.23 | 4.52 | 4.36 | 4.42 | 4.27 | 4.52 | 4.35 | 4.24 | 4.19 | 4.57 | 490 |
|  | Sample size | 147 | 199 | 321 | 235 | 432 | 359 | 308 | 85 | 57 | 313 | 354 | 667 |

Note: Scores are averages based on a scale of 0–6 with a higher score implying a greater degree of the emotion

n/a not applicable

[a]Computed only on valid cases with no missing income information

- *Social/Recreation:* Socializing, relaxing, leisure, sports, exercise, and recreation
- *Shopping:* Consumer purchases
- *Work:* Work and work-related activities
- *Travel:* Traveling
- *Personal Enrichment:* Caring for and helping non-household members, education, religious and spiritual activities, and volunteer activities
- *Other:* Telephone calls and activities that could not be coded into a single activity type

Travel episodes are considered to be exclusively performed outside home, and the very small number of travel episodes that were reported to be undertaken inside home were removed from the analysis. As expected, discretionary leisure activities are associated with the greatest levels of happiness. Eat meal, social/recreational, shopping, and personal enrichment activities are associated with high levels of happiness. In general, activities engender greater degrees of happiness when conducted outside home (thus necessitating travel) than when undertaken inside home. An interesting finding, however, is that younger individuals aged 18–34 years (the millennials) show some anomalies to this general pattern. For example, they actually report a higher average happiness score for eat meal activities inside home than outside home (although the difference is very small). Likewise, they report higher levels of happiness for shopping activities inside home (presumably online shopping) than shopping activities undertaken outside home, and for personal and household maintenance activities undertaken inside home than outside home. Although these differences are small, the fact that they are unique and unusual (compared to the pattern in the rest of the table) is noteworthy—and may explain, at least to some degree, the lower levels of travel proclivity among this age group that has been reported by others (e.g., McDonald 2015).

Among the varied patterns that can be discerned from this table, the one that is noteworthy in the context of this chapter is that travel episodes, in general, engender a very similar level of happiness as episodes of other activity types. The average happiness rating for travel episodes is well above 4.0 for all demographic groups; it is on par with the rating for shopping and personal and household maintenance activity types, lower than for eat meal and social/recreational activity types, and better than for work episodes. In other words, travel is not particularly onerous or unpleasant and is not viewed all that unfavorably when compared with other routine household and personal activities that are undertaken to maintain or fulfill the needs of the person and/or the household. Morris and Guerra (2015) report similar findings and suggest that, for the most part, travel is not necessarily viewed as an activity that is undesirable and the mood of an individual is no worse during travel than on average.

This analysis of travel-related emotions indicates that the feelings of well-being that people generally associate with travel episodes are not very different from those associated with other activity types. Thus, it appears that travel is not necessarily increasing or decreasing overall subjective well-being or quality of life in a manner that is incongruent with the way in which other activities affect well-being. Travel essentially affects overall wellness and quality of life to the same degree and in the same way that other routine activity episodes, such as personal and household maintenance or shopping, do.

## 2.4   Influence of Travel Satisfaction on Subjective Well-Being

The potential contribution of transportation to SWB has long been recognized (e.g., Kitamura et al. 1997; Vella-Brodrick and Stanley 2013; Nordbakke and Schwanen 2014). With respect to the five avenues of that contribution identified by De Vos et al. (2013) and others, most discussions have focused on the role of transportation in providing access to activities that contribute to SWB, and to its symbolic value as a marker of self-reliance and freedom (the *motility* concept), with less-common references to the intrinsic positive utility of travel (e.g., Delbosc 2012; Reardon and Abdallah 2013; Abou-Zeid and Ben-Akiva 2014). It is only relatively recently, however, that scholars have conceptualized travel satisfaction as a key construct in its own right, which directly influences SWB (Ettema et al. 2010).

Within the past decade, several studies have empirically investigated the influence of travel satisfaction per se on SWB. The geographic contexts for these studies include *Sweden* (Bergstad et al. 2011; Eriksson et al. 2013; Olsson et al. 2013) and the *United States* (Cao 2013). They vary in how they measure SWB, with time scales including *life in general* (Bergstad et al. 2011; Cao 2013), *last month* (Olsson et al. 2013), and *right after the trip and the day as a whole* (Eriksson et al. 2013). With respect to travel satisfaction, two used the *five-item Satisfaction with Travel Scale* (Bergstad et al. 2011; Cao 2013) and two used the *nine-item STS* (Eriksson et al. 2013; Olsson et al. 2013). Types of travel included *daily* (Bergstad et al. 2011; Cao 2013) and *commuting* (Eriksson et al. 2013; Olsson et al. 2013). Most allow for only one direction of causality—*travel satisfaction influences SWB*—but Cao (2013) tested each direction (one at a time), and found similar goodness of fit for the two formulations. (By contrast, Schwanen and Wang 2014 tested each direction when investigating "episode well-being" for out-of-home activities among Hong Kong residents, and found substantially better fit for the model in which *life satisfaction influences episode well-being*).

Collectively, these and other studies highlight a number of issues associated with the effort to assess the impacts of travel satisfaction on SWB. Mokhtarian (2017) discusses such issues in the broader context of travel; drawing on that discussion, we offer here a succinct synopsis, tailored to the travel satisfaction construct in particular:

- A mismatch in time frame or specificity between travel satisfaction and SWB could attenuate the estimated relationship between them.
- Focusing on the direct impact of travel satisfaction on SWB is likely to miss the key indirect role that travel plays, e.g. in offering access to activities that themselves increase SWB. The travel itself may be unsatisfactory and thus appear

to have a negative contribution to SWB, but that may be substantially outweighed by the positive contribution of the activities accessed by the travel.

- Even as an instrument for accessing activities, a focus on travel per se excludes consideration of home-based activities and information/communication technology substitutes for face-to-face activities involving travel.
- Even if positive, the *direct* impact of travel satisfaction on overall SWB is likely to be small—other life domains such as health and social relationships could be expected to play larger roles.
- Even if travel satisfaction *does* have a statistically significant and meaningfully large impact on SWB, we currently have no idea how much each of the five avenues identified in Sect. 2.2.1 contributes to that satisfaction.
- It is important to disentangle directions of causality: SWB is at least as likely to influence travel behavior, and thence satisfaction, as the converse. Only specifying one direction of causality in the model could badly distort estimates of the influence of one factor on the other.

## 2.5  Concluding Comments

A considerable body of empirical evidence exists on the subject of travel satisfaction and its relation to well-being. Although numerous factors are associated with variations in travelers' satisfaction, the overall picture that emerges is that most people are relatively satisfied with their travel and that travel episodes do not necessarily engender emotional feelings or moods that are all that different from those associated with other activity episode types. In fact, based on an analysis of the 2013 American Time Use Survey (ATUS), emotions are generally more positive for activity episodes that are undertaken outside home (regardless of activity type), suggesting that individuals continue to desire out-of-home activity experiences that entail travel. This does not necessarily mean that people are eager to travel more for its own sake, but at a minimum it suggests that they are not necessarily eager to travel less. The ATUS data show that for the most part, travel as a car passenger engenders the most positive emotions while—consistent with several other studies—travel by public transit engenders the least positive emotions. It is clear that public transit continues to face an uphill battle in its quest to offer a high degree of travel satisfaction and become a preferred mode of transportation for many.

Despite the evidence accumulated to date, much remains to be learned about how best to measure travel satisfaction, the factors that drive travel satisfaction, the manner in which travel satisfaction affects well-being, and the way in which well-being affects travel satisfaction. In an era of rapidly emerging transportation technologies and disruptive shared mobility services that leverage the convenience of mobile platforms and ubiquitous connectivity, it is likely that feelings of well-being derived from travel experiences are going to continue to evolve in very substantial ways. Traveling in an autonomous vehicle of the future—where the traveler is free of the guidance and navigation tasks of driving, has the privacy and safety of an individual vehicle, and has the ability to pursue any other activity during the travel episode—is likely to be very different from traveling in any of the private or public transport modes of today. It would be of value to understand the relative contribution of various elements of the travel experience to feelings of satisfaction and well-being; such an understanding would, in turn, help illuminate the far-reaching implications of increasingly automated mobility platforms and vehicular technologies.

**Acknowledgements** The authors thank Venu Garikapati of the National Renewable Energy Laboratory for his assistance in compiling tabulations of emotional measures using data from the 2013 well-being module of the American Time Use Survey Data. The authors also gratefully acknowledge partial support provided by the Center for Teaching Old Models New Tricks (TOMNET), a University Transportation Center sponsored by the US Department of Transportation through Grant No. 69A3551747116.

# References

## Service Quality-Based Satisfaction Measures

Cronin, J. J., Jr., & Taylor, S. A. (1994). SERVPERF versus SERVQUAL: Reconciling performance based and perceptions-minus-expectations measurement of service quality. *Journal of Marketing, 58*(1), 125–131.

Eboli, L., & Mazzulla, G. (2009). A new customer satisfaction index for evaluating transit service quality. *Journal of Public Transportation, 12*(3), 21–37.

Eiro, T., & Martinez, L. M. (2014). Modeling daily mobility satisfaction using a structural equation model. In J. F. de Sousa & R. Rossi (Eds.), *Computer-based modelling and optimization in transportation* (pp. 391–403). Cham: Springer.

Hensher, D. A., & Prioni, P. (2002). A service quality index for area-wide contract performance assessment. *Journal of Transport Economics and Policy, 36*(1), 93–113.

Hill, N., Brierley, J., & MacDougall, R. (2003). *How to measure customer satisfaction* (2nd ed.). Hampshire: Gower Publishing Limited.

Parasuraman, A., Zeithaml, V. A., & Berry, L. L. (1985). A conceptual model of service quality and its implications for future research. *Journal of Marketing, 49*(4), 41–50.

Teas, R. K. (1993). Expectations, performance evaluation, and consumers' perceptions of quality. *Journal of Marketing, 57*(4), 18.

## Subjective Well-Being-Based Satisfaction Measures

Abou-Zeid, M., Witter, R., Bierlaire, M., Kaufmann, V., & Ben-Akiva, M. (2012). Happiness and travel mode switching: Findings from a Swiss public transportation experiment. *Transport Policy, 19*(1), 93–104.

Bergstad, C. J., Gamble, A., Gärling, T., Hagman, O., Polk, M., Ettema, D., Friman, M., & Olsson, L. E. (2011). Subjective well-being related to satisfaction with daily travel. *Transportation, 38* (1), 1–15.

Cao, J. (2013). The association between light rail transit and satisfactions with travel and life: Evidence from twin cities. *Transportation, 40*(5), 921–933.

Cao, J., & Ettema, D. (2014). Satisfaction with travel and residential self-selection: How do preferences moderate the impact of the Hiawatha light rail transit line? *Journal of Transport and Land Use, 7*(3), 93–108.

De Vos, J., Schwanen, T., van Acker, V., & Witlox, F. (2015). How satisfying is the Scale for Travel Satisfaction? *Transportation Research Part F, 29*, 121–130.

De Vos, J., Mokhtarian, P. L., Schwanen, T., van Acker, V., & Witlox, F. (2016). Travel mode choice and travel satisfaction: Bridging the gap between decision utility and experienced utility. *Transportation, 43*, 771–796.

Diab, E. I., & El-Geneidy, A. M. (2014). Transitory optimism: Changes in passenger perception following bus service improvement over time. *Transportation Research Record, 2415*, 97–106.

Eriksson, L., Friman, M., & Gärling, T. (2013). Perceived attributes of bus and car mediating satisfaction with the work commute. *Transportation Research A, 47*, 87–96.

Ettema, D., Gärling, T., Olsson, L. E., & Friman, M. (2010). Out-of-home activities, daily travel, & subjective well-being. *Transportation Research A, 44*, 723–732.

Ettema, D., Gärling, T., Eriksson, L., Friman, M., Olsson, L. E., & Fujii, S. (2011). Satisfaction with travel and subjective well-being: development and test of a measurement tool. *Transportation Research F, 14*, 167–175.

Ettema, D., Friman, M., Gärling, T., Olsson, L. E., & Fujii, S. (2012). How in-vehicle activities affect work commuters' satisfaction with public transport. *Journal of Transport Geography, 24*, 215–222.

Ettema, D., Gärling, T., Olsson, L. E., Friman, M., & Moerdijk, S. (2013). The road to happiness: Measuring Dutch car drivers' satisfaction with travel. *Transport Policy, 27*, 171–178.

Friman, M., Fujii, S., Ettema, D., Gärling, T., & Olsson, L. E. (2013). Psychometric analysis of the satisfaction with travel scale. *Transportation Research A, 48*, 132–145.

Gatersleben, B., & Uzzell, D. (2007). Affective appraisals of the daily commute: Comparing perceptions of drivers, cyclists, walkers, and users of public transport. *Environment and Behavior, 39*(3), 416–431.

Lucas, J. L., & Heady, R. B. (2002). Flextime commuters and their driver stress, feelings of time urgency, and commute satisfaction. *Journal of Business and Psychology, 16*(4), 565–571.

Manaugh, K., & El-Geneidy, A. M. (2013). Does distance matter? Exploring the links among values, motivations, home location, and satisfaction in walking trips. *Transportation Research A, 50*, 198–208.

Olsson, L. E., Friman, M., Pareigis, J., & Edvardsson, B. (2012). Measuring service experience: Applying the satisfaction with travel scale in public transport. *Journal of Retailing and Consumer Services, 19*(4), 413–418.

Olsson, L. E., Gärling, T., Ettema, D., Friman, M., & Fujii, S. (2013). Happiness and satisfaction with work commute. *Social Indicators Research, 111*(1), 255–263.

Sirgy, M. J., Kruger, P. S., Lee, D.-J., & Yu, G. B. (2010). How does a travel trip affect tourists' life satisfaction? *Journal of Travel Research, 50*(3), 261–275.

Smith, O. (2017). Commute well-being differences by mode: Evidence from Portland, Oregon, USA. *Journal of Transport and Health, 4*, 246–254.

St-Louis, E., Manaugh, K., van Lierop, D., & El-Geneidy, A. (2014). The happy commuter: A comparison of commuter satisfaction across modes. *Transportation Research F, 26*, 160–170.

Susilo, Y. O., & Cats, O. (2014). Exploring key determinants of travel satisfaction for multi-modal trips by different traveler groups. *Transportation Research A, 67*, 366–380.

Suzuki, H., Fujii, S., Gärling, T., Ettema, D., & Olsson, L. E. (2014). Rules for aggregated satisfaction with work commutes. *Transportation, 41*(3), 495–506.

Taniguchi, A., Grääs, C., & Friman, M. (2014). Satisfaction with travel, goal achievement, and voluntary behavioral change. *Transportation Research F, 26*, 10–17.

Ye, R., & Titheridge, H. (2017). Satisfaction with the commute: The role of travel mode choice, built environment and attitudes. *Transportation Research D, 52*, 535–547.

## Other Travel Satisfaction Measures

Abou-Zeid, M., & Ben-Akiva, M. (2012). Well-being and activity-based models. *Transportation, 39*(6), 1189–1207.

Choo, S., Collantes, G. O., & Mokhtarian, P. L. (2005). Wanting to travel, more or less: Exploring the determinants of the deficit and surfeit of personal travel. *Transportation, 32*, 135–164.

Circella, G., Salgado, J. R., Mokhtarian, P. L., Diana, M. (in progress, available from the authors). The impact of activities while traveling on the subjective valuation of travel time.

Duarte, A., Garcia, C., Giannarakis, G., Limão, S., Polydoropoulou, A., & Litinas, N. (2010). New approaches in transportation planning: Happiness and transport economics. *Netnomics, 11*(1), 5–32.

Etezady, A., Circella, G., & Mokhtarian, P. L. (2017). *Investigating the satisfaction with travel amounts: A comparison of commuters and noncommuters in California.* Unpublished manuscript, available from the authors.

Frei, C., Mahmassani, H. S., & Frei, A. (2015). Making time count: Traveler activity engagement on urban transit. *Transportation Research Part A, 76*, 58–70.

Lyons, G., Jain, J., & Weir, I. (2016). Changing times—a decade of empirical insight into the experience of rail passengers in Great Britain. *Journal of Transport Geography, 57*, 94–104.

Mokhtarian, P. L., Papon, F., Goulard, M., & Diana, M. (2015). What makes travel pleasant and/or tiring? An investigation based on the French National Travel Survey. *Transportation, 42*(6), 1103–1128.

Ory, D. T., & Mokhtarian, P. L. (2005). When is getting there half the fun? Modeling the liking for travel. *Transportation Research A, 39*(2–3), 97–123.

Paez, A., & Whalen, K. (2010). Enjoyment of commute: A comparison of different transportation modes. *Transportation Research A, 44*, 537–549.

Pedersen, T., Friman, M., & Kristensson, P. (2011). The role of predicted, on-line experienced and remembered satisfaction in current choice of public transport use. *Journal of Retailing and Consumer Services, 18*, 471–475.

Susilo, Y. O., Lyons, G., Jain, J., & Atkins, S. (2012). Rail passengers' time use and utility assessment: 2010 findings from Great Britain with multivariate analysis. *Transportation Research Record, 2323*, 99–109.

## Other References

Abou-Zeid, M., & Ben-Akiva, M. (2014). Satisfaction and travel choices. In T. Gärling, D. F. Ettema, & M. Friman (Eds.), *Handbook of sustainable travel* (pp. 53–65). Dordrecht: Springer. Available at https://link.springer.com/chapter/10.1007%2F978-94-007-7034-8_4. Accessed 27 June 2017.

Brickman, P., Coates, D., & Janoff-Bulman, R. (1978). Lottery winners and accident victims: Is happiness relative? *Journal of Personality and Social Psychology, 36*(8), 917–927.

Chen, C.-C., & Petrick, J. F. (2013). Health and wellness benefits of travel experiences. *Journal of Travel Research, 52*(6), 709–719.

De Vos, J., Schwanen, T., van Acker, V., & Witlox, F. (2013). Travel and subjective well-being: a focus on findings, methods and future research needs. *Transport Reviews, 33*(4), 421–442.

Delbosc, A. (2012). The role of well-being in transport policy. *Transport Policy, 23*, 25–33.

Evans, G. W., Wener, R. E., & Phillips, D. (2002). The morning rush hour: Predictability and stress. *Environment and Behaviour, 34*(4), 521–530.

Kaufman, V., Bergman, M. M., & Joye, D. (2004). Motility: Mobility as capital. *International Journal of Urban and Regional Research, 28*(4), 745–756.

Kitamura, R., Fujii, S., & Pas, E. I. (1997). Time-use data, analysis and modeling: Toward the next generation of transportation planning methodologies. *Transport Policy, 4*(4), 225–235.

McDonald, N. (2015). Are millennials really the "Go-Nowhere" generation? *Journal of the American Planning Association, 81*(2), 90–103.

Mokhtarian, P. L. (2017). *Subjective well-being and travel: Retrospect and prospect.* Under review; available from the author.

Mokhtarian, P. L., & Salomon, I. (2001). How 'derived' is the demand for travel? Some conceptual and measurement considerations. *Transportation Research A, 35*, 695–719.

Morris, E. A., & Guerra, E. (2015). Mood and mode: Does how we travel affect how we feel? *Transportation, 42*(1), 25–43.

Nordbakke, S., & Schwanen, T. (2014). Well-being & mobility: A theoretical framework and literature review focusing on older people. *Mobilities, 9*(1), 104–129.

Novaco, R. W., & Gonzalez, O. I. (2009). Commuting and well-being. In Y. Amichai-Hamburger (Ed.), *Technology and psychological well-being* (pp. 174–205). Cambridge: Cambridge University Press. https://doi.org/10.1017/CBO9780511635373.008.

Reardon, L., & Abdallah, S. (2013). Well-being and transport: Taking stock and looking forward. *Transport Reviews, 33*(6), 634–657.

Schwanen, T., & Wang, D. (2014). Well-being, context, and everyday activities in space and time. *Annals of the American Association of Geographers, 104*(4), 833–851.

Shaw, F. A., Malokin, A., Mokhtarian, P. L., & Circella, G. (2018). *Outcomes of travel-based multitasking: Reported benefits and disadvantages of conducting activities while commuting.* Paper presented at the 2018 annual meeting of the transportation research board; available from the authors.

Stradling, S. G., Anable, J., & Carreno, M. (2007). Performance, importance & user disgruntlement: A six-step method for measuring satisfaction with travel modes. *Transportation Research A, 41*(1), 98–106.

Vella-Brodrick, D. A., & Stanley, J. (2013). The significance of transport mobility in predicting well-being. *Transport Policy, 29*, 236–242.

Waterhouse, J., Reilly, T., & Edwards, B. (2004). The stress of travel. *Journal of Sports Sciences, 22*(10), 946–965.

# Chapter 3
# Travel and Feelings

Tommy Gärling

**Abstract** Frequent observations showing that travel influences satisfaction with life suggest that transport policy making and planning would increase society's welfare by taking this influence into account. To do this requires detailed knowledge of how travel influences satisfaction with life. Two routes of influence have been proposed and empirically confirmed, one through the facilitation of out-of-home activities that are important for satisfaction with life, and the other through reducing negative feelings caused by hassles associated with daily travel. The latter route is the focus of the chapter. A theoretical framework is proposed that makes quantitative predictions of the impacts of transient feelings (emotional responses) on enduring feelings (mood) with consequences for well-being during and after travel. Positive and negative emotional responses are assumed to be evoked by both transient critical incidents (e.g. disruptions) and non-transient factors (e.g. noise) during travel. Numerical experiments illustrate the quantitative predictions of changes in mood during and after travel for both types of evoking factors. It is also shown how emotion regulation may moderate effects of transient factors as well as how hedonic adaptation and desensitization associated with non-transient factors may affect mood after travel. The conclusion is that measurement of mood at different points in time should be a valuable complement to or sometimes a substitute for retrospective self-reports of satisfaction with travel that are likely to be more susceptible to systematic errors.

**Keywords** Travel · Satisfaction · Feeling · Emotional response · Mood · Emotional well-being · Theoretical framework · Numerical experiment

T. Gärling (✉)
University of Gothenburg, Göteborg, Sweden

Karlstad University, Karlstad, Sweden
e-mail: Tommy.Garling@psy.gu.se

## 3.1  Introduction

An increasing number of studies has in recent years investigated satisfaction with urban travel (for reviews, see De Vos et al. 2013; Ettema et al. 2016; Mokhtarian 2016). A point of departure of these studies is research on satisfaction with life in general as well as satisfaction with different domains of life (e.g. job, family life, leisure) (Diener et al. 1999; Dolan et al. 2008; Veenhofen 2008) demonstrating consequences for longevity and success in life (Diener and Chan 2011; Lyubomirski et al. 2005). If travel influences satisfaction with life, transport policy making and planning may increase society's welfare by taking this influence into account. This requires knowledge of how travel influences satisfaction with life.

Satisfaction with travel has been defined as a domain-specific satisfaction based on how travelers evaluate any type of travel (Ettema et al. 2010). Yet, most empirical studies have investigated commute trips by different modes (e.g. Ettema et al. 2012; Gatersleben and Uzzell 2007; Martin et al. 2014; Olsson et al. 2013; St-Louis et al. 2014). An exception is Friman et al. (2017a) who measured satisfaction with all daily travel. The results of previous research show that satisfaction with travel decreases with travel time and crowdedness/congestion, is higher for active modes and driving than public transport, increases with social interactions as well as meaningful solitary activities (e.g. job-related web surfs) during public transport, and is negatively influenced by bad weather.

Several studies have also demonstrated that satisfaction with travel influences satisfaction with life. Morris (2015) found that satisfaction with life increases with travel time per day, in particular for time spent walking or bicycling in connection with recreational activities. Jakobsson Bergstad et al. (2011) showed that satisfaction with life was positively influenced by satisfaction with travel directly as well as indirectly through positive feelings associated with participation in out-of-home activities. Olsson et al. (2013) reported that satisfaction with work commutes has a weak positive effect on satisfaction with life but a stronger effect on feelings.

The question of how satisfaction with travel influences satisfaction with life has still not yet been satisfactorily answered. Two routes of this influence were proposed by Ettema et al. (2010) and empirically confirmed by Jakobsson Bergstad et al. (2011), one through the facilitation of out-of-home activities that are important for satisfaction with life and the other through reducing negative feelings caused by hassles associated with daily travel. The latter is the focus of this chapter.

Previous research of the role of satisfaction with travel has largely failed to study feelings evoked by travel and residual effects of these feelings influencing activities subsequent to travel. In the next section some theoretical constructs are presented that were developed in basic emotion research. These constructs will be used in the subsequent sections. A following section discusses how travel-related feelings have been conceptualized and measured retrospectively. After this another view is presented of how travel-related feelings should be conceptualized and measured.

## 3.2  Feeling Constructs

In this section a distinction is first made between *evaluation* and *feeling*, then between transient feelings, referred to as *emotional responses*, usually attributable to some external event, and less transient feelings, referred to as *mood*, primarily dependent on an individual's internal state. In general, emotional responses are stronger than mood and when occurring they become the focus of consciousness, whereas mood resides in the background. If events evoke transient emotional responses, their strength may still depend on mood such that a negative emotional response is weakened by a positive mood or exaggerated by a negative mood. Emotional responses may also change mood. Residual effects on mood of emotional responses would then be likely to influence subsequent activities.

Events may be evaluated as good or bad. Evaluations are however distinct from feelings (Russell 2003). As proposed by Carver and Scheier (1990), Lazarus (1991), and Oatley (2009), evaluations invoke feelings if and only if they are personally relevant. For instance, a delay of travel may be evaluated as negative. Feelings would still not be evoked unless the delay has personally relevant consequences such a being late for an appointment.

In the theory proposed by Russell (2003), emotions are constructed from different mental ingredients although core affects are elemental building blocks of all emotions. A core affect is a "neurophysiological state consciously accessible as the simplest raw (nonreflective) feeling evident in moods and emotions" (p. 148). Core affects are always accessible, either being neutral or having any other value in a dimensional system defined by the orthogonal axes pleasure-displeasure and activation-deactivation (Russell 1980, 2003; Yik et al. 2011).[1] Corroboration comes from neuro-imaging research (Posner et al. 2009; Wilson-Mendenhall et al. 2013). Mood is in Russell's (2003) theory conceived of as a prolonged core affect.

Figure 3.1 displays the two-dimensional system of pleasure-displeasure and activation-deactivation referred to as the affect grid (Yik et al. 2011). Others have posited that emotions are discrete (e.g. Lazarus 1991; Lerner et al. 2015). As shown in the figure, discrete emotions may be conceptualized as combinations of values on the pleasure and activation dimensions.

The affect grid as well as Russell's (2003) theory of core affects have played an important role in research beyond the study of emotion including also travel research.

---

[1]Several different methods have been used to measure core affects including self-reports, startle responses, peripheral physiology, face expressions assessed by automated picture recognition systems or electrical muscle potentials, and brain measures. A dimensional description of core affects is supported by these methods, although not all converge on the two orthogonal pleasure-displeasure and activation-deactivation dimensions (Mauss and Robinson 2009).

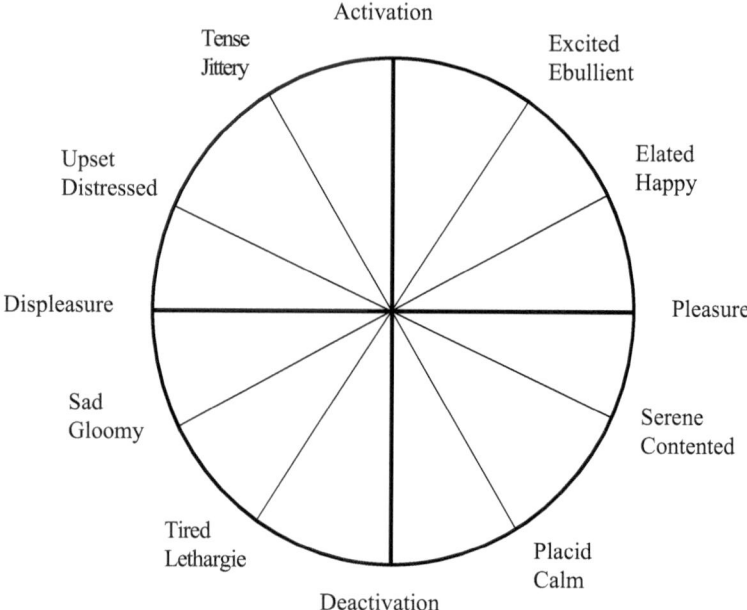

**Fig. 3.1** The affect grid (Reprinted from Yik et al. 2011, with permission BY American Psychological Association)

## 3.3 Conceptualization and Retrospective Measurements of Travel-Related Feelings

Travel-related feelings are by definition related to any feature of any type of travel. In order to have bearings on applications, the focus here will be on feelings related to such features and types of travel that are investigated in travel behavior research. These include emotional responses to discrete events such as various disruptions of travel as well as influences on mood of continuous aspects such as travel time. A causal effect is usually assumed although it may frequently be mediated by other factors. Measurement methods have been developed and applied in order to investigate emotional responses or influences on mood.

In related research on subjective well-being (Busseri and Sadava 2011), methods are used to retrospectively measure the frequency or duration and intensity of different feelings during a specified time interval. In retrospective measurements people report from memory how they have felt during a past period. Conventional self-report rating scales such as the *Positive Affect and Negative Affect Scale* (PANAS, Watson et al. 1988) or the *Swedish Core Affect Scale* (SCAS, Västfjäll et al. 2002; Västfjäll and Gärling 2007) have been used for this purpose. Although these scales may be used to measure both dimensions in the affect grid, it is common to limit measurement to the valence dimension ranging from positive to negative. The affect balance is an index constructed to aggregate positive and negative feelings, either as the ratio of the frequencies of positive and negative feelings (Diener et al. 1991), the difference between the average intensity of positive feelings and the average intensity of negative feelings (Kahneman et al. 2004), or the difference between duration-weighted positive and negative feeling intensities (Krueger and Schkade 2008).

Emotional responses evoked by events during travel as well as changes in mood would potentially influence the affect balance. In support Kahneman et al. (2004) found that in retrospective measures of emotional responses, commuting was less associated with positive feelings and more associated with negative feelings when compared to other activities. Morris and Guerra (2015a) obtained an aggregate measure of mood (based on 0-to-6 ratings of happiness, sadness, tiredness, pain, and stress) during the preceding day. Excluding purely recreational travel, the results showed that daily travel accounted for a few percent of the variance in mood. Stone and Schneider (2016) found that commuting episodes during a day were, compared to other activities on the same day, retrospectively rated high in stress and tiredness and low in meaningfulness. Commutes to work were found to have less negative effects on tiredness than commutes home, while longer commutes increased stress and tiredness. Olsson et al. (2013) showed that retrospectively self-reported positive feelings decreased with the duration of work commutes. Morris and Guerra (2015b) confirmed the negative association between travel time and mood, primarily because of increased stress, fatigue, and sadness during longer journeys. Gatersleben and Uzzell (2007) asked university employees to retrospectively report their feelings associated with work commutes. They found that to car users (drivers and passengers) the commutes were more stressing than to walkers or cyclists to whom the commutes were more relaxing, whereas to public transport users the commutes were more boring than to the others to whom the commutes were more exciting.

Other research has used the *Satisfaction with Travel Scale* (STS) (Ettema et al. 2011; Friman et al. 2013). Feelings measured by the STS varies along two dimensions that are orthogonal to each other and oblique to the valence and activation dimensions in the affect grid (Västfjäll et al. 2002; Västfjäll and Gärling 2007), one ranging from positive activation (positive valence, high activation) to negative deactivation (negative valence, low activation) and the other ranging from positive deactivation (positive valence, low activation) to negative activation (negative valence, high activation). The STS may therefore primarily measure less transient feelings (e.g. stress, relaxation, boredom, enthusiasm) commonly experienced during travel (e.g., Gatersleben and Uzzell 2007), although Friman et al. (2017b) recently showed that the STS also correlates with self-reported events that evoked either positive or negative emotional responses during work commutes. This is to be expected if emotional responses change mood.

Does the STS or any other retrospective self-report method provide a valid measure of feelings during travel? There are three reasons to doubt this. First, since memory of evaluations during travel is susceptible to forgetting, frequently only the last part of a journey and the peak or bottom (the best or worst evaluation) may influence the ratings. This is referred to as the peak-end rule which has been demonstrated in many laboratory experiments (e.g. Schreiber and Kahneman 2000;

for review, see Fredrickson 2000) although not as clearly in field studies (Kemp et al. 2008; Miron-Shatz 2009) when memory presumably is more accurate. A travel behavior example is Suzuki et al. (2014) who showed that satisfaction with commute trips to and from work is proportional to the average of duration-weighted satisfaction with the different stages of the trips (e.g. walking to the bus stop, riding the bus, walking to the work place). A caveat is that the ratings of the stages were made retrospectively at the same time as the retrospective ratings of the whole trip were made. Second, it is questionable whether the memory of even the peak/bottom and end is accurate. If feelings are difficult to recall (which Robinson and Clore 2002, argue is common), memory is likely to be influenced by stereotypical beliefs associated with memory of evaluations or factors evoking evaluations, for instance, the emotional response to a disruption may not be remembered but inferred from what is believed to have been felt. A long trip may be remembered as more boring than it was experienced. Third, if memory is difficult to recall after a journey, the reported feelings during the journey may be influenced by how one feels at the moment of recall after the journey (Friman et al. 2017b).

## 3.4 Conceptualization and Instantaneous Measurement of Travel-Related Feelings

Are there any alternatives to retrospective measures of feelings during travel if these have limited validity due to inaccurate recall from memory? In a chapter entitled "Objective happiness" Kahneman (1999) argues that instantaneous measures of mood (also referred to as instant utility) are preferable. But some minimal time to integrate information is still needed. Are instantaneous self-report measures therefore not free of memory bias?

In self-reports time to integrate information is thus necessary and must rely on recall of the information. Susceptibility to recall errors should still be substantially reduced in instantaneous compared to retrospective self-reports such that they for practical purposes can be ignored. Another issue raised by Kahneman (1999) is whether instantaneous measures are possible to aggregate. He shows that an objectively aggregated measure would have desirable interval or ratio scale properties. It is also clear that retrospective self-reports made according to the peak-end rule would not lead to the same result. Which one should then be chosen?

But are instantaneous measures feasible? In travel behavior research on-line methods such as observations, surveys (e.g. on-board interviews), and physiological measures (e.g. excretion of stress hormones, heart rate) have been applied in past research. With new advanced and portable technology, these methods are improved (e.g. Echeverri 2005; Pareigis et al. 2011) by the use of video-recordings of naturally occurring events combined with think-aloud protocols documenting users' experiences. Several studies have also for a long time used time-sampling or event-sampling techniques to obtain instantaneous self-report from people of how they feel (Stone et al. 1999). In one recent travel behavior study using such a technique, Ettema and Smajic (2015) used smartphone questionnaires to measure feelings during walking. It was found that negative feelings are evoked in places with many people and on-going activities, but also that more quiet places foster positive feelings, in particular in the presence of natural elements such as trees and water. Dunlop et al. (2015) sent self-report questionnaires to passengers' smartphones every sixth minutes during public transport journeys. Heightened anxiety and discomfort were observed when participants experienced undesirable conditions. Ettema et al. (2017) and Friman et al. (2017b) obtained self-reports from smartphones before, immediately after, and 1 h after morning commutes to work. The results showed that self-reported positive emotional responses evoked by events during travel (e.g. light traffic, seat availability, warm temperature) were related to mood changes directly after the commute but not later in the day.

Even though instantaneous measures are relatively free from recall biases, they are not continuous. Thus, at what time to measure feelings is an issue that needs to be addressed. An alternative to the investigator choosing the time is to leave the choice to respondents. Respondents may be asked during a time interval such as a journey to report pre-defined events (Flanagan 1954; Friman 2004; Gremler 2004), for instance events perceived as negative or positive, positive or negative emotional responses, or changes in mood in a positive or negative direction.

In the remainder of this section I will discuss the possibility to measure *mood* to infer the effects of events evoking emotional responses. Measurements of mood need to be made minimally at two points in time and preferably more frequently. This method reduces recall errors and imposes minimal load on respondents. At the same time inferences rely on several theoretical assumptions. The basic one is that mood is influenced by emotional responses such that its measurement would reflect residual effects. Olsson et al. (2017) recently provided empirical support for this assumption but additional research is needed to verify the findings of their laboratory experiments.

In order to understand how mood is influenced by events evoking emotional responses, Gärling et al. (2017) proposed the following model of how changes in mood depend on emotional responses. The model is consistent with statements made in the section on feeling constructs although for simplicity it is posited that mood varies along a single dimension ranging from maximally negative to maximally positive through neutral.[2] It is consistent with the model that emotional responses are stronger and more transient than mood, that evaluations not invariably evoke emotional responses (although the necessary conditions are not specified in the model), and that the influence of emotional responses on mood depends on the

---

[2]Kahneman (1999) argues that this is the most important evaluative dimension (by him referred to as Good-Bad evaluations) although activation would augment or attenuate such evaluations. Västfjäll et al. (2001) showed how the pleasure-displeasure and activation-deactivation dimensions may be collapsed into a unidimensional dimension of positive versus negative feelings. See also the related discussion in Kuppens et al. (2013) of different conceptualizations of the relation between pleasure-displeasure and activation-deactivation.

mood at the time of influence. The model is represented by the following equation relating current mood ($CM_i$) at time $i$ ($\in$ 1, 2,..., n) to mood at time $i - 1$ if the evaluation ($E_i$) of an event at time $i$ evokes an emotional response that has an impact on mood ($\phi_i$),

$$CM_i = \begin{cases} CM_{i-1} + (CM_{max} - CM_{i-1})(1 - \exp(-\phi_i E_i)) & E_i \geq 0; 0 \leq \phi_i \leq 1 \\ CM_{i-1} - (CM_{i-1} - CM_{min})(1 - \exp(-\phi_i E_i)) & E_i < 0 \end{cases}$$

(3.1)

The impact on current mood $CM_i$ increases with how good or bad the evaluation $E_i$ is and its impact $\phi_i$ on mood that varies from no impact (0) to maximal impact (1). The degree of change is limited by $CM_{max} = -CM_{min} > 0$. Equation 3.1 thus implies that current mood at any point in time changes in the same direction as an emotional response ($\phi_i > 0$) evoked by evaluations of an event. The change is in general less than proportional to the emotional response ($\phi_i < 1$). It also depends on the current mood if it deviates from being neutral such that the effect of the same emotional response is weaker in the same direction and stronger in the reverse direction.

Equation 3.1 applies both to events that are discrete and events that vary on some relevant dimension, for instance, intensity or duration. If events during travel vary along such a single dimension denoted $X$, evaluations ($E$) as positive or negative are posited to be related to $X$ by prospect theory's value function (Kahneman and Tversky 1979),[3] where $c$ is an adaptation level (Baucells et al. 2011) which determines whether $X$ is evaluated as positive ($c < X$), negative ($c > X$) or neutral ($X = c$). Thus,

$$E = \begin{cases} -a_P |X - c|^b & c > X; a_P, b > 0 \\ a_N (X - c)^b & c \leq X; a_N, b > 0 \end{cases}$$

(3.2)

$a_N$ and $a_P$ are slope constants and $b$ a measure of the curvature of the function. In prospect theory (Tversky and Kahneman 1992) the value function is upwards concave and downwards convex for $b$ approximately equal to 0.75. The slope is approximately twice as steep for $X < c$ than for $X > c$ ($a_p \approx a_N/2$).

Next the numerical experiments reported in Gärling (2017) are described with the aim of showing quantitatively how discrete events and continuous factors influence positive and negative mood during and immediately after travel. The main question I raise is under which conditions changes in current mood caused by emotional responses have residual effects on feelings directly after travel. This is a demonstration of how Eqs. 3.1 and 3.2 may be used to make quantitative predictions of residual travel-related feelings. Current mood is calculated according to Eqs. 3.1 and 3.2 for different parameter values. The basic set-up is that current mood is neutral at the start

---

[3]Prospect theory is currently used in many models of travel behavior (Li and Hensher 2011; Van De Kaa 2010). Note however that prospect theory accounts for evaluations of quantitative information but not for emotional responses or influences on mood. Equation 3.1 is thus a necessary complement.

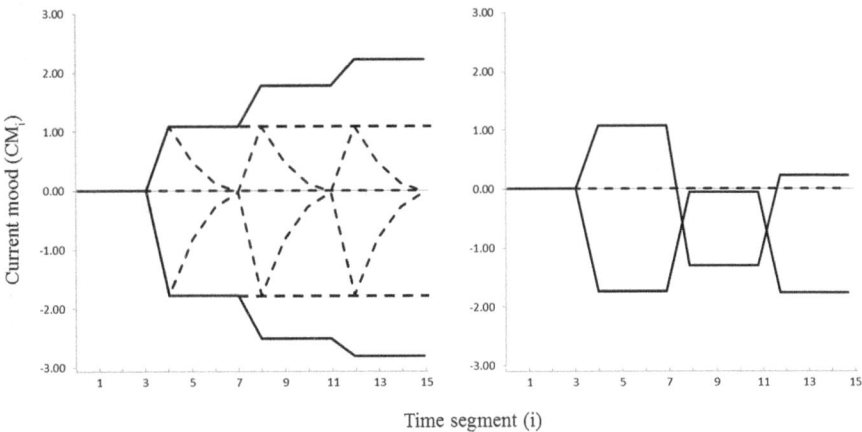

**Fig. 3.2** Changes in current mood over time (solid lines) and hypothetical adjustments (broken lines) due to discrete events evoking positive and negative emotional responses during travel (Reprinted from Gärling 2017, www.tandfonlie.com, with permission by Taylor & Francis Ltd.)

of a journey consisting of neutral time segments. It is then shown how current mood is changed by discrete events and continuous factors evoking emotional responses.

Figure 3.2 shows current mood ($CM_i$) plotted against 15 ($i = 1, \ldots 15$) time segments of a journey.[4] Assume that every time segment except three ($i = 4, 8, 12$) are evaluated as neutral ($X - c = 0$) and that current mood is neutral ($CM_0 = 0$) at the start of the journey. In the left graph all three time segments are either all evaluated as positive ($X - c > 0$) or negative ($X - c < 0$). The parameter $\phi_i$ representing the degree of impact of the emotional response on current mood is given a positive value (0.75) for these segments, $CM_{max} = -CM_{min} = 3$ and the parameters in Eq. 3.2 are set to $a_P = a_N/2 = 1$ and $b = 0.75$.[5] The right graph illustrates how an emotion-evoking negative event moderates the effects of two emotion-evoking positive events and the reverse. In all plots, residual effects on current mood are observed.

In general, a neutral or positive current mood that has changed to negative may not remain negative. A vast research literature on mood regulation (e.g. Erber et al. 2004) suggests that people actively attempt to regain a neutral or positive mood. A positive mood may similarly not necessarily remain positive due to negative emotion impacts of events not related to travel. This has been indicated by the broken lines in the left graph of Fig. 3.2. If mood regulation or mood-inducing events unrelated to travel neutralizes the emotion impacts of events during travel, no residual mood changes would remain. This is still unlikely to occur if the emotion impacts are substantial. If measurements are made at shorter intervals it is even more unlikely.

---

[4]For simplicity the effects on current mood are analyzed at the last time segment of the journey.
[5]The values of the parameters $a_B$, $a_G$, and $b$ are selected to be approximately consistent with the findings in empirical studies (e.g. Carter and McBride 2013; Tversky and Kahneman 1992).

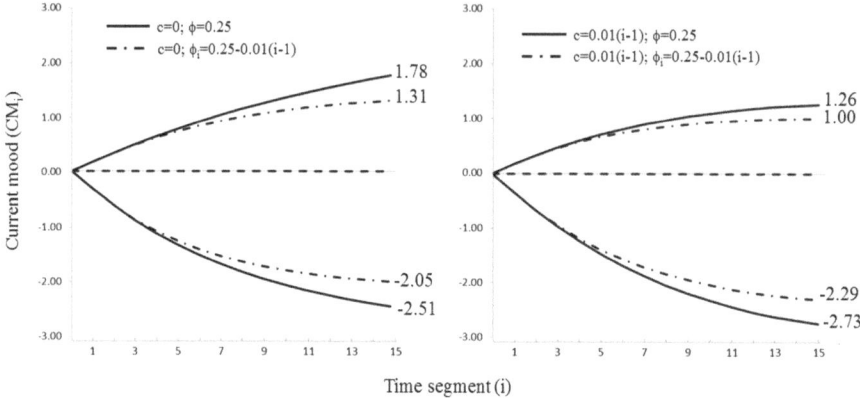

**Fig. 3.3** Changes in current mood due to continuous factors evoking positive and negative emotional responses during travel when evaluations (c) and impact of the emotional responses (φ) change over time (Reprinted from Gärling 2017, www.tandfonlie.com, with permission by Taylor & Francis Ltd.)

Continuous factors may also influence current mood during travel. Examples include in-vehicle noise, crowdedness or an activity during travel (e.g. reading). A continuous factor is however not likely to be perceived as such. As shown in several laboratory experiments (Ariely and Zauberman 2000, 2003; Ariely and Carmon 2000), people may due to attentional shifts instead experience it intermittently. If thus assuming that a continuous factor consist of a series of separate events, a single evaluation would be made of each. If all these evaluations are the same and have the same emotional impact, then current mood would change as shown by the solid curves in the left graph of Fig. 3.3 where $X - c$ is either positive or negative for a constant value of $\phi_i$ (0.25). Other parameter values are the same as in Fig. 3.2. The graphs show that current mood changes towards the positive or negative asymptotic values. At the end current mood has changed compared to before the journey.

Repeated evaluations tend to become less positive for non-changing circumstances (equal evaluations of each event). This is referred to as hedonic adaptation (Fredericks and Loewenstein 1999). After some time positive evaluations may therefore be evaluated as neutral. However, as noted by Wilson and Gilbert (2008), over time negative evaluations seem to remain negative or even become more negative. The solid curves in the right graph of Fig. 3.3 compared to the solid curves in the left graph show how current mood changes if $c$ increases linearly with time. The changes towards the asymptotic values are slower, more for positive than negative impacts of emotional responses on mood. It is noteworthy that the residual mood effects still remain.

Another change is desensitization (Fredericks and Loewenstein 1999) implying that emotional responses are gradually weakened. If as the broken curves in the left graph show, the mood impact ($\phi_i$) decreases linearly with time, the residual effects remain although the changes in both positive and negative current moods are reduced. Finally, the broken curves in the right graph show that if $c$ increases and $\phi_i$ decreases linearly with $i$, the results only differ from the broken curves in the left graph by changing more slowly and thus resulting in weaker residual effects. Taken together, for continuous influencing factors both changes in the evaluations and mood impacts over time have effects on current mood during travel but do not eliminate any residual mood effects.

The results of the numerical experiments may now be summarized as follows: (i) Residual effects are demonstrated for three discrete events evoking emotional responses during travel. Eqs. 3.1 and 3.2 may in empirical studies be used to predict such effects given information or assumptions about the occurrences of the events and the emotional responses they evoke. (ii) Continuous factors are due to attentional shifts evaluated intermittently. Unlike discrete events the evaluations do not remain the same but change over time, becoming less positive than initially or more negative than initially. Emotional responses to the evaluations are also weakened over time. As a consequence, both positive and negative residual feelings are weaker. (iii) How active mood regulation may neutralize mood effects of events evoking negative emotional responses is illustrated qualitatively. If aggregated across individuals such effects may be treated as random influences.

## 3.5  Discussion

The message from the research on the affect balance in everyday life is not that it is desirable that people are in a positive mood all the time. First of all, as noted by Diener and Chan (2011) it is not beneficial for people since they may be less cautious than they ought to be.[6] It may, for instance, foster unhealthy life styles. And people may ignore symptoms of illness. Second, the downs need to be part of life for people to appreciate the ups. For this and other reasons (e.g. personal integrity) research studies should not aim at measuring mood at all times but to focus on critical circumstances when it is important that people do not have negative feelings. A case in point is long commutes to and from work in crowded public transport vehicles which millions of people undertake every weekday.

If people are not feeling positive during commutes, does this have effects carried over to subsequent activities at the work place or at home? Several US studies document negative such effects. Schaeffer et al. (1988) and Novaco et al. (1979) found that automobile commuting resulted in worse post-travel proof-reading performance which is a common measure of stress after-effects. Wener et al. (2003)

---

[6]It may however be noted that cross-cultural research shows that worldwide people tend to be in a mild to moderate positive mood in the absence of important negative circumstances (Diener et al. 2015). Thus, the set-point is a positive rather than a neutral mood. Evolutionary arguments are invoked as an explanation, partly based on that a positive mood increases the likelihood of adaptive behaviors such as creativity, planning, mating, and sociality, partly based on the observation that a positive affect balance increases longevity and success in life (Diener and Chan 2011; Lyubomirski et al. 2005). This relationship may however be non-linear with the largest positive effects for a lower than the maximal affect balance.

demonstrated better post-travel proof-reading performance after improvements of public transport that shortened travel time. White and Rotton (1998) reported reduced persistence to completing unsolvable puzzles (another measure of stress after-effects) after both automobile and bus commuting. Another study (Van Rooy 2006) showed that longer distances and higher traffic congestion led automobile commuters to more negatively evaluate unqualified job candidates at the work place. In a similar vein Hennessy (2008) found increased aggression at work after automobile commuting. Novaco et al. (1991) observed that home commutes had negative effects on activities at home. It remains to empirically connect research findings (e.g. Ettema et al. 2017; Friman et al. 2017b) showing residual travel-related mood effects to these observations of impaired performance but also to positive effects on performance. Would positive influences on mood of, for instance, sunshine and a moderately warm temperature during walking or bicycling to work improve work performance?

It may also in this connection be asked what the relation is between mood during travel (as, for instance, measured recurrently by Dunlop et al. 2015, or Ettema and Smajic 2015) and satisfaction with travel as measured after travel by, for instance, the STS (Ettema et al. 2011; Friman et al. 2013). Although this issue has not been subject to extensive research, Kahneman (1999) concludes from some laboratory experiments that a retrospective evaluation is more likely to influence repeat choices. Yet, it would be hasty to generalize this to applications of travel policy making and planning. It should be equally important how people feel during travel as how satisfied they are after travel, in part because how people feel during travel may, as reviewed in the preceding paragraph, have carry-over effects, and in part because people should not need to experience negative travel-related feelings during travel. Note also that people are not necessarily aware of influences on mood during travel, whereas retrospectively they are aware of their satisfaction with travel. Influences on mood are furthermore in general more accurately measured as current mood than retrospective self-reports of satisfaction and merit attention also for this reason. Therefore, as argued, measurements of mood are more likely to permit valid inferences of "objective satisfaction" free of biased self-report.

**Acknowledgements** My co-authored research reported in this chapter has been financially supported by grant #2014-05335 from the Swedish Governmental Agency for Innovation Systems awarded to the SAMOT VINN Excellence Center in public transport at Karlstad University, Sweden. I thank the Editors for their research collaboration as well as comments on the chapter. I also thank Michael Ståhl for assisting me with the numerical experiments.

# References

Ariely, D., & Carmon, Z. (2000). Gestalt characteristics of experiences: The defining features of summarized events. *Journal of Behavioral Decision Making, 13*, 191–201.

Ariely, D., & Zauberman, G. (2000). On the making of an experience: The effects of breaking and combining experiences on their overall evaluation. *Journal of Behavioral Decision Making, 13*, 219–232.

Ariely, D., & Zauberman, G. (2003). Differential partitioning of extended experiences. *Organizational Behavior and Human Decision Processes, 91*, 128–139.

Baucells, M., Weber, M., & Welfens, F. (2011). Reference-point formation and updating. *Management Science, 57*, 506–519.

Busseri, M. A., & Sadava, S. W. (2011). A review of the tripartite structure of subjective well-being: Implications for conceptualization, operationalization, analysis, and synthesis. *Personality and Social Psychology Review, 15*, 290–314.

Carter, S., & McBride, M. (2013). Experienced utility: Putting the 'S' in satisfaction. *The Journal of Socio-Economics, 42*, 13–23.

Carver, C. S., & Scheier, M. F. (1990). Origins and functions of positive and negative affect: A control-process view. *Psychological Review, 97*, 19–35.

De Vos, J., Schwanen, T., Van Acker, V., & Witlox, F. (2013). Travel and subjective well-being: A focus on findings, methods, and future research needs. *Transport Reviews, 33*, 421–442. https://doi.org/10.1080/01441647.2013.815665.

Diener, E., & Chan, M. Y. (2011). Happy people live longer: Subjective well-being contributes to health and longevity. *Applied Psychology: Health and Well-Being, 3*, 1–43. https://doi.org/10.1111/j.1758-0854.2010.01045.x.

Diener, E., Sandvik, E., & Pavot, W. (1991). Happiness is the frequency, not the intensity, of positive versus negative affect. In F. Strack, M. Argyle, & N. Schwarz (Eds.), *Subjective well-being: An interdisciplinary perspective* (pp. 119–139). New York: Pergamon.

Diener, E., Suh, E. M., Lucas, R. E., & Smith, H. L. (1999). Subjective well-being: Three decades of progress. *Psychological Bulletin, 125*, 276–302. https://doi.org/10.1037/0033-2909.125.2.276.

Diener, E., Kanazawa, S., Suh, E. M., & Oishi, S. (2015). Why people are in a generally good mood. *Personality and Social Psychology Review, 19*, 235–256. https://doi.org/10.1177/1088868314544467.

Dolan, P., Peasgood, T., & White, M. P. (2008). Do we really know what makes us happy? A review of the economic literature on the factors associated with subjective well-being. *Journal of Economic Psychology, 29*, 94–122. https://doi.org/10.1016/j.joep.2007.09.001.

Dunlop, I. N., Casello, J. M., & Doherty, S. T. (2015). *Tracking the transit rider experience: Using smartphones to measure comfort and wellbeing throughout the trip.* Transportation Research Board 94th Annual Meeting of Compendium of Papers #15-5944. Washington, DC: Transportation Research Board.

Echeverri, P. (2005). Video-based methodology: Capturing real-time perceptions of customer processes. *International Journal of Service Industry Management, 16*, 199–209.

Erber, R., Erber, M. W., & Poe, J. (2004). Mood regulation and decision-making: Is irrational exoberance really a problem? In I. Brocas & J. D. Carrilo (Eds.), *The psychology of economic decisions* (Vol. 2, pp. 197–210). New York: Oxford University Press.

Ettema, D., & Smajic, I. (2015). Walking, places and wellbeing. *Geographical Journal, 181*, 102–109. https://doi.org/10.1111/geoj.12065.

Ettema, D., Gärling, T., Olsson, L. E., & Friman, M. (2010). Out-of-home activities, daily travel, and subjective well-being. *Transportation Research Part A, 44*, 723–732. https://doi.org/10.1016/j.tra.2010.07.005.

Ettema, D., Gärling, T., Eriksson, L., Friman, M., Olsson, L. E., & Fujii, S. (2011). Satisfaction with travel and subjective wellbeing: Development and tests of a measurement tool. *Transportation Research Part F, 14*, 167–175. https://doi.org/10.1016/j.trf.2010.11.002.

Ettema, D., Friman, M., Gärling, T., Olsson, L. E., & Fujii, S. (2012). How in-vehicle activities affect work commuters' satisfaction with public transport. *Journal of Transport Geography, 24*, 215–222. https://doi.org/10.1016/j.jtrangeo.2012.02.007.

Ettema, D., Gärling, T., Friman, M., & Olsson, L. E. (2016). Travel mode use, travel mode shift, and subjective well-being: Overview of theories, empirical findings, and policy implications. In D. Wang & S. He (Eds.), *Mobility, sociability and wellbeing of urban living* (pp. 129–150). New York: Springer. https://doi.org/10.1007/978-3-662-48184-4_7.

Ettema, D., Friman, M., Olsson, L. E., & Gärling, T. (2017). Season and weather effects on travel-related mood and travel satisfaction. *Frontiers in Psychology: Environmental Psychology, 8,* 140. https://doi.org/10.3389/fpsyg.2017.00140.

Flanagan, J. C. (1954). The critical incident technique. *Psychological Bulletin, 51,* 327–357.

Fredericks, S., & Loewenstein, G. (1999). Hedonic adaptation. In D. Kahneman, E. Diener, & N. Schwartz (Eds.), *Well-being: The foundations of hedonic psychology* (pp. 302–329). New York: Russell Sage Foundation.

Fredrickson, B. L. (2000). Extracting meaning from past affective experiences: The importance of peaks, ends, and specific emotions. *Cognition and Emotion, 14,* 577–606. https://doi.org/10.1080/026999300402808.

Friman, M. (2004). The structure of affective reactions to critical incidents. *Journal of Economic Psychology, 25,* 331–353. https://doi.org/10.1016/S0167-4870(03)00012-6.

Friman, M., Fujii, S., Ettema, D., Gärling, T., & Olsson, L. E. (2013). Psychometric analysis of the satisfaction with travel scale. *Transportation Research Part A, 48,* 132–145. https://doi.org/10.1016/j.tra.2012.10.012.

Friman, M., Gärling, T., Ettema, D., & Olsson, L. E. (2017a). How does travel affect emotional well-being and life satisfaction? *Transportation Research Part A, 106,* 170–180.

Friman, M., Olsson, L. E., Ståhl, M., Ettema, D., & Gärling, T. (2017b). Travel and residual emotional well-being. *Transportation Research Part F, 49,* 159–176.

Gärling, T. (2017). Travel-related feelings: Review, theoretical framework, and numerical experiments. *Transportation Letter.* https://doi.org/10.1080/19427867.2017.1300399.

Gärling, T., Ettema, D., Friman, M., & Olsson, L.E. (2017). *Updated current mood: A conceptualization of aggregation of instant utilities.* Unpublished paper.

Gatersleben, B., & Uzzell, D. (2007). Affective appraisals of the daily commute: Comparing perceptions of drivers, cyclists, walkers and users of public transport. *Environment and Behavior, 39,* 416–431.

Gremler, D. D. (2004). The critical incident technique in service research. *Journal of Service Research, 7,* 65–89. https://doi.org/10.1177/1094670504266138.

Hennessy, D. A. (2008). The impact of commuter stress on workplace aggression. *Journal of Applied Social Psychology, 38,* 2315–2335. https://doi.org/10.1111/j.1559-1816.2008.00393.x.

Jakobsson Bergstad, C., Gamble, A., Hagman, O., Polk, M., Gärling, T., Ettema, D., Friman, M., & Olsson, L. E. (2011). Subjective well-being related to satisfaction with daily travel. *Transportation, 38,* 1–15. https://doi.org/10.1007/s11116-010-9283-z.

Kahneman, D. (1999). Objective happiness. In D. Kahneman, E. Diener, & N. Schwartz (Eds.), *Well-being: The foundations of hedonic psychology* (pp. 3–25). New York: Russell Sage Foundation.

Kahneman, D., & Tversky, A. (1979). Prospect theory: An analysis of decision under risk. *Econometrika, 47,* 263–291.

Kahneman, D., Krueger, A. B., Schkade, D., Schwarz, N., & Stone, A. (2004). A survey method for characterizing daily life experience: The Day Reconstruction Method (DRM). *Science, 306,* 1776–1780. https://doi.org/10.1126/science.1103572.

Kemp, S., Burt, C. D., & Furneaux, L. (2008). A test of the peak-end rule with extended autobiographical events. *Memory & Cognition, 36,* 132–139.

Krueger, A. B., & Schkade, D. (2008). The reliability of subjective well-being measures. *Journal of Public Economics, 92,* 1833–1845. https://doi.org/10.1016/j.jpubeco.2007.12.015.

Kuppens, P., Tuerlinckx, F., Russell, J. A., & Feldman Barret, L. (2013). The relation between valence and arousal in subjective experience. *Psychological Bulletin, 139,* 917–940. https://doi.org/10.1037/a0030811.

Lazarus, R. S. (1991). *Emotion and adaptation.* New York: Oxford University Press.

Lerner, J. S., Li, Y., Valdesolo, P., & Kassam, K. S. (2015). Emotion and decision making. *Annual Review of Psychology, 66,* 799–823.

Li, Z., & Hensher, D. A. (2011). Prospect theoretic contributions in understanding traveler behaviour: A review and some comments. *Transport Reviews, 31*(1), 97–115. https://doi.org/10.1080/01441647.2010.498589.

Lyubomirski, S., King, L., & Diener, E. (2005). The benefits of frequent positive affect: Does happiness lead to success? *Psychological Bulletin, 131*, 803–855. https://doi.org/10.1037/0033-909.131.6.803.

Martin, A., Goryakin, Y., & Suhrcke, M. (2014). Does active commuting improve psychological wellbeing? Longitudinal evidence from eighteen waves of the British Household Panel Survey. *Preventive Medicine, 69*, 296–303.

Mauss, I. B., & Robinson, M. D. (2009). Measures of emotion: A review. *Cognition and Emotion, 23*, 209–237. https://doi.org/10.1080/02699930802204677.

Miron-Shatz, T. (2009). Evaluating multi episode events: Boundary conditions for the peak-end rule. *Emotion, 9*, 206–213. https://doi.org/10.1037/a0015295.

Mokhtarian, P. L. (2016). *Subjective well-being and travel: Retrospect and prospect.* Unpublished paper.

Morris, E. A. (2015). Should we all stay at home? Travel, out-of-home activities, and life satisfaction. *Transportation Research Part A, 78*, 519–536. https://doi.org/10.1016/j.tra.2015.06.009.

Morris, E. A., & Guerra, E. (2015a). Mood and mode: Does how we travel affect how we feel? *Transportation, 42*, 25–43. https://doi.org/10.1007/s11116-014-9521-x.

Morris, E. A., & Guerra, E. (2015b). Are we there yet? Trip duration and mood during travel. *Transportation Research Part F, 33*, 38–47. https://doi.org/10.1016/j.trf.2015.06.003.

Novaco, R., Stokols, D., Campbell, J., & Stokols, J. (1979). Transportation, stress, and community psychology. *American Journal of Community Psychology, 7*, 361–380. https://doi.org/10.1007/BF00894380.

Novaco, R. W., Kliewer, W., & Brouet, A. (1991). Home environmental consequences of commute travel impedance. *American Journal of Community Psychology, 19*, 881–909. https://doi.org/10.1007/BF00937890.

Oatley, K. (2009). Communication to self and others: Emotional experience and its skill. *Emotion Review, 1*, 206–213. https://doi.org/10.1177/1754073909103588.

Olsson, L. E., Gärling, T., Ettema, D., Friman, M., & Fujii, S. (2013). Happiness and satisfaction with work commute. *Social Indicators Research, 111*, 255–263. https://doi.org/10.1007/s11205-012-0003-2.

Olsson, L. E., Gärling, T., Ettema, D., Friman, M., & Ståhl, M. (2017). Current mood and recalled impacts of current moods after exposures to sequences of potential monetary outcomes. *Frontiers in Psychology: Cognition, 8*, 66. https://doi.org/10.3389/fpsyg.2017.00066.

Paregis, J., Edvardsson, B., & Enquist, B. (2011). Exploring the role of the service environment in forming customer's service experience. *International Journal of Quality and Service Sciences, 3*, 110–124.

Posner, J., Russell, J. A., Gerber, A., Gorman, D., Colibazzi, T., Yu, S., Wang, Z., Kangarlum, A., Zhu, H., & Peterson, B. S. (2009). The neurophysiological basis of emotion: An fMRI study of the affective circumplex using emotion-denoting words. *Human Brain Mapping, 30*, 883–895. https://doi.org/10.1002/hbm.20553.

Robinson, M. D., & Clore, G. L. (2002). Belief and feeling: Evidence for an accessibility model of emotional self-report. *Psychological Bulletin, 128*, 934–960. https://doi.org/10.1037/0033-2909.128.6.934.

Russell, J. A. (1980). A circumplex model of affect. *Journal of Personality and Social Psychology, 39*, 1161–1178. https://doi.org/10.1037/h0077714.

Russell, J. A. (2003). Core affect and the psychological construction of emotion. *Psychological Review, 110*, 145–172. https://doi.org/10.1037/0033-295X.110.1.145.

Schaeffer, M. H., Street, S. W., Singer, J. E., & Baum, A. (1988). Effects of control on the stress reactions of commuters. *Journal of Applied Social Psychology, 18*, 944–957. https://doi.org/10.1111/j.1559-1816.1988.tb01185.x.

Schreiber, C. A., & Kahneman, D. (2000). Determinants of the remembered utility of aversive sounds. *Journal of Experimental Psychology: General, 129*, 27–42. https://doi.org/10.1037/0096-3445.129.1.27.

St-Louis, E., Manaugh, K., van Lierop, D., & El-Geneidy, A. (2014). The happy commuter: A comparison of commuter satisfaction across modes. *Transportation Research Part F, 26*, 160–170.

Stone, A. A., & Schneider, S. (2016). Commuting episodes in the United States: Their correlates with experiential wellbeing from the American Time Use Survey. *Transportation Research Part F, 42*, 117–124. https://doi.org/10.1016/j.trf.2016.07.004.

Stone, A. A., Shiffman, S. S., & DeVries, M. W. (1999). Ecological momentary assessment. In D. Kahneman, E. Diener, & N. Schwarz (Eds.), *Well-being: The foundations of hedonic psychology* (pp. 26–39). New York: Russell-Sage.

Suzuki, H., Fujii, S., Gärling, T., Ettema, D., Olsson, L. E., & Friman, M. (2014). Rules for aggregating satisfaction with work commute. *Transportation, 41*, 495–506. https://doi.org/10.1007/s11116-013-9484-3.

Tversky, A., & Kahneman, D. (1992). Advances in prospect theory: Cumulative representation of uncertainty. *Journal of Risk and Uncertainty, 5*, 297–323.

Van De Kaa, J. E. (2010). Applicability of an extended prospect theory to travel behaviour research: A meta-analysis. *Transport Reviews, 30*(6), 771–804. https://doi.org/10.1080/01441647.2010.486907.

Van Rooy, D. L. (2006). Effects of automobile commute characteristics on affect and job candidate evaluations: A field experiment. *Environment and Behavior, 38*, 626–655. https://doi.org/10.1177/0013916505280767.

Västfjäll, D., & Gärling, T. (2007). Validation of a Swedish short self-report measure of core affect. *Scandinavian Journal of Psychology, 48*, 233–238. https://doi.org/10.1111/j.1467-9450.2007.00595.x.

Västfjäll, D., Gärling, T., & Kleiner, M. (2001). Does it make you happy feeling this way? A core affect account of preference for current mood. *Journal of Happiness Studies, 2*, 337–354.

Västfjäll, D., Friman, M., Gärling, T., & Kleiner, M. (2002). The measurement of core affect: A Swedish self-report measure. *Scandinavian Journal of Psychology, 43*, 19–31. https://doi.org/10.1111/1467-9450.00265.

Veenhofen, R. (2008). Sociological theories of subjective well-being. In M. Eid & R. J. Larsen (Eds.), *The science of subjective well-being* (pp. 44–61). New York: Guilford Press.

Watson, D., Clark, L. A., & Tellegen, A. (1988). Development and validation of brief measures of positive and negative affect: The PANAS scales. *Journal of Personality and Social Psychology, 47*, 1063–1070. https://doi.org/10.1037/0022-3514.54.6.1063.

Wener, R. E., Evans, G. W., Phillips, D., & Nadler, N. (2003). Running for the 7:45: The effects of public transit improvements on commuter stress. *Transportation, 30*, 203–220. https://doi.org/10.1023/A:1022516221808.

White, S. M., & Rotton, J. (1998). Type of commute, behavioral after effects, and cardiovascular activity: A field experiment. *Environment and Behavior, 30*, 763–780. https://doi.org/10.1177/001391659803000602.

Wilson, T. D., & Gilbert, D. T. (2008). Explaining away: A model of affective adaptation. *Perspectives on Psychological Science, 3*, 370–386.

Wilson-Mendenhall, C. D., Feldman Barret, L., & Barsalou, L. W. (2013). Neural evidence that human emotions share core affective properties. *Psychological Science, 25*, 947–956.

Yik, M., Russell, J. A., & Steiger, J. H. (2011). A 12-point circumplex structure of core affect. *Emotion, 11*, 705–731. https://doi.org/10.1037/a0023980.

# Chapter 4
# Accessibility and Exclusion Related to Well Being

**Alexa Delbosc and Graham Currie**

**Abstract** Contemporary research linking transport, social exclusion and well-being has developed through a number of leading studies over the last decade. In this chapter we explore these links using a review of the research literature. The chapter includes a discussion about the difference between mobility (actual travel) and accessibility (the quality of opportunities to engage in activities) and how this distinction is conceptualised in the literature on transport and well-being. The chapter will also bring together factors influencing access, social exclusion and well-being into a conceptual framework. It also introduces the question of 'how much transport is enough' to support social inclusion and well-being. A major aim of the work is to reflect on where research has taken us and to identify where future research needs to focus. The chapter identifies a number of gaps in existing research, including: only one project looked at the interrelationships between transport, social exclusion and well-being; very few studies explore the relationship between accessibility and well-being; very few studies explore the relationship between transport and eudemonic well-being. To date, many hypothesised links between transport, accessibility, mobility, subjective well-being and social exclusion remain unexplored, providing fertile ground for future research.

**Keywords** Well-being · Accessibility · Mobility · Social exclusion · Transport · Quality of life · Hedonic well-being · Eudemonic well-being

## 4.1 Introduction

Travel is one of the most important facilitators of life and has been widely acknowledged as a prerequisite for economic and social activity. Contemporary research linking transport, social exclusion and well-being has developed through a number

A. Delbosc · G. Currie (✉)
Monash University, Clayton, VIC, Australia
e-mail: alexa.delbosc@monash.edu; Graham.Currie@monash.edu

© Springer International Publishing AG, part of Springer Nature 2018
M. Friman et al. (eds.), *Quality of Life and Daily Travel*, Applying Quality of Life
Research, https://doi.org/10.1007/978-3-319-76623-2_4

of leading studies over the last decade. Although this research field is beginning to mature, we have yet to take stock of the current state of knowledge.

In this chapter we aim to explore the links between transport accessibility, social exclusion and psychological well-being using a review of the research literature. The chapter includes a discussion about the difference between mobility (actual travel) and accessibility (the quality of opportunities to engage in activities) and how this distinction is conceptualised in the literature on transport and well-being. The chapter will also bring together factors influencing access, social exclusion and well-being into a conceptual framework. It also introduces the question of 'how much transport is enough' to support social inclusion and well-being. A major aim of the work is to reflect on where research has taken us and to identify where future research needs to focus.

The chapter starts with a review of research approaches in this area. This establishes differences between studies measuring transport mobility and transport accessibility which is the topic of the following discussion. The chapter then considers the question of how much transport is enough, then concludes with a summary of key findings of the review and implications for policy and research futures.

## 4.2   Transport, Social Exclusion and Well-Being

Transport is an important facilitator to activities that promote societal and individual well-being. It comes as no surprise, then, that a considerable body of research has explored the impact that transport (or the lack of transport) has on social exclusion and well-being. Table 4.1 is a synthesis of published research papers that have explored how constraints to transport are associated with social exclusion or psychological well-being.[1] The work is divided into studies of transport and well-being, transport and social exclusion and studies of transport, social exclusion and well-being. Only one set of analyses from Australia considered all three components together (Currie and Delbosc 2010; Delbosc and Currie 2011b; Stanley et al. 2011). There is also a great deal of variation in how each of these three components is defined and measured.

**Social exclusion** is a concept that developed when it was recognised that a focus on poverty neglected the key interconnections between different areas of disadvantage such as insufficient housing, poor health, low levels of education and insufficient social support (Stanley 2011b). Crucially, discourses around social exclusion emphasise the importance of participating in society rather than focussing purely on income or material resources (Hodgson and Turner 2003).

---

[1]Note that this table excludes papers that measure travel satisfaction (see Chap. 2) or how mode choice influences well-being (see Chap. 5).

**Table 4.1** Selected review of studies on transport, social exclusion and/or well-being

| Study | Population | Transport measures | | | Well being measures | | Social exclusion measures |
|---|---|---|---|---|---|---|---|
| | | Accessibility | Mobility | Transport disadvantage | Hedonic | Eudemonic | |
| Transport and social exclusion studies | | | | | | | |
| Church et al. (2000) | General pop. Mapping | ✓ | | | n/a | n/a | Spatial |
| Schonfelder and Axhausen (2003) | General population | ✓ | | | n/a | n/a | Demographic, economic |
| Hine (2004) | General population | ✓ | | | n/a | n/a | Demographic, economic |
| Xiao et al. (2017) | Disadvantaged mapping | ✓ | | | n/a | n/a | Demographic, economic |
| Hurni (2007) | Sole parents/unemployed youth | ✓ | | | n/a | n/a | Demographic |
| Casas (2007) | Disabled persons | | ✓ | | n/a | n/a | Spatial, demographic |
| Casas et al. (2009) | Children | | ✓ | | n/a | n/a | Spatial, demographic, economic |
| Engels and Liu (2011) | Elderly | | ✓ | | n/a | n/a | Spatial, demographic |
| Lucas (2011)[a] | Excluded populations | | | ✓ | n/a | n/a | Demographic |
| Shay et al. (2016) | General population mapping | | | ✓ | n/a | n/a | Demographic, economic |
| Xia et al. (2016) | Elderly, no-car and low-income | | | ✓ | n/a | n/a | Demographic, economic |
| Özkazanç and Sönmez (2017) | General population mapping | | | ✓ | n/a | n/a | Demographic, economic |
| Wasfi et al. (2017) | Disabled persons | | | ✓ | n/a | n/a | Demographic |

(continued)

**Table 4.1** (continued)

| Study | Population | Transport measures | | | Well being measures | | Social exclusion measures |
|---|---|---|---|---|---|---|---|
| | | Accessibility | Mobility | Transport disadvantage | Hedonic | Eudemonic | |
| *Transport and well being studies* | | | | | | | |
| Musselwhite and Haddad (2010)[a] | Elderly | ✓ | ✓ | | QoL | | n/a |
| Doi et al. (2008) | General population | ✓ | | | QoL, indicators | | n/a |
| Banister and Bowling (2004) | Elderly | | ✓ | | QoL | | n/a |
| Mollenkopf et al. (2005) | Elderly | | ✓ | | Affect, SWL | | n/a |
| Spinney et al. (2009) | Elderly | | ✓ | | Affect, SWL | | n/a |
| Bergstad et al. (2012) | General population | | ✓ | | Affect, SWL | | n/a |
| Archer et al. (2013) | General population | | ✓ | | Affect | | n/a |
| Ravulaparthy et al. (2013) | Elderly | | ✓ | | SWB | | n/a |
| Vella-Brodrick and Stanley (2013) | General population | | | ✓ | SWB | PWB | n/a |
| Delbosc and Vella-Brodrick (2015) | Young adults | | | ✓ | SWB | PWB[b] | n/a |
| *Transport, social exclusion and well being studies* | | | | | | | |
| Currie and Delbosc (2010), (Delbosc and Currie 2011b) | General population | | | ✓ | SWB | | Indicators (economic and participation) |
| Stanley et al. (2011) | General population | | ✓ | | SWB | | Indicators (economic & participation) |

*QoL* quality of life, *PWB* psychological well-being (eudemonic), *SWB* subjective well-being, *SWL* satisfaction with life
[a]These studies were conducted with qualitative interviews
[b]Only included the 'autonomy' sub-scale

Some groups in society are more likely to be at risk of social exclusion, including the young, the aged, those with a disability, ethnic minorities, the geographically isolated and people with a poor education (Stanley 2011b). For this reason, many studies on transport and social exclusion have focussed on specific segments of the population (e.g. Casas 2007; Hurni 2007; Titheridge and Solomon 2008; Engels and Liu 2011). Others have taken a more empirical approach by defining and measuring social exclusion using indicators such as income, employment status, levels of social support, activity participation and political activity (Stanley 2011a). As the research field developed, others have categorised a range of ways that transport can contribute to social exclusion including physical barriers, geographical distance, fear, lack of time, constrained economic resources, and exclusion from facilities and spaces (Church et al. 2000).

Research that focuses on the impact of transport limitations on well-being use various measurements such as affect (mood), subjective well-being, satisfaction with life, and quality of life. Other authors in this volume have given a more comprehensive definition and discussion of well-being measures used in transport (see Chaps. 1, 2, and 3) and also (Nordbakke and Schwanen 2014). One important distinction is that some researchers have emphasised the importance of differentiating between hedonic measures (related to happiness and fulfilling wants) and eudemonic measures (related to autonomy, self-actualisation and fulfilling a purpose) (Ryan and Deci 2001; Shliselberg and Givoni 2017).

Finally, the transport dimension of this relationship has been defined in a range of ways depending on the research context. In the literature on transport and social exclusion, the dialogue often refers to the need to address 'transport disadvantage'. Definitions of transport disadvantage are complex and varied; it is sometimes used synonymously with concepts such as transport stress, transport poverty and transport exclusion (Currie and Delbosc 2011; Pyrialakou et al. 2016). For the purpose of this chapter, a working definition for transport disadvantage is *a set of conditions that results in difficulties accessing the transport system.* These barriers may stem from the land use and transport system, institutional arrangements or characteristics of the person (car ownership, low income, physical ability, age, etc.) (Lucas 2012).

Ultimately, however, transport disadvantage is reflected either in constraints to **accessibility** (e.g. reduced opportunities to travel) or reduced **mobility** (fewer trips and therefore fewer out-of-home activities) (Lucas 2012; Pyrialakou et al. 2016). The distinction between these two facets is important in the context of understanding research in the field.

## 4.3 Accessibility vs Mobility

As shown in Table 4.1, the literature linking transport and well-being overwhelmingly measures **mobility** in its various forms (number of trips, time use or out-of-home activities). This may be expected, as mobility is still the primary means to reach desired destinations that support participation in life's essential activities.

Furthermore, the act of travel itself can instil benefits through improving health, reinforcing social connections and capital on the journey, or deriving pleasure from the journey itself (Stanley et al. 2010; Jones et al. 2012; Morris and Guerra 2015). Only one study focussed exclusively on accessibility but it associated it with population-level quality of life indicators such as traffic crashes, employment rates and spatial amenity (Doi et al. 2008). To the authors' knowledge, to date there are no studies which attempt to link destination accessibility to individual well-being.

And yet it has been argued that **accessibility** places a value on a wider set of mobility choices, beyond what is actually chosen (or not). Furthermore, a number of scholars have recognized that the *potential* to travel (motility) can also have implications for well-being (De Vos et al. 2013). Indeed, most hypothetical models of how transport influences well-being make a case for the importance of accessibility as distinct from mobility. Ettema et al. (2010), perhaps the earliest hypothetical model in this space, focussed solely on mobility's impact on well-being; accessibility was not considered in this model. But then Delbosc (2012) emphasised the role of accessibility in facilitating satisfaction with activities; it also considered the indirect impact of transport infrastructure on well-being through externalities such as pollution and noise. Reardon and Abdallah (2013) took a broader view of how the transport system could influence well-being through its impacts on the economy, environment, social relationships (including social inclusion) and the individual. All of these models discussed the impact on 'well-being' somewhat generally without distinguishing between hedonic or eudemonic well-being.

De Vos et al. (2013) progressed the dialogue by developing a theoretical framework that more explicitly distinguishes between the role of accessibility and mobility through their diverging impact on hedonic and eudemonic well-being (see Fig. 4.1). They hypothesised that accessibility and mobility contribute to eudemonic well-being, or the ability to lead a full and meaningful life. Although mobility can contribute to eudemonic well-being, Shliselberg and Givoni (2017) argue that it primarily services short-term hedonic well-being and mood.

It is curious that no research has ever been undertaken to explore empirical relationships between accessibility and eudemonic well-being (Table 4.1). In part this may be an issue with measurement; we were only able to uncover two papers to date that has used a measure of eudemonic well-being (Vella-Brodrick and Stanley 2013), and one of those only incorporated the 'autonomy' aspect of a eudemonic scale (Delbosc and Vella-Brodrick 2015). Or perhaps these relationships are too long-term and complex to measure quantitatively. However there has been qualitative work that suggests these relationships are worth further exploration. For example, there is a rich body of work on older people facing driving cessation. It finds that a car does not just provide instrumental mobility; the motility (potential to travel) offered by a car also provides important psychological benefits (Musselwhite and Haddad 2010).

In contrast to well-being-transport studies, many social exclusion-transport studies adopt the lens of accessibility to understand dimensions of transport disadvantage (see Table 4.1). For example, Church et al. (2000) used London Transport's travel time estimation model to illustrate the degree of accessibility for economically

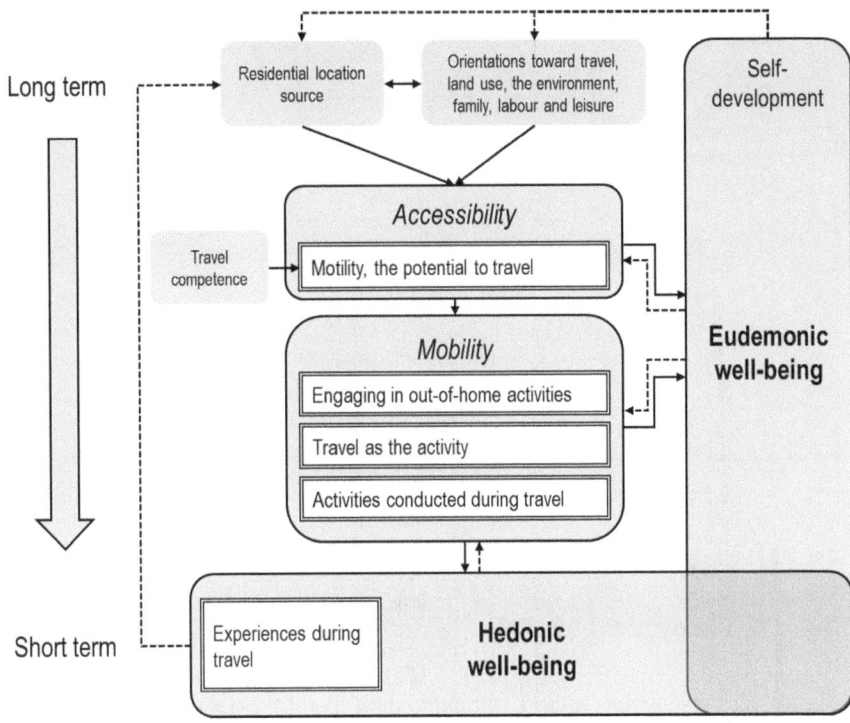

**Fig. 4.1** Links between accessibility, mobility and well-being (Source: Adapted from De Vos et al. 2013 and Mokhtarian 2015)

deprived areas of the city. Similarly, Casas (2007) mapped out the potential activity spaces for disabled persons and later compared time-space prisms and cumulative opportunity for children (Casas et al. 2009). Other authors focussed on transit accessibility or transit supply as the key indicator of access (Hurni 2007; Xia et al. 2016). Still others used composite measures of multiple indicators of access, such as subjective travel distance thresholds (Engels and Liu 2011) or a combination of destination accessibility, transit stops and road density (Xiao et al. 2017). All of these studies found some degree of association between social exclusion and problems with accessibility, often through identifying key regions of a city in need of greater access.

In contrast, fewer studies attempted to link social exclusion to mobility (realised travel). In urban Scotland, Hine (2004) found that women and people without cars took longer to access activities, although there was no consideration for the number of trips taken. Stanley et al. (2011) found that fewer daily trips was associated with a greater risk of social exclusion. Interestingly, one study that attempted to associate mobility with social exclusion through activity spaces and found *no association* between activity spaces and social exclusion (Schonfelder and Axhausen 2003), although the authors suggest this may be due to their travel survey method failing to recruit sufficiently disadvantaged populations.

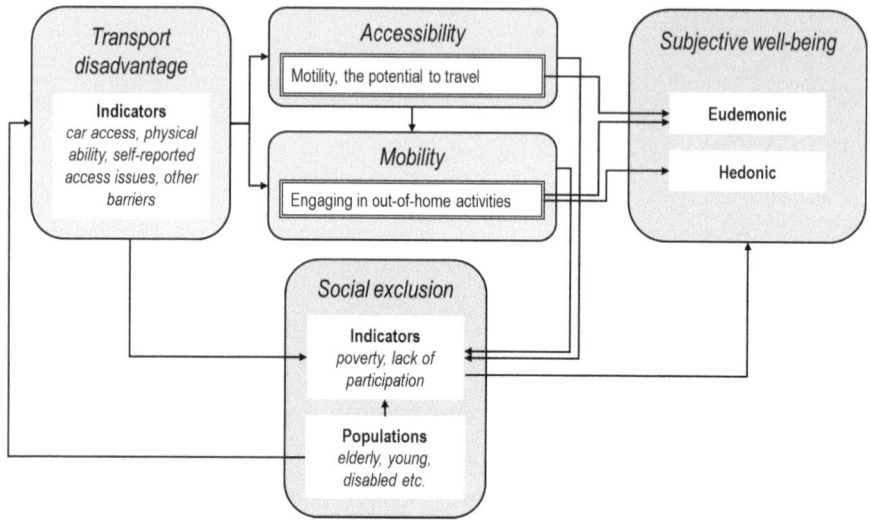

**Fig. 4.2** Links between transport, social exclusion and well-being

## 4.4 A Theoretical Model

Figure 4.2 presents the authors' thoughts on a likely theoretical framework which links the relevant components in the nexus between transport disadvantage, social exclusion and well-being. Accessibility and mobility both likely have an impact on social exclusion and well-being. Mobility is a function of accessibility, yet this link is rarely explored in the social exclusion, transport and well-being literature. Table 4.1 suggests only a single study has explored both accessibility and mobility and this was a qualitative study (Musselwhite and Haddad 2010).

The other key element of Fig. 4.2 is the separate consideration given to the eudemonic and hedonic aspects of well-being. As our review in Table 4.1 shows, eudemonic well-being is hardly researched and a fertile area for exploration.

## 4.5 How Much Transport Is Enough?

Until this point, our discussion of the relationships between transport, social exclusion and well-being has implicitly assumed that more transport (in whatever form) will improve outcomes in a more or less linear fashion. If low access/mobility causes social exclusion or lower well-being, then providing more access/mobility should improve the situation.

Yet we postulate that it is plausible that this relationship is non-linear: that 'more transport' will not always result in 'more inclusion' or 'more well-being.' There is likely a threshold effect, after which one more journey or one more potentially accessible destination is unlikely to improve one's situation. Although to our knowledge there are no studies that directly examine whether a threshold effect exists, there is indirect evidence that suggests a need for further exploration. For example there is evidence of satiation effects for activity duration, at least among the elderly (Ravulaparthy et al. 2016), where after a certain duration of activity well-being actually *decreases*.

It is also worth noting that the strongest relationships between transport and well-being are found among the most disadvantaged groups. It is no coincidence that most studies of transport's impact on social exclusion and well-being are conducted on the elderly, disabled, young adults or other disadvantaged groups; these are the groups that face the most restrictions on their travel. Consequently, these are the groups that stand to benefit the most from improvements to transport.

Studies that attempt to link these concepts across the general population have mixed success. For example, the earliest work attempting to empirically link self-reported transport disadvantage, social exclusion and well-being in the general population could not establish a statistically significant link between transport and well-being; instead, it acted through its impact on social exclusion and time poverty (Currie and Delbosc 2010). A later update of this model, which included a larger sample of disadvantaged populations, found a direct relationship between transport disadvantage and well-being (Delbosc and Currie 2011b). Further work in this area found that the relationship between transport and well-being was strongest in peri-urban and regional areas (Delbosc and Currie 2011c), the unemployed (Delbosc and Currie 2011a), among people who lack social support or rely on others for transport (Delbosc and Currie 2011d; Delbosc and Currie 2011a).

At the other end of the spectrum, there is growing evidence that excess travel can have a negative impact on individuals; so can transport and well-being be *negatively* linked in some cases? One study has found that longer commute times are associated with lower subjective well-being (Choi et al. 2013), although another study found that time spent travelling is positively associated with life satisfaction (Morris 2015). The negative impacts that excessive (generally car-based) mobility has on *society* are now well documented: congestion, pollution, road trauma and physical inactivity. One of the justifications for implementing road pricing is that if roads are priced correctly, trips that are less valuable to an individual will be reduced (Litman 2017), which will have follow-on benefits to society.

Yet there is an emerging discourse about the dark side of excess mobility on individuals. A new term, 'hypermobility', has been coined to describe excess travel (generally associated with business and frequent air travel). Although negative impacts are not likely to be as significant as the barriers faced by the transport disadvantaged, the glamorization of hypermobile lives may be masking the negative personal costs (Cohen and Gössling 2015). Frequent air travel contributes to fatigue, chronic jet lag, deep vein thrombosis and exposure to radiation. It can also contribute to time stress, social dislocation and alienation from family and the local community (Cohen and Gössling 2015). If excess long-distance travel has a negative side, is it feasible that negative social and psychological impacts could occur following 'excessive' shorter-distance daily travel?

Another potentially negative association between travel and well-being may occur when travel facilitates exposure to potentially harmful activities. For example, remote Australian aboriginal communities have strong family and social networks in their home communities. Transport facilitates access to jobs and essential services, but it also facilitates easier access to drugs and alcohol which can have devastating impacts on these communities (Brady 2000). In a similar vein, it has been argued that gaining a driving license exposes teenagers and young adults not just to the dangers of crash risk but also greater opportunities for sexual risk-taking, alcohol and drug use (Voas and Kelley-Baker 2008).

Overall these discussion points are important as they have significant implications for how 'equitable access' is integrated into policy and public discourse. For example some governments are moving away from using journey time savings as the primary valuation method and toward improving access to basic services (Wee and Geurs 2011). These policies may focus on horizontal equity (providing equal resources to all regardless of ability) or contain elements of vertical equity (providing additional resources to historically under-serviced groups). Overall, the focus is on how to minimise differences between people.

Yet if mobility and access provide only diminishing returns on well-being, perhaps a different perspective is in order. The ethical principle of 'sufficientarianism' proposes that everyone should live above a certain minimum threshold which is sufficient to meet their basic needs (Lucas et al. 2016). At present it is largely a political choice to decide how much access is 'sufficient' – how many jobs within 30 min is 'sufficient'? How many grocery stores? – although there may be a role for research to inform this choice.

## 4.6   Taking Stock and Looking Forward

This chapter provided an overview of existing research related to accessibility, exclusion and well-being and aimed to identify where future research needs to focus. A range of approaches to these topics have been undertaken but there are significant gaps in research to date:

- Only one research program to date has explored transport, social exclusion and also well-being using a quantitative framework. Most research explores either the transport-well-being or transport-social exclusion nexus.
- Although accessibility is a growing focus for policy and research, hardly any research in the transport and well-being area has used an accessibility-based approach. This is a fertile topic for future research.
- Almost all studies in the field have focussed on hedonic based aspects of well being; there is much scope to explore aspects of well-being in the eudemonic sphere.

Our narrative has also shown that almost all studies show some degree of association between transport, social inclusion and well-being and that in general these links are assumed to be linear. However we speculate that in practice some thresholds between travel, social exclusion and well-being are likely but again no research has confirmed this to date. Indeed we have also speculated that in some cases, *negative* links may existing between travel and well-being although these might be specific to a given context, social group or area.

The general policy implication of research to date is that transport has a significant social role and is important to the quality of life of humanity. This was probably already accepted, however it has never been fully explored quantitatively and this has been a major achievement of the contemporary research reviewed in this chapter.

The significance of this achievement should not be under-played; transport policy has spent a century understanding travel time and its economic implications for business and the community. The implications for human flourishing seem to be a more fundamentally important outcome for society than travel time, yet we only began to explore this in research over the last few decades. Despite this importance, one cannot help but consider the field to be somewhat immature; many hypothesised links between fundamental transport and well-being (Fig. 4.2) remain unexplored. There is clearly much scope to address this in future research in this field.

# References

Archer, M., Paleti, R., Konduri, K., Pendyala, R., & Bhat, C. (2013). Modeling the connection between activity-travel patterns and subjective well-being. *Transportation Research Record: Journal of the Transportation Research Board, 2382*, 102–111.

Banister, D., & Bowling, A. (2004). Quality of life for the elderly: The transport dimension. *Transport Policy, 11*, 105–115.

Bergstad, C. J., Gamble, A., Hagman, O., Polk, M., Garling, T., Ettema, D., Friman, M., & Olsson, L. E. (2012). Influences of affect associated with routine out-of-home activities on subjective well-being. *Applied Research in Quality of Life, 7*(1), 49–62.

Brady, M. (2000). Alcohol policy issues for indigenous people in the United States, Canada, Australia and New Zealand. *Contemporary Drug Problems, 27*(3), 435–509.

Casas, I. (2007). Social exclusion and the disabled: An acessibility approach. *The Professional Geographer, 59*(4), 463–477.

Casas, I., Horner, M. W., & Weber, J. (2009). A comparison of three methods for identifying transport-based exclusion: A case study of children's access to urban opportunities in Erie and Niagara Counties, New York. *International Journal of Sustainable Transportation, 3*(4), 227–245.

Choi, J., Coughlin, J., & D'Ambrosio, L. (2013). Travel time and subjective well-being. *Transportation Research Record: Journal of the Transportation Research Board, 2357*, 100–108.

Church, A., Frost, M., & Sullivan, K. (2000). Transport and social exclusion in London. *Transport Policy, 7*(3), 195–205.

Cohen, S. A., & Gössling, S. (2015). A darker side of hypermobility. *Environment and Planning A, 47*(8), 166–1679.

Currie, G., & Delbosc, A. (2010). Modelling the social and psychological impacts of transport disadvantage. *Transportation, 37*(6), 953–966.

Currie, G., & Delbosc, A. (2011). Transport disadvantage: A review. In *New perspectives and methods in transport and social exclusion research*. Bingley: Emerald.

De Vos, J., Schwanen, T., Van Acker, V., & Witlox, F. (2013). Travel and subjective well-being: A focus on findings, methods and future research needs. *Transport Reviews, 33*(4), 421–442.

Delbosc, A. (2012). The role of well-being in transport policy. *Transport Policy, 23*(0), 25–33.

Delbosc, A., & Currie, G. (2011a). Exploring the relative influences of transport disadvantage and social exclusion on well-being. *Transport Policy, 18*(4), 555–562.

Delbosc, A., & Currie, G. (2011b). Piecing it together: A structural equation model of transport, social exclusion and well-being. In G. Currie (Ed.), *New perspectives and methods in transport and social exclusion research.* Bingley: Emerald.

Delbosc, A., & Currie, G. (2011c). The spatial context of transport disadvantage, social exclusion and well-being. *Journal of Transport Geography, 19*(6), 1130–1137.

Delbosc, A., & Currie, G. (2011d). Transport problems that matter – Social and psychological links to transport disadvantage. *Journal of Transport Geography, 16*(1), 170–178.

Delbosc, A., & Vella-Brodrick, D. (2015). The role of transport in supporting the autonomy of young adults. *Transportation Research Part F: Traffic Psychology and Behaviour, 33*, 97–105.

Doi, K., Kii, M., & Nakanishi, H. (2008). An integrated evaluation method of accessibility, quality of life, and social interaction. *Environment and Planning B: Planning and Design, 35*(6), 1098–1116.

Engels, B., & Liu, G.-J. (2011). Social exclusion, location and transport disadvantage amongst non-driving seniors in a Melbourne municipality, Australia. *Journal of Transport Geography, 19*(4), 984–996.

Ettema, D., Gärling, T., Olsson, L. E., & Friman, M. (2010). Out-of-home activities, daily travel, and subjective well-being. *Transportation Research Part A: Policy and Practice, 44*(9), 723–732.

Hine, J. (2004). Transport disadvantage and social exclusion in Urban Scotland. *Built Environment, 30*(2), 161–171.

Hodgson, F. C., & Turner, J. (2003). Participation not consumption: The need for new participatory practices to address transport and social exclusion. *Transport Policy, 10*, 265–272.

Hurni, A. (2007). Marginalised groups in Western Sydney: The experience of sole parents and unemployed young people. In G. Currie, J. Stanley, & J. Stanley (Eds.), *No way to go: Transport and social disadvantage in Australian communities.* Melbourne: Monash University.

Jones, A., Steinbach, R., Roberts, H., Goodman, A., & Green, J. (2012). Rethinking passive transport: Bus fare exemptions and young people's wellbeing. *Health & Place, 18*(3), 605–612.

Litman, T. (2017). *Socially optimal transport prices and markets: Principles, strategies and impacts.* Victoria: Victorian Transport Policy Institute.

Lucas, K. (2011). Making the connections between transport disadvantage and the social exclusion of low income populations in the Tshwane Region of South Africa. *Journal of Transport Geography, 19*(6), 1320–1334.

Lucas, K. (2012). Transport and social exclusion: Where are we now? *Transport Policy, 20*, 105–113.

Lucas, K., van Wee, B., & Maat, K. (2016). A method to evaluate equitable accessibility: Combining ethical theories and accessibility-based approaches. *Transportation, 43*(3), 473–490.

Mokhtarian, P.L. (2015). Subjective well-being and travel: Retrospect & prospect. In *International association for travel behaviour research.* Windsor.

Mollenkopf, H., Baas, S., Marcellini, F., Oswald, F., Ruoppila, I., Szeman, Z., Tacken, M., & Wahl, H.-W. (2005). Mobility and quality of life. In H. Mollenkopf, F. Marcellini, I. Ruoppila, Z. Szeman, & M. Tacken (Eds.), *Enhancing mobility in later life: Personal coping, environmental resources and technical support.* Amsterdam: IOS Press.

Morris, E. A. (2015). Should we all just stay home? Travel, out-of-home activities, and life satisfaction. *Transportation Research Part A: Policy and Practice, 78*, 519–536.

Morris, E. A., & Guerra, E. (2015). Mood and mode: Does how we travel affect how we feel? *Transportation, 42*(1), 25–43.

Musselwhite, C., & Haddad, H. (2010). Mobility, accessibility and quality of later life. *Quality in Ageing and Older Adults, 11*(1), 25–37.

Nordbakke, S., & Schwanen, T. (2014). Well-being and mobility: A theoretical framework and literature review focusing on older people. *Mobilities, 9*(1), 104–129.

Özkazanç, S., & Sönmez, F. N. Ö. (2017). Spatial analysis of social exclusion from a transportation perspective: A case study of Ankara metropolitan area. *Cities, 67*, 74–84.

Pyrialakou, V. D., Gkritza, K., & Fricker, J. D. (2016). Accessibility, mobility, and realized travel behavior: Assessing transport disadvantage from a policy perspective. *Journal of Transport Geography, 51*, 252–269.

Ravulaparthy, S., Yoon, S., & Goulias, K. (2013). Linking elderly transport mobility and subjective well-being. *Transportation Research Record: Journal of the Transportation Research Board, 2382*, 28–36.

Ravulaparthy, S. K., Konduri, K. C., & Goulias, K. G. (2016). Fundamental linkages between activity time use and subjective well-being for the elderly population. *Transportation Research Record: Journal of the Transportation Research Board, 2566*, 31–40.

Reardon, L., & Abdallah, S. (2013). Well-being and transport: Taking stock and looking forward. *Transport Reviews, 33*(6), 634–657.

Ryan, R. M., & Deci, E. L. (2001). On happiness and human potentials: A review of research on hedonic and eudaimonic well-being. *Annual Review of Psychology, 52*, 141–166.

Schonfelder, S., & Axhausen, K. (2003). Activity spaces: Measures of social exclusion? *Transport Policy, 10*, 273–286.

Shay, E., Combs, T. S., Findley, D., Kolosna, C., Madeley, M., & Salvesen, D. (2016). Identifying transportation disadvantage: Mixed-methods analysis combining GIS mapping with qualitative data. *Transport Policy, 48*, 129–138.

Shliselberg, R., & Givoni, M. (2017). Motility as a policy objective. *Transport Reviews*, 1–19.

Spinney, J. E. L., Scott, D. M., & Newbold, K. B. (2009). Transport mobility benefits and quality of life: A time-use perspective of elderly Canadians. *Transport Policy, 16*(1), 1–11.

Stanley, J. (2011a). Measuring social exclusion. In G. Currie (Ed.), *New perspectives and methods in transport and social exclusion research*. Bingley: Emerald.

Stanley, J. (2011b). Social Exclusion. In G. Currie (Ed.), *New perspectives and methods in transport and social exclusion research*. Bingley: Emerald.

Stanley, J., Stanley, J., Vella-Broderick, D., & Currie, G. (2010). The place of transport in facilitating social inclusion via the mediating influence of social capital. *Research in Transportation Economics, 29*, 280–286.

Stanley, J. K., Hensher, D. A., Stanley, J. R., & Vella-Broderick, D. (2011). Mobility, social exclusion and well-being: Exploring the links. *Transportation Research Part A, 45*, 789–801.

Titheridge, H., & Solomon, J. (2008). Social exclusion, accessibility and lone parents. In *UK-Ireland planning research conference*. Belfast.

Vella-Brodrick, D. A., & Stanley, J. (2013). The significance of transport mobility in predicting well-being. *Transport Policy, 29*(0), 236–242.

Voas, R., & Kelley-Baker, T. (2008). Licensing teenagers: Nontraffic risks and benefits in the transition to driving status. *Traffic Injury Prevention, 9*, 89–97.

Wasfi, R., Steinmetz-Wood, M., & Levinson, D. (2017). Measuring the transportation needs of people with developmental disabilities: A means to social inclusion. *Disability and Health Journal, 10*(2), 356–360.

Wee, B., & Geurs, K. (2011). Discussing equity and social exclusion in accessibility evaluations. *European Journal of Transport and Infrastructure Research, 11*(4).

Xia, J. C., Nesbitt, J., Daley, R., Najnin, A., Litman, T., & Tiwari, S. P. (2016). A multi-dimensional view of transport-related social exclusion: A comparative study of greater perth and Sydney. *Transportation Research Part A: Policy and Practice, 94*, 205–221.

Xiao, R., Wang, G., & Wang, M. (2017). *Social indicators research*. https://doi.org/10.1007/s11205-017-1616-2

# Part III
# Case-Study Applications

# Chapter 5
# Commuting and Happiness: What Ways Feel Best for What Kinds of People?

**Sascha Lancée, Martijn Burger, and Ruut Veenhoven**

**Abstract** How happy we are, depends partly on how we live our life and part of our way of life is how we commute between home and work. In that context, we are faced with the question of how much time spent on commuting is optimal happiness wise and with what means of transportation we will feel best. Decisions about commuting are typically made as a side issue in job choice and there are indications that we are bad in predicting how such decisions will work out on our happiness in the long-run. For that reason, it is helpful to know how commuting has worked out on the happiness of other people and on people like you in particular. Several cross-sectional studies found lower happiness among long-distance commuters and among users of public transportation. Yet these differences could be due to selection effects, such as unhappy people opting more often for distant jobs without having a car. Still another limitation is that earlier research has focused on the average effect of commuting, rather than specifying what is optimal for whom. Data of the Dutch 'Happiness Indicator' study was analyzed, in the context of which 5000 participants recorded what they had done in the previous day and how happy they had felt during these activities. This data allows comparison between how the same person feels at home and during commute, which eliminates selection effects. The number of participants is large enough to allow a split-up between different kinds of people, in particular among the many well-educated women who participated in this study. People feel typically less happy when commuting than at home, and that the negative

An extended version of this paper was published in Transportation Research Part A 104C (2017) pp. 195–208, DOI: 10.1016/j.tra.2017.04.025

S. Lancée · M. Burger
Erasmus Happiness Economics Research Organization (EHERO), Erasmus University Rotterdam, Rotterdam, The Netherlands
e-mail: mburger@ese.eur.nl

R. Veenhoven (✉)
Erasmus Happiness Economics Research Organization (EHERO), Erasmus University Rotterdam, Rotterdam, The Netherlands

Opentia Research Program, North-West University, Potchefstroom, South Africa
e-mail: veenhoven@ese.eur.nl

difference is largest when commuting with public transportation and smallest when commuting by bike. It is not per se the commuting time that causes happiness loss, but specific combinations of commuting time and commuting mode. Increasing commuting times can even lead to a gain in happiness for certain types of women, when the commute is by bike. Split-up by different kinds of people shows considerable differences, such as an optimal commute alone or even by public transport for some highly educated women. Optimal ways of commuting for different kinds of people are presented in a summary table, from which individuals can read what will fit them best. The differences illustrate that research focusing on average effects of happiness will not help individuals in making a more informed choice.

**Keywords** Happiness · Hedonic level of affect · Mood during commute · Day Reconstruction Method (DRM)

## 5.1   Introduction

The last few decades show a rising interest in happiness, also known as 'life satisfaction' and 'subjective wellbeing'. This topic has been around since antiquity in Western society and has been much debated ever since. Happiness was once an object of theoretical speculation, now it is an object of empirical research in the social sciences and increasingly in economics (Layard 2005; Frey and Stutzer 2002). The rise of scientific interest in happiness is part of a wider cultural change, in which 'quality of life' gains prominence relative to traditional values such as religious devotion and societal success (Veenhoven 2016).

Empirical research on happiness has shown that most people are happy, at least in contemporary developed nations (Veenhoven 2015a). Research in modern societies has also shown that greater happiness is possible for most people and that an individual's happiness depends to a considerable degree on the choices that one makes in life (Lyubomirsky 2008). As people typically want to live a happy life, there is a demand for information on the effects of choices on happiness. This information demand reflects in soaring sales of 'how to be happy books' and the development of the life-coaching business. Although much of this advice is based on folk-wisdom, empirical happiness research is increasingly used to support the informed pursuit of happiness (Veenhoven 2015c).

One of the choices we make is how we travel between work and home, an important aspect of modern life, which takes up a lot of time of daily life. Even in a small country such as the Netherlands, commuting is a surprisingly time-consuming activity with an average commuting time of 34.5 min one way (ANWB 2015), while at the same time commuting time and distances increased considerably over the past decades (Van Wee et al. 2006; Susilo and Maat 2007). To make a well-informed choice on this matter it is helpful to know how different aspects of commuting have affected the happiness of other people in general and of people like us in particular.

Hence, the question addressed in this paper is '*What does optimal commuting look like to enhance happiness for whom?*' To answer this question, three related sub-questions will be answered.

1. Does commuting affect happiness? If so, how much?
2. Which aspects of commuting influence happiness most and least?
3. How different are these effects across persons and situations?

## 5.2 Previous Research

Commuting is an important and increasing part of how workers use their time. For instance, Koslowsky et al. (1995) note that psychologists have long recognized the possible negative effects of commuting on psychological health and found that commuting is often experienced as an unpleasant experience that has delayed effects on health and family life. Amongst others, commuting leads to increased anxiety and hostility (Koslowsky et al. 1995). Since Koslowsky et al. (1995), more and more research has looked into the relationship between commuting and happiness, which in general states that commuting has a negative effect on life satisfaction, also known as subjective well-being (Pfaff 2014; Dolan et al. 2006; Frey and Stutzer 2014). Moreover, Kahneman et al. (2003) found that commuting appears to be the daily activity that generates the lowest level of positive affect and a high level of negative affect. Important negative aspects of commuting are boredom and increased social isolation, which leads to unhappiness (Gatersleben and Uzzell 2007; Putnam 2000).

### 5.2.1 Topics

Several aspects of commuting in specific add to the negative consequences of commuting while others help diminish these effects. These aspects will now be discussed.

*Commuting Time* Stutzer and Frey (2008) have researched the effects of commuting on subjective well-being in Germany in a study of 14 years. Their research found that people with a longer commuting time systematically indicate that they have a lower subjective well-being. In a replication study, Studer and Winkelmann (2011) found similar results. However, they also found that very satisfied people are less affected by an increasing commuting time than people who are dissatisfied with their life. Research by the Office for National Statistics (ONS) in the United Kingdom indicates that each successive minute of travel decreases the level of life satisfaction. Average levels of happiness significantly drop after 15 min of commuting and life satisfaction after 45 min of commuting. In general, the worst effects come from commuting times between 60 and 90 min (ONS 2014). Van der Meer and Wielers (2013) indicate that commuting times defined as short and long have larger negative effect on happiness than moderate commuting times. Commuting time is also negatively associated with satisfaction with the environment, health satisfaction and satisfaction with spare time (Kahneman et al. 2003).

*Commuting Mode* Research on commuting mode and subjective wellbeing has generally found that cycling and walking to work contribute to higher levels of subjective wellbeing compared to motorized travel (Duarte et al. 2010; Friman et al. 2013; Olsson et al. 2013; Ettema and Smajic 2014; Morris and Guerra 2015; Chng et al. 2016). In particular, Ettema and Smajic (2014) found that the level of physical activity involved in walking increases mental health and enhances the mood, indicating that commuting modes involving physical activity might have a lower negative or even positive effect on happiness. On a different note, several studies have reported that commuting by car generates higher levels of subjective wellbeing than commuting by public transportation or transit (Mokhtarian and Solomon 2001; Ettema et al. 2011; Abou-Zeid et al. 2012; Morris and Guerra 2015; Olsson et al. 2013). As pointed out by Morris and Guerra (2015), the difference in subjective wellbeing of car and public transport commuters can be explained by factors such as prestige, self-esteem, convenience, comfort, reliability, and greater control over one's environment.

*Travelling Alone or Together* According to Ettema et al. (2012) the strongest positive effect on satisfaction with travel is talking to others during the travel. This indicates how travelling alone or together can influence the commuters' happiness.

*Rush Hour* Commuting can be a major cause of stress due to its unpredictability and perceived loss of control (Roberts et al. 2011). When people do not have control over certain factors that can occur during driving, commuting is experienced as more stressful and leads people to report lower experienced well-being. Drivers generally experience a lesser feeling of control during rush hours when environmental stressors are the highest and the driver needs a higher level of concentration to focus on his task.

*To Work or Back Home* Ettema et al. (2012) examined the difference between commuting to work and from work on satisfaction with travel. It appears that commuters have different mindsets when travelling to and from work. While commuters on the way to work prepare themselves for a working day, on the way home the prospect of private time enables them to be more open to enjoying the commute. This is also shown for ICT use in public transport, which has a negative effect on well-being on the way to work when ICT use is possibly work related, whereas it has a positive effect on well-being on the way home when ICT is possibly used to coordinate private time (Ettema et al. 2012). This indicates that the experienced happiness when commuting may also be different to and from work. See also Olsson et al. (2013). In contrast, Koslowsky et al. (1995) found that commuting always leads to a bad temper, either when arriving at work or at home.

*Differences in Effects*  Robert et al. (2011) mainly looked into gender differences in the effects of commuting on psychological health and found that although women tend to commute less, they are more influenced by the negative effects of commuting than men. It is argued that this is because women have a greater responsibility for the household. Within their wide variety of tasks besides work, commuting is another competing demand on a woman's time and thus a greater psychological burden.

## 5.2.2   Limitations

Although the existing literature has produced a rich body of knowledge on subjective well-being and transportation, several issues have remained unaddressed in this literature. First, selection effects are often not well-covered. For example, several cross-sectional studies found lower subjective wellbeing among long-distance commuters and among users of public transportation; however, these differences could be due to selection effects, such as unsuccessful unhappy workers settling more often for a job far away. Another point not taken into account is that people have different determined set points (Lykken and Tellegen 1996) and personality traits (e.g. Furnham and Cheng 1999) that largely affect their mood level.[1]

Another limitation is that earlier research has focused on the average effect of commuting, rather than addressing the heterogeneous relationship between commuting and well-being and specifying what is optimal for whom. Commuting is likely to work out differently for different people and the question is rather how relations differ in subgroups of the general population. For example, where for some people travelling by car can be conducive to their level of affect, for other types of people more active transport modes such as biking or walking have a positive impact on well-being. This is worth knowing, not only for individual commuters, but also for policy makers in the field of transportation.

In our exploratory analysis, we address both selection effects and the heterogeneous relationship between commuting and well-being, where we examine what way of travel feels best for what kind of people.

## 5.3   Approach of This Study

### 5.3.1   Concept of Happiness

The term 'happiness' has been around since antiquity in Western society, but its meaning has been continuously debated ever since. For this paper, we use the definition of overall happiness developed by Veenhoven (2012:334). Happiness is

---

[1]For an exception see Morris and Guerra (2015).

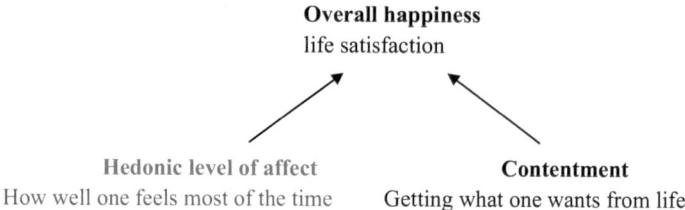

**Fig. 5.1** Components of happiness

*'the degree to which an individual judges the overall quality of his/her own life-as-a-whole favorably'*. Simply put: how much one likes the life one leads.

Veenhoven distinguishes between 'overall' happiness and the different 'components' of happiness, which function as 'sub-totals' in the overall evaluation of life (Veenhoven 1984, 2009). First, there is the affective component, called 'hedonic level of affect'. This entails how well we feel most of the time. Second, there is the cognitive component, called 'contentment', which is the degree to which we think we have what we want in life. These components of happiness are visually represented in Fig. 5.1. The weight of the two sources of happiness is variable, though hedonic level tends to dominate (Veenhoven 2009). The affective component, hedonic level of affect, is central to this study.

## 5.3.2  Research Method: Day Reconstruction Method

The data is gathered using the Day Reconstruction Method (DRM). Respondents first 'reconstruct' the previous day, listing all the activities that they engaged in and recording with whom they did these activities and where. Next, they rate how well they felt during each of these activities. Thus, DRM is a combination of time-use study and a mood diary. Contrary to traditional survey research, it captures momentary experience rather than global memories and provides a comprehensive view of the day.

DRM is a rather new tool, which was developed by Kahneman et al. (2003). The DRM is an appropriate tool to measure instant happiness over the course of one day by combining features of time-budget measurement and experience sampling. Time-budget studies assess how people spend their time and typically uses diaries (e.g. Juster and Stafford 1991). Experience sampling techniques capture mood of the moment and often use cell phones for that purpose (e.g. Shiffman et al. 2008).

### 5.3.3   Data Source

The data was collected through a website called *Happiness Indicator* (2016), which is available at http://happinessindicator.com. The Dutch variant is named 'GeluksWijzer' (2011 http://www.gelukswijzer.nl). The *Happiness Indicator* is a combination of a self-help website and a long-term follow up study on happiness. The Happiness Indicator involves an on-line application of the above-mentioned Day Reconstruction Method, in that context called the 'Happiness Diary'.

The *Happiness Indicator* aims to foster happiness in two ways. In the short term by making people more aware of how happy they are and how much they enjoy their daily activities. Respondents not only get a better view of how they feel most of the time, but can also compare with how similar respondents feel. This informs them about chances of getting happier and how. The long-term goal is to get a view on the effects of mayor life choices on happiness, such as having children or early retirement and in particular how such choices work out for different kinds of people. This information should then be used for evidence based happiness education.

The *Happiness Indicator* is an initiative of health-insurance company VGZ and the Erasmus University Rotterdam. The website has been online in the Netherlands since 2009.

### 5.3.4   Variables

#### 5.3.4.1   Demographics

Respondents were recruited by using client communications of the health-insurance company and free publicity. Interested individuals visited the website and created an account. Next, they enter information about their age, gender, education, income, job specifics, chronic illness, pets, alcohol and tobacco use, height and weight. This 'profile' is used later for comparing with similar respondents.

#### 5.3.4.2   Commuting and Happiness Measured Using the Happiness Diary

Happiness for this data was measured through the *Happiness Diary*. The happiness diary is an internet application of the Day Reconstruction Method as described above. In the happiness diary, you can indicate your activities per half hour of the day and then rate your experienced happiness during these activities on a scale from 1 to 10 as shown in Figs. 5.2, 5.3, and 5.4.

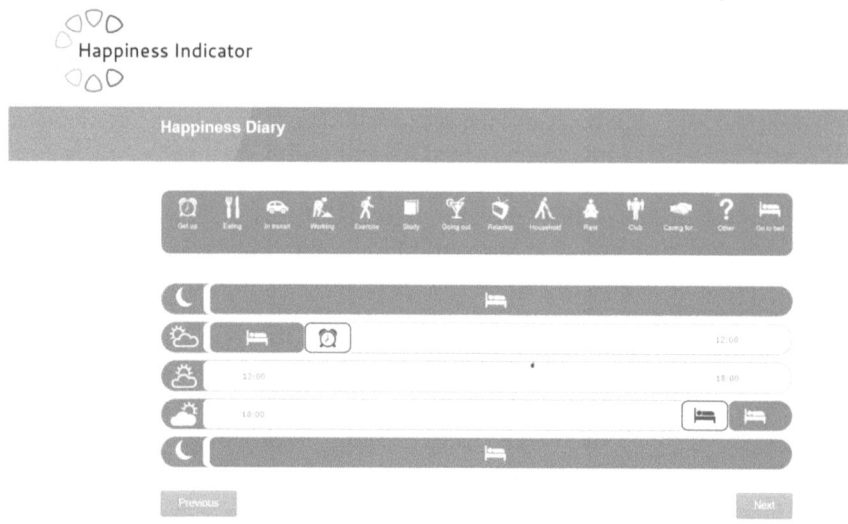

**Fig. 5.2** Example of a happiness diary

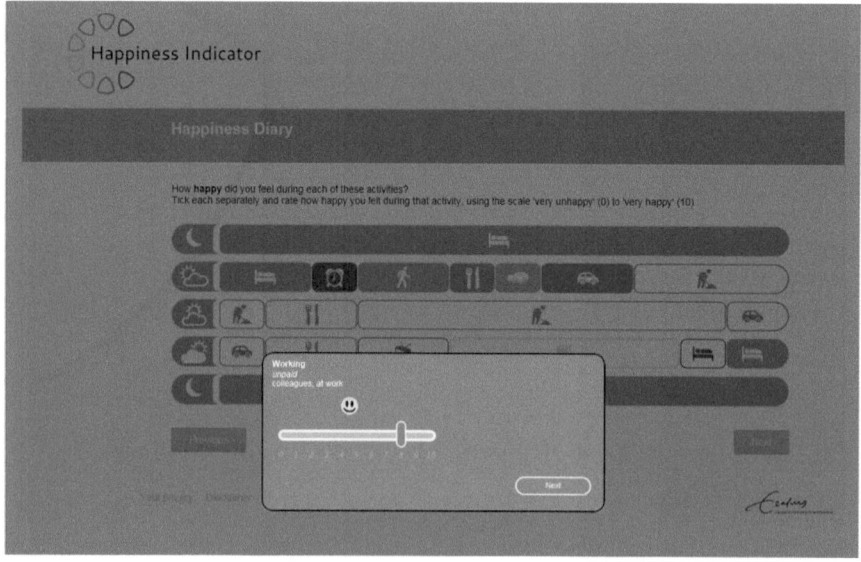

**Fig. 5.3** Rating of happiness during daily activities

One of the activities is 'in transit'. When that activity takes place before or after work we assume it is 'commuting'. The respondents then indicate with whom they were in transit. Then they indicate with which transport mode they commuted. From

**Your Happiness Diary**

The Happiness Diary shows how much happiness you derive from everyday things and activities. If you fill in the diary more often, you will get more information about your lifestyle and your happiness. With this information you can start looking for the lifestyle that best suits you.

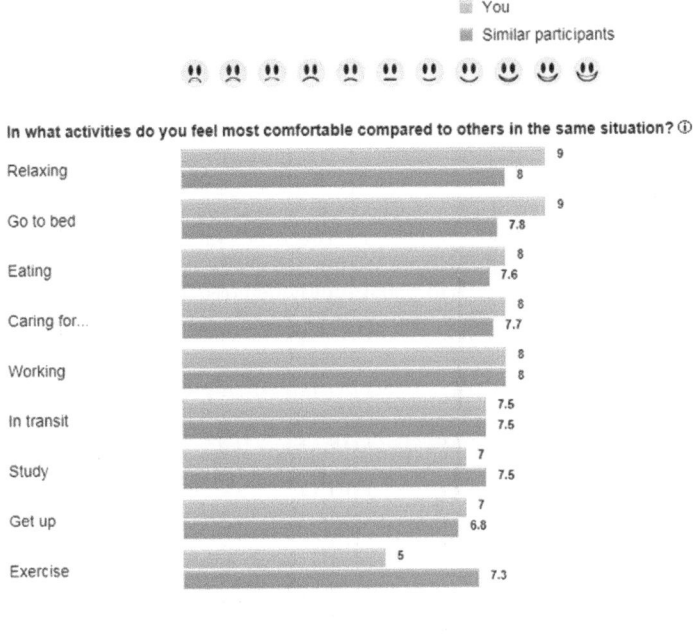

**Fig. 5.4** Comparison of an individual's mood during activities with the average of similar people

the questions, we can thus find if people commute, how long they commute, with what commuting mode, if they commute alone or together and what their mood is during the commute. The hours of their commute show us if this was in or out of rush hour (06:30–09:00 and 16:00–18:30 ANWB 2015; NS 2015) and if they were commuting to work (morning) or back from work (evening).

The happiness diary can then compare your experienced happiness during different activities with others 'like you' as shown in Fig. 5.4. The average happiness grade for all activities on one day combined represent the average daily mood. The average happiness grade for all activities at home, indicated by the question where this activity found place, represent the average mood at home.

It should be noted that data collected online has some well-known limitations, such as problems with the representativeness of the sample and quality of the data. However, given the goal of the *'Happiness Indicator'*, representativeness is not really a problem. The *'Happiness Indicator'* gathers information **on** particular people, **for** particular people, in this case mainly on and for well-educated women interested in getting happier than they are. Representativeness' for the general population is therefore not required. What is required is representativeness for the specific goal-group.

In total, the happiness diary provided about 100.000 data points, which allow comparison over time of some 5000 participants.

### 5.3.5  Descriptive Statistics

#### 5.3.5.1  Demographics

The demographic characteristics of the respondents are shown in Table 5.1. Most of the participants were female (82%), had paid employment (87%), and were highly educated (62%). In terms of living-situation 24% of them lived alone and 38% had children living at home. On average, the participants worked 4.13 days or 30.7 h per week. The majority of the participants was active in the non-profit sector.

Obviously, the participants are not representative of Dutch society and the results of this study can therefore not be generalized to the general population in the Netherlands. We do not see this as a major problem, since the goal of this study was to generate information *on particular people, for particular people,* namely those who would like to improve their happiness through a self-help website.

**Table 5.1**  Demographic characteristics of respondents

| Variable | $N$ | Mean | Median | Min. | Max. | S.D. |
|---|---|---|---|---|---|---|
| **Gender** (1 = male, 2 = female) | 1328 | 1.82 | 2 | 1 | 2 | .385 |
| **Education** (1 = Primary, 2 = VMBO, 3 = MBO, 4 = HAVO, 5 = VWO, 6 = HBO, 7 = University) | 1328 | 5.2 | 6 | 1 | 7 | 1.69 |
| **Family income** (1 = below average, 2 = average, 3 = above average) | 1327 | 2.16 | 2 | 1 | 3 | .78 |
| **Living situation** (1 = alone, 2 = together, 3 = two parent family with children, 4 = one parent family with children, 5 = living group, 6 = intramural, 7 = living with parents, 8 = different, 9 = divorced) | 1328 | 3.04 | 2 | 1 | 9 | 2.14 |
| **Chronic disease** (1 = no, 2 = yes) | 1328 | 1.13 | 1 | 1 | 2 | .42 |
| **Paid work** (1 = yes, 2 = no) | 1316 | 1.13 | 1 | 1 | 2 | .33 |
| **Sector** (1 = government, 2 = education, 3 = healthcare, 4 = cultural services, 5 = business and financial services, 6 = transportation, 7 = retail, 8 = hospitality and recreation, 9 = other) | 1144 | 4.39 | 3 | 1 | 9 | 2.64 |
| **Working days** | 1161 | 4.12 | 4 | 0 | 7 | 1.12 |
| **Working hours** | 1162 | 30.61 | 32 | 0 | 70 | 10.5 |

*N = 1450*

**Table 5.2** Frequencies for the commuting aspects

| Variable | Time | Car | Public | Bike | Multimodal with walking | Multimodal without walking | With someone | In rush hour | To work | Back from work |
|---|---|---|---|---|---|---|---|---|---|---|
| N | 4354 | 2009 | 582 | 1258 | 238 | 164 | 634 | 3066 | 2495 | 1878 |

$N = 33,281$

Representativeness for the general population was therefore not required; what was required is exemplification of a specific goal-group.

### 5.3.5.2  Commuting Time and Mode

The frequencies for all the commuting aspects are given in Table 5.2. The participants commuted on average 45 min one way, with a standard deviation of 27 min. Most participants indicated that they commuted for approximately 30 min. The car (48%) and bike (27%) were the most used transport modes, followed by public transport (13%). The category 'Other/Multimodal' represents commuting using other or multiple transportation modes. The most often mentioned commuting modes that fell into this category were combinations of the active modes of commuting and public transportation (77%). Over half of the commuting trips (58%) took place during rush hours, while most respondents (89%) travelled alone to work.

### 5.3.5.3  Mood

The descriptive statistics for the well-being variables are given in Table 5.3. The average daily mood of respondents at the first time of participation was a 6.7, which is slightly below average affect scores around 7.0 reported in Dutch surveys (see Veenhoven 2015b). During 37% of the activities the mood level was rated 6 or lower. This indicates that the *Happiness Indicator* website particularly attracts individuals who are less happy than the average citizen is and probably therefore would like to work on their happiness.

Participants feel mostly happier during other times of the day than while commuting. On average, average affect during commuting was rated a 6.5, which is lower than the 'average mood at home'.

The mean affect level for the main different activities during the working day is shown in Fig. 5.5. From the graph, it becomes clear that commuting is, on average, disliked more than other activities, particularly leisure and eating. Likewise, travel for other purposes is evaluated more positively than commuting. At the same time, the average mood level for commuting indicates that most people do not have the most terrible time when commuting.

**Table 5.3** Descriptive statistics for happiness variables

| Variable | $N$ | Mean | Median | Min. | Max. | S.d. |
|---|---|---|---|---|---|---|
| Average daily mood | 33,281 | 7.69 | 7.88 | 1 | 11 | 1.22 |
| Mood during commute | 4345 | 7.45 | 8.00 | 1 | 11 | 1.56 |
| Average mood at home | 33,281 | 7.65 | 7.88 | 1 | 11 | 1.30 |
| Difference in mood during commute and at home | 4345 | −.20 | −.14 | −7.09 | 5.21 | 1.21 |

$N = 33,281$

## 5.4 Results

The main question of this paper is: *What does optimal commuting look like to enhance happiness for whom?*' and this question was broken down into the following sub-questions:

1. Does commuting affect happiness? If so, how much?
2. Which aspects of commuting influence happiness most and least?
3. How different are these effects across persons and situations? (cf. Sect. 5.1)

What answers to these questions do our data allow?

### 5.4.1  Does Commuting Affect Happiness? If So How Much?

The effect of commuting on happiness is captured by the difference in mood during travel and at home. These effects tend to be negative, as can be seen in Table 5.4, which presents average differences in happiness by aspects of commuting. Likewise, the correlation matrix in Table 5.5 links between commuting and happiness.

These statistical relations indicate a causal effect of commuting on happiness. Reversed causation is unlikely to be involved since happiness is measured by with-in person differences. Even if trait-unhappy persons are more likely to commute by public transportation that will not affect this within-person difference in mood during commute and at home. Neither is response bias likely to be involved. If trait happy people tend to have a rosier look on life, that will influence their rating of mood during commuting about as much as their rating of how they feel at home.

Table 5.6 provides also an answer the question of *how much* commuting affects happiness. The differences in mood during commute and at home vary between +.05 (traveling with someone) to −.70 (travel to between 30 and 60 min), that is between 0,5% and 7% on this 0–10 scale. When all commute variables are entered together in a regression analysis, an explained variance of 3% appears (Table 5.6). A more sophisticated econometric analysis, reported in Lancee et al. (2017), showed that, on average, mood during commuting is 0.28 points lower compared to average mood during the day.

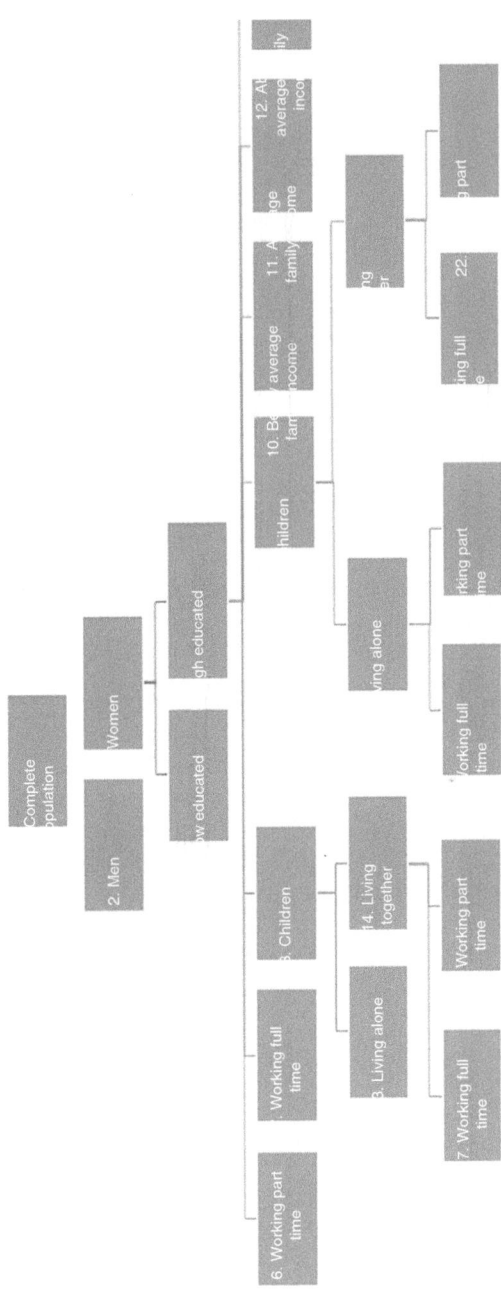

**Fig. 5.5** Average affect levels during main activities of the working day

**Table 5.4** Commuting and mood: means on scale 0–10 for the entire population

| | | Difference in mood during commute and at home | N data points |
|---|---|---|---|
| Time | <30 (0) | −.34 | 41 |
| | 30 | −.70 | 2739 |
| | 60 | −.22 | 1115 |
| | 90 | −.41 | 308 |
| | 120 | −.35 | 77 |
| Mode | Car | −.21 | 1995 |
| | Public | −.50 | 577 |
| | Bike | −.08 | 1253 |
| | Multimodal with walking | −.27 | 238 |
| | Multimodal without walking | −.06 | 161 |
| Travel with someone | | +.05 | 629 |
| Rush hour | | −.21 | 2882 |
| Travel to work | | −.29 | 2478 |
| Travel back from work | | −.08 | 1867 |

Data points: $N = 33{,}465$

### 5.4.2 Which Aspects of Commuting Influence Happiness Most and Least?

The averages presented in Table 5.6 show that public transport goes with the greatest loss in happiness of about half a point (−.50). Commuting by car involves a much smaller loss of happiness and commute by bike the least. The most positive effect was found by a commute with someone for both the comparison of means (+.05), and the correlation matrix (+.09, p < .05).

Split-up by commuting time in Table 5.7 hardly changes that picture, but reveals a small positive effect of commuting by bike for about an hour. Surprisingly, we observed little effect of commuting time as such; the loss is more in the mode of transportation than in the duration of transportation. This is illustrated by the size of the happiness dip in public transportation, which is deepest with the shortest commuting time.

### 5.4.3 What Way of Commuting Is Optimal for Whom?

Average effects of commuting on happiness may veil substantial differences across kinds of people; for instance, a zero correlation may result from a strong positive effect in one-half of a sample and an equally strong positive effect in the other. Since we aim at tailored advice, we split-up in subgroups as far as the allowed. These sub-groups are presented in Fig. 5.6. As higher educated women are well represented among the participants we could differentiate most in this category.

**Table 5.5** Correlation matrix

| Variable | M | S.D. | 1 | 2 | 3 | 4 | 5 | 6 | 7 | 8 | 9 | 10 |
|---|---|---|---|---|---|---|---|---|---|---|---|---|
| 1. Time (in min.) | 45 | 27 | 1 | | | | | | | | | |
| 2. Car | – | – | -.09 | 1 | | | | | | | | |
| 3. Public | – | – | +.26 | -.03 | 1 | | | | | | | |
| 4. Bike | – | – | -.23 | -.05 | -.03 | 1 | | | | | | |
| 5. Multimodal with walking | – | – | +.15 | -.02 | -.01 | -.02 | 1 | | | | | |
| 6. Multimodal without walking | – | – | +.15 | -.02 | -.01 | -.01 | -.01 | 1 | | | | |
| 7. Travelling with someone | .02 | .14 | +.06 | +.20 | +.14 | +.23 | +.05 | +.03 | 1 | | | |
| 8. Rush hour | .09 | .29 | -.08 | +.49 | +.27 | +.41 | +.16 | +.14 | +.32 | 1 | | |
| 9. To work | .07 | .26 | -.02 | +.47 | +.24 | +.39 | +.15 | +.14 | +.26 | +.62 | 1 | |
| 10. Back from work | .06 | .23 | +.02 | +.42 | +.22 | +.31 | +.15 | +.11 | +.23 | +.42 | -.07 | 1 |
| 11. Difference mood when commuting and at home | -.20 | 1.21 | -.02 | -.03 | -.10 | +.06 | -.01 | +.02 | +.09 | -.01 | -.09 | +.09 |

Notes: In bold = $p < 0.05$, $N = 33{,}465$

**Table 5.6** Explained variance of the different regression analyses

|  | Average daily mood | | Mood during commute | | Mood at home | | Difference in mood during commute and at home | |
|---|---|---|---|---|---|---|---|---|
| Variable | M1 | M2 | M1 | M2 | M1 | M2 | M1 | M2 |
| $R^2$ | .04 | .05 | .02 | .05 | .04 | .05 | .01 | .03 |
| Adjusted $R^2$ | .04 | .05 | .02 | .05 | .04 | .05 | .00 | .03 |

**Table 5.7** Mean loss or gain of happiness combining commuting time and mode for the entire population

|  | Commuting time | | | | | |
|---|---|---|---|---|---|---|
|  | 30 (min) | N | 60 (min) | N | 90–120 (min) | n |
| Commuting mode |  |  |  |  |  |  |
| Car | −**.19** | 1348 | −.22 | 473 | −.34 | 141 |
| Public transport | −**.66** | 141 | −**.37** | 274 | −.59 | 153 |
| Bike | −**.11** | 1040 | **+.04** | 183 | +.06 | 17 |
| Multimodal with walking | −.22 | 78 | −**.38** | 93 | −.13 | 62 |
| Multimodal without walking | −.14 | 35 | −.02 | 81 | −.01 | 39 |

$N = 33,465$

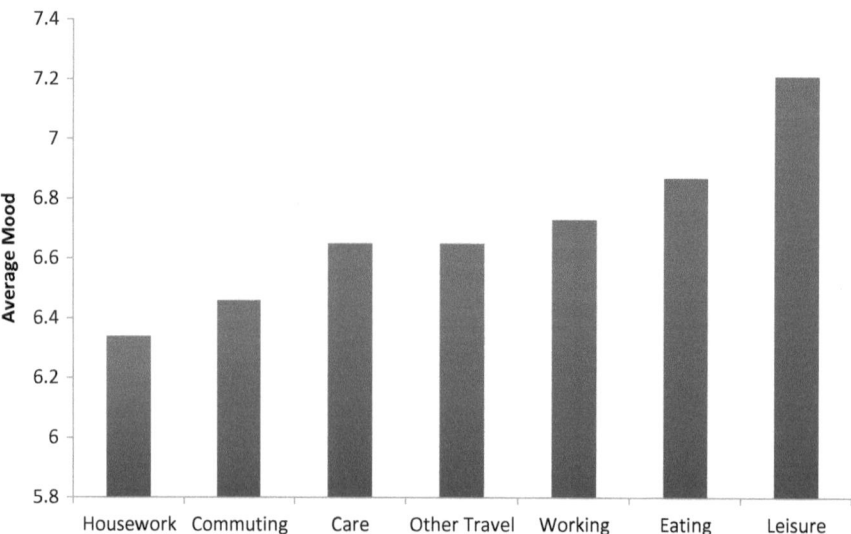

**Fig. 5.6** Overview of sub-groups

Overall the most optimal commuting mode for highly educated women is most often the bike, and the least optimal commuting mode public transport. However, this is actually the opposite for women living alone without children and working part time.

The most optimal commute is more often a commute with someone, but for several types of highly educated women feel better when commuting alone. Half of highly educated women should commute out of rush hour for an optimal commute, while the other half should commute in rush hour for an optimal commute.

The effects of different commuting modes for each of these subgroups are summarized on Table 5.8, in which an '+' stands for the commuting aspect that should be used to enhance happiness and a '−' stands for a commuting aspect that should not be used when one wants to enhance happiness. When a '↓' is given for the commuting time >0, this indicates that as commuting time increases, the loss of happiness increases.

Elsewhere we reported an econometric analysis of these differences (Lancee et al. 2017), which revealed striking differences between groups for the different commuting modes. While for men, older, higher-income and higher-educated people the active modes appear to be conducive for mood, this does not hold for the women, young, lower-income and lower-educated; the active modes (walking and biking) do not boost the mood of these latter people. These differences can be explained by differences in lifestyle and location of residence, which need further examination.

Travelling with someone has less effect on the mood of people with children. Apparently when children are the ones on board, e.g., they are being brought to school on a multipurpose commuting trip, travelling with someone is less satisfying than when travelling with partner, colleagues or friends.

## 5.5   Discussion

### 5.5.1   Main Findings

Analysis of the Happiness Indicator dataset confirms earlier studies that observed a negative effect of commuting on happiness. Beyond that, the within-person comparison shows that the negative effect is causal, that is, not due to selection bias or reversed causality. The analysis has also revealed that the effect of different ways of commuting differ considerably across different kinds of people, even among different kinds of highly educated women.

### 5.5.2   Agenda for Further Research

This exploratory study does not allow generalization of the results, not even to the many highly educated women participating in this study and certainly not to the

**Table 5.8** The optimal commute for sub-groups

| Sub-group | All | | | | | | | | | | | Highly educated women only | | | | | | | | | |
|---|---|---|---|---|---|---|---|---|---|---|---|---|---|---|---|---|---|---|---|---|---|
|  | 1. Men | 2. Women | 3. Lower educated women | 4. Highly educated women | 5. Working part time | 6. Working full time | 7. With children | 8. Without children | 9. With a family income below average | 10. With an average family income | 11. With a family income above average | 12. With children living alone | 13. With children living together | 14. Without children living alone | 15. Without children living together | 16. With children living together working full time | 17. With children living together working part time | 18. Without children living alone working full time | 19. Without children living alone working part time | 20. Without children living together working full time | 21. Without children living together working part time |
| **N observations** | 5777 | 25170 | 10918 | 20029 | 10294 | 16497 | 11257 | 15822 | 7606 | 10933 | 12396 | 3651 | 7808 | 7686 | 8163 | 2326 | 2207 | 1969 | 1383 | 1383 | 1969 |
| **Time** minutes, one way | | | | | | | | | | | | | | | | | | | | | |
| >0 | → | → | → | → | → | | → | → | → | → | → | → | → | → | → | → | → | → | | → | → |
| 30–60 | | – | | | | | + | | + | | | | + | + | + | + | | | | | |
| 60–90 | | + | | | | | + | | + | | | | + | + | | + | | | | | |
| **Mode** | | | | | | | | | | | | | | | | | | | | | |
| Car | – | – | – | – | – | | – | – | – | | – | – | – | | | – | | + | + | | |
| Public | + | + | | + | + | + | + | + | | + | + | + | + | – | + | + | + | – | – | – | + |
| Bike | | | | | | – | | | | – | | | | | | | | + | | + | – |
| Multimodal with walking | + | | + | | | | | | | – | | | | | – | | | | | | – |
| Multimodal without walking | + | | | | | | | | + | – | | | | + | – | | | | | | |
| **With whom** | | | | | | | | | | | | | | | | | | | | | |
| With someone | + | + | + | + | + | + | + | | + | + | + | | + | + | | + | + | + | | | |
| Alone | | | | | | | | | | | | + | | | + | | | | | | + |
| **When** | | | | | | | | | | | | | | | | | | | | | |
| In rush hour | | + | + | | + | + | + | | + | | | | + | + | | + | + | | | | |
| Out of rush hour | | | | | | | | + | | | | + | | | | | | + | + | + | + |

general population in the Netherlands. So next the step is replication of this study using probability samples, be it probability samples of the general population or specific publics, such as highly educated women. Testing of hypothesis and assessing statistical significance will be useful in that context, but was not apt in this exploratory study.

These data used her set limitations. Some information is not available at all, and some information is not represented by a sufficient amount of entries, both limiting specification. Even in some of the specifications that are included in this thesis, several commuting aspects fall away as they are not represented by the minimum of 25 entries. This especially limits the possibilities to combine commuting time and mode, which shows promising results.

The data did not allow to explore several of the commuting aspects extensively. For one, it was not possible to make a distinction between different means of public transportation. Also, the results show that some types of highly educated women do better travelling out of rush hour, and others in rush hour. This raises the question why travelling in rush hour would enhance happiness for certain kinds of highly educated women. Previous research cannot answer this question and the data does not allow to explore this matter further.

Earlier research has focused on general tendencies and has tried to assess pure effect using regression analysis with many control variables. The wisdom aimed at, is typically a 'best-practice' applicable to all. However, this analysis shows that there are no such general tendencies. The effects of commuting are typically contingent, causing the effects to be different for different kinds of people. There is no one best way for everybody. This is why specification should be more central in future in happiness research.

## 5.6   Conclusions

There is no one-way of commuting that is optimal for everybody. Although public transport is the commuting mode that most commonly causes larges negative effects, it is actually the most optimal commuting mode for highly educated women without children living alone and working part time. For highly educated women it also varies widely if commuting in or out of rush hour, and commuting alone or together leads to the optimal commute. Especially highly educated women with a family income below average, benefit from a commute with others.

## References

Abou-Zeid, M., Witter, R., Bierlaire, M., Kaufmann, V., & Ben-Akiva, M. (2012). Happiness and travel mode switching: Findings from a Swiss public transportation experiment. *Transport Policy, 19*(1), 93–104.

ANWB. (2015). *Dagelijkse drukke trajecten ochtend en avondspits*. [online]. Available at: http://www.anwb.nl/verkeer/nederland/verkeersinformatie/dagelijkse-drukke-trajecten. Accessed 10 June 2015.

Chng, S., White, M., Abraham, C., & Skippon, S. (2016). Commuting and wellbeing in London: The roles of commute mode and local public transport connectivity. *Preventive Medicine, 88*(1), 182–188.

Dolan, P., Peasgood, T., & White, M. P. (2006). *Review of research on the influences on personal well-being and application to policy making*. Report for Defra, UK.

Duarte, A., Garcia, C., Giannarakis, G., Limão, S., Polydoropoulou, A., & Litinas, N. (2010). New approaches in transportation planning: Happiness and transport economics. *NETNOMICS: Economic Research and Electronic Networking, 11*(1), 5–32.

Ettema, D., & Smajic, I. (2014). Walking, places and wellbeing. *The Geographical Journal, 181*(2), https://doi.org/10.1111/geoj.12065.

Ettema, D., Gärling, T., Eriksson, L., Friman, M., Olsson, L. E., & Fujii, S. (2011). Satisfaction with travel and subjective well-being: Development and test of a measurement tool. *Journal of Transportation Research Part F, 14*, 167–175.

Ettema, D., Friman, M., Gärling, T., Olsson, L.E., & Fujii, S. (2012). How in-vehicle activities affect work commuters' satisfaction with public transport. *Journal of Transport Geography*. https://doi.org/10.1016/j.jtrangeo.2012.02.007.

Frey, B. S., & Stutzer, A. (2002). What can economists learn from happiness research? *Journal of Economic Literature, XL*, 402–435.

Frey, B. S., & Stutzer, A. (2014). Economic consequences of mispredicting utility. *Journal of Happiness Studies, 15*, 937–956.

Friman, M., Fujii, S., Ettema, D., Gärling, T., & Olsson, L. E. (2013). Psychometric analysis of the satisfaction with travel scale. *Transportation Research Part A, 48*, 132–145.

Furnham, A., & Cheng, H. (1999). Personality as predictor of mental health and happiness in East and West. *Personality and Individual Differences, 27*, 395–403.

Gatersleben, B., & Uzzell, D. (2007). Affective appraisals of the daily commute: comparing perceptions of drivers, cyclists, walkers, and users of public transport. *Environment and Behavior, 39*(3), 416–431.

Gelukswijzer: Gereedschap voor werken aan geluk. (2011). Erasmus University Rotterdam, Happiness Economics Research Organization. Available at: https://www.gelukswijzer.nl

Happiness Indicator. (2016). Erasmus University Rotterdam, Erasmus Happiness Economics Research Organization EHERO. Available at: http://happinessindicator.com

Juster, F. T., & Stafford, F. P. (1991). The allocation of time: Empirical findings, behavioral models, and problems of measurement. *Journal of Economic Literature, 29*(2), 471–522.

Kahneman, D., Krueger, A. B., Schkade, D. A., Schwarz, N., & Stone, A. A. (2003). *A survey method for characterizing daily life experience: The Day Reconstruction Method (DRM)*. Mimeo, Princeton University.

Koslowsky, M., Kluger, A. M., & Reich, M. (1995). *Commuting stress: Causes, effects, and methods of coping*. New York: Plenum Press.

Lancee, S., Burger, M., & Veenhoven, R. (2017). Mood during commute in the Netherlands. *Transportation Research Part A, 104C*(2017), 195–208.

Layard, R. (2005). *Happiness: Lessons of a new science*. New York: Penguin.

Lykken, D. T., & Tellegen, A. (1996). Happiness is a stochastic phenomenon. *Psychological Science, 7*, 186–189.

Lyubomirsky, S. (2008). *The how of happiness: A scientific approach to getting the life that you want*. New York: Penguin Press.

Mokhtarian, P. L., & Salomon, I. (2001). How derived is the demand for travel? Some conceptual and measurement considerations. *Transportation Research Part A: Policy and Practice, 35*(8), 695–719.

Morris, E. A., & Guerra, E. (2015). Mood and mode: Does how we travel affect how we feel? *Transportation, 42*(1), 25–43.

NS. (2015). *Wat zijn daluren?* Available at: http://www.ns.nl/reizigers/klantenservice/klantenservice/voorwaardenenfolders/daluren.html. [Accessed 10 Jun. 2015].

Olsson, L. E., Gärling, T., Ettema, D., Friman, M., & Fujii, S. (2013). Happiness and satisfaction with work commute. *Social Indicators Research, 111*(1), 255–263.

ONS. (2014). *Commuting and personal well-being.* London: Office for National Statistics.

Pfaff, S. (2014). Pendelenfernung, Lebenszufriedenheit und Entlohnung: Eine Längsschnittuntersuchung mit den Daten des SOEP von 1998 bis 2009. *Zeitschrift für Soziologie, 43*, 113–130.

Putnam, R. D. (2000). *Bowling alone: The collapse and revival of the American community.* New York: Simon & Schuster.

Roberts, J., Hodgson, R., & Dolan, P. (2011). "It's driving her mad": Gender differences in the effects of commuting on psychological health. *Journal of Health Economics, 30*(5), 1064–1076.

Shiffman, S., Stone, A. A., & Hufford, M. R. (2008). Ecological momentary assessment. *Annual Review of Clinical Psychology, 4*, 1–32.

Studer, R., & Winkelmann, R. (2011). *Specification and estimation of rating scale models: With an application to the determinants of life satisfaction* (SOEP Paper no. 372). Berlin, Germany.

Stutzer, A., & Frey, B. S. (2008). Stress that doesn't pay: The commuting paradox. *Scandinavian Journal of Economics, 110*(2), 339–366.

Susilo, Y. O., & Maat, K. (2007). The influence of built environment to the trends in commuting journeys in the Netherlands. *Transportation, 34*(5), 589–609.

*The Happiness Indicator: A self-help website and a scientific follow-up study.* Erasmus University Rotterdam, Happiness Economics Research Organization. Available at: http://happinessindicator.com.

Van der Meer, P. H., & Wielers, R. (2013). What makes workers happy? *Applied Economics, 45* (357), 368.

Van Wee, B., Rietveld, P., & Meurs, H. (2006). Is average daily travel time expenditure constant? In search of explanations for an increase in average travel time. *Journal of Transport Geography, 14*(2), 109–122.

Veenhoven, R. (1984). *Conditions of happiness.* Dordrecht: Springer.

Veenhoven, R. (2009). How do we assess how happy we are? Tenets, implications and tenability of three theories. In A. Dutt & B. Radcliff (Eds.), *Happiness, economics and politics: Towards a multi-disciplinary approach* (1st ed., pp. 45–69). Cheltenham: Edward Elger Publishers.

Veenhoven, R. (2012). Cross-national differences in happiness: Cultural measurement bias or effect of culture? *International Journal of Wellbeing, 2*(4), 333–353.

Veenhoven, R. (2015a). *Distributional findings on happiness in nations.* World Database of Happiness, Erasmus University Rotterdam, the Netherlands. [Online]. Available at: http://worlddatabaseofhappiness.eur.nl. Accessed 21 July 2015.

Veenhoven, R. (2015b). *Happiness in Netherlands (NL).* World Database of Happiness, Erasmus University Rotterdam, the Netherlands. [Online]. Available at: http://worlddatabaseofhappiness.eur.nl. Accessed 21 July 2015.

Veenhoven, R. (2015c). *Evidence based pursuit of happiness: What should we know, do we know and can we get to know?* Erasmus Happiness Economics Research Organization. White paper nr. 1. Erasmus University Rotterdam. [Online]. Available at: http://www2.eur.nl/fsw/research/veenhoven/Pub2010s/2012j-full.pdf. Accessed 3 Aug 2015.

Veenhoven, R. (2016) Happiness, history of the concept. In J. Wright (Ed.), *International Encyclopaedia of social and behavioural sciences* (2nd ed., Vol. 10, pp. 521–525). Oxford Elsevier.

# Chapter 6
# Dynamic Modeling of Activity Happiness: An Investigation of the Intra-activity Hedonic Treadmill

Isabel Viegas de Lima, Maya Abou-Zeid, Ronny Kutadinata, Zahra Navidi, Stephan Winter, Fang Zhao, and Moshe Ben-Akiva

**Abstract** While travel has traditionally been considered a means to reach activities, researchers have begun to investigate the effect it has on well-being. Improved surveying methods enabled by mobile phone applications, leveraging GPS, GSM, accelerometer, and WiFi, allow researchers to collect more complete data and test hypotheses related to individuals' happiness with travel and activities. This chapter describes a data collection effort that took place in Melbourne, Australia using Future Mobility Sensing, a mobile phone application and web-based platform. Throughout the study, users were asked twice daily to report on happiness for a single activity, including travel. The chapter develops a dynamic Ordinal Logit Model based on the collected data and discusses the estimation results in the context of Hedonic Theory. The deviation of the reported happiness for an activity observation and an individual Set Point, defined as the median reported happiness of a user, is modeled as a function of covariates. The results show how different activity types (work, education, personal, discretionary, travel, staying at home, and other) affect individuals' experienced happiness. It is found that educational activities, followed by work and travel, are the most disliked. Discretionary actives—which include social activities, meals, recreation, etc.—and other activities are seen to lead to more positive experiences of happiness. The model is used to test for the presence of an intra-activity Hedonic Treadmill Effect. It is found that people remember their

I. Viegas de Lima · M. Ben-Akiva
Massachusetts Institute of Technology, Cambridge, MA, USA
e-mail: iviegas@mit.edu; mba@mit.edu

M. Abou-Zeid (✉)
American University of Beirut, Beirut, Lebanon
e-mail: ma202@aub.edu.lb

R. Kutadinata · Z. Navidi · S. Winter
The University of Melbourne, Melbourne, VIC, Australia
e-mail: ronny.kutadinata@advi.org.au; z.navidikashani@student.unimelb.edu.au;
winter@unimelb.edu.au

F. Zhao
Singapore-MIT Alliance for Research and Technology, Singapore, Singapore
e-mail: fang.zhao@smart.mit.edu

© Springer International Publishing AG, part of Springer Nature 2018
M. Friman et al. (eds.), *Quality of Life and Daily Travel*, Applying Quality of Life Research, https://doi.org/10.1007/978-3-319-76623-2_6

activities as more neutral in later reports of happiness. The implications for the measurement of happiness data are discussed.

**Keywords** Hedonic treadmill · Real-time happiness · Retrospective happiness · Duration neglect · Smartphone data · Future mobility sensing · Dynamic ordinal logit model

## 6.1 Introduction

Travel has traditionally been thought of as a means to reach specific activities. Within the last decade, researchers have begun looking at how these activities affect people's well-being, which in turn helps generate individuals' demand to perform such activities. Raveau et al. (2015) describes how well-being has been studied by transportation researchers over time. A number of studies have looked at users' self-reported subjective well-being associated with performed, current, or anticipated activities (Kahneman et al. 1999). While some studies—such as Abou-Zeid and Ben-Akiva (2012) and Bergstad et al. (2012)—measure well-being associated with activities in general, others developed measurements to understand the well-being of individuals during travel. These include studies such as Ory and Mokhtarian (2005), who modeled the additional well-being derived from travel itself; Duarte et al. (2008), who looked at leisure and work trips; Ettema et al. (2011), who looked at satisfaction with travel; and Ravulaparthy et al. (2013), who measured the well-being of elderly travel. This study adds to the first case, analyzing the subjective happiness of individuals during and after different activities.

Data collection for transportation surveys has significantly improved in past years by leveraging the increase in smartphone ownership. By using GPS, GSM, accelerometer, and WiFi sensors, smartphone applications have the capacity to collect and process travel information without user intervention. These applications mitigate a number of issues associated with pen-and-paper travel surveys, such as under-reporting of activities and rounding of activity durations. Recent studies that have used smartphone capabilities to collect travel diaries include the *Quantified Traveler* (Jariyasunan et al. 2012), which collected travel data for 135 participants and then calculated their travel footprint. The objective of the study was to relay the personal information back to the users to modify their travel patterns and aid in more sustainable behavior. Furthermore, smartphones have also been used to collect data on happiness. Killingsworth and Gilbert (2010) developed an iPhone application called *Track Your Happiness*. The application asked users about their current happiness, their current activity, and they were thinking about anything unrelated and, if so, what it was. The study collected data from 5000 people from 83 different countries, leading to half a million sample points. Similarly, Baumeister et al. (2016) followed 500 people in Chicago. They were pinged throughout their day to inquire what they were thinking about and how it made them feel. Passive ways of capturing the happiness of people have become possible as well: sentiment analysis of social media reveals happiness related to activities or locations (Giachanou and Crestani 2016; Sinnott and Cui 2016). This study utilizes these developed capabilities.

Different methods have been applied to understanding and quantifying a person's subjective well-being. While hedonic theory is vast, a number of developed concepts apply directly to this study, mainly those pertaining to Hedonic Adaptation. Frederick and Loewenstein (1999) summarize Hedonic Adaptation as the process by which individuals adapt their expectations to reduce overly positive and overly negative experiences throughout their day. Also known as the Hedonic Treadmill Effect, the process involves both an individual's cognitive ability to transform situations and neurochemical processes that desensitize the brain's reaction to negative and positive stimuli. To measure this, the concept of an Adaptation Level was originally developed by Helson (1964). This Adaptation Level, also known as a Set Point, is a moving average of a person's stimulus levels. Therefore, a person's Hedonic State is the difference between a given stimulus and their Set Point. Parducci (1968) went on to argue that the stimulus should be compared to the range and to the median. He developed measurements for the Set Point that weighed distinct activity purposes differently and used medians. More complex models were later introduced by Ryder and Heal (1973), March (1988), and Hardie et al. (1993), among others. These models are time-dependent and consider differences between positive and negative stimuli. Fujita and Diener (2005), on the other hand, argue that people have a stable Set Point, against which they understand their Life Satisfaction (LS). However, Diener (1984) also highlights that there are a number of issues when measuring happiness. Measurements that are done on single-item scales are easier to compare over time, yet more likely to be skewed towards *happy* categories (Andrews and Withey 1976).

Another major component of hedonic theory is the concept of Duration Neglect. Kahneman (1999) distinguishes between moment-utility—the Hedonic State during an activity—and the Remembered Utility, which is the remembered Hedonic State. Kahneman cites a number of studies that show that people do not consider the whole activity when recalling their experience of an activity. Instead, they remember the feeling during the peak of the activity and the end of the activity, known as the Peak-End Rule. Furthermore, the length of an activity does not affect an individual's perception of their Hedonic State during an activity, which is known as Duration Neglect.

The motivation of this study was to elaborate on the one developed by Raveau et al. (2015), which modeled reported happiness data collected from a convenience sample. This chapter develops a dynamic Ordinal Logit Model (OLM) using a larger sample from Melbourne, Australia, and ties its results back to the Hedonic Theory. Using happiness data collected over time for the same activities, the model is used to test whether an intra-activity Hedonic Treadmill exists. An intra-activity Hedonic Treadmill refers to the change in perception of the remembered experienced happiness for a specific activity instance over time. The model results extend the understanding that the experienced happiness changes over time from specific uncomfortable situations—such as colonoscopies (Kahneman et al. 1993), inflicted pain (Ariely 1998), and annoying noises (Ariely and Zauberman 2000)—and travel

(Pedersen et al. 2011; Abou-Zeid and Ben-Akiva 2012), generalizing it to a number of activities in individuals' day-to-day lives. The chapter presents the data collection methodology and describes the sample. Then it proceeds to specify the dynamic OLM and present the model estimation. Finally, it discusses the estimation results, the implications for the measurement of happiness, and the limitations of the study.

## 6.2    Data Collection and Sample Statistics

Data for this study was collected through the *Future Mobility Sensing* (FMS) mobile phone application (Cottrill et al. 2013; Raveau et al. 2015). FMS leverages increasing smartphone penetration to collect travel information and disseminate surveys. The application uses sensing technology built in phones, as well as machine learning algorithms in the backend server, to infer individual travel patterns. Data collected through mobile phone sensors are sent to the server database, where they are analyzed and stored. Users have access to their processed data for validation through web- and phone-based interfaces. Furthermore, the user interface allows researchers to ask additional questions about users' activities throughout the day and during validation.

The mobile application is designed to efficiently run in the background of users' phones. Available for Android and iOS, it collects data using GPS, GSM, accelerometer, and WiFi sensors. In addition, it is designed to consume little memory. Collected data is sent to the database either by WiFi or cellular network, where they are interpreted by the backend server. Activities—such as going to work, shopping, or staying at home—and travel modes are inferred based on sensors, contextual transportation and location data, and user-specific previously validated data. The user interfaces allow individuals to validate their data over a web-based interface or on a mobile app. Validation includes confirming inferred patterns, completing missing data, correcting incorrect inferences, and indicating activity purposes when necessary.

FMS was used in this survey to collect socio-demographic characteristics through a pre-survey and daily activity information, and to disseminate questions about happiness. Users were prompted to give information on their happiness with regard to a certain activity at two different points: once throughout the day on their phone while performing the activity and once during subsequent validation of the activity. They were alerted of the question on their phone at a randomly chosen time after movement was detected at the beginning of a day and before 9:00 PM, and could answer the mobile question anytime until a new question became available the following day. If the user did not respond within 30 min of the mobile alert, the question that appeared on their phone was modified from *"How happy are you with your current activity?"* to *"How happy were you with your activity ___ hours ago?"*. Both questions—the one appearing on the phone and the one appearing during subsequent validation of the activity—asked users about their experienced happiness regarding the same activity in a given day, such that each activity may

**Table 6.1** Individual demographics and socioeconomic characteristics

| Category | Percentage |
|---|---|
| **Gender** | |
| Male | 47% |
| Female | 53% |
| **Age** | |
| 18–29 | 40% |
| 30–49 | 51% |
| 50–69 | 9% |
| 70+ | 0% |
| **Education** | |
| Year 12 or under | 19% |
| Bachelor | 31% |
| Master's or Postgraduate Degree | 24% |
| Doctorate | 12% |
| Other | 14% |
| **Employment** | |
| Any employment | 80% |
| Not employed | 20% |
| **Household income (per week)** | |
| $1–599 | 11% |
| $600–1249 | 15% |
| $1250–1999 | 15% |
| $2000+ | 40% |
| Missing income | 18% |
| **Marital status** | |
| Single | 43% |
| Married | 53% |
| Divorced | 4% |

have one or two happiness reports. Happiness was reported on a 7-point scale, ranging from "*Very Unhappy*" to "*Very Happy*."

The data collection took place in Melbourne, Australia, namely the University of Melbourne. To encourage participation, users who fulfilled certain requirements—such as age restriction and residence address (Roddis 2016)—and finished a full 14-day survey were remunerated with AU$50 e-vouchers. Of the 437 registered users, participating over varying lengths of periods, 114 answered happiness questions. Tables 6.1 and 6.2 provide summaries of the respondents' demographic and socioeconomic characteristics.

The gender profile of the participants is similar to that from the local household travel survey, the Victorian Integrated Survey of Travel and Activity (VISTA) (The Victorian Department of Transport 2011), in which 52% of the respondents are female. Being over 18 years old was a prerequisite to participate in the survey, such that there are no participants under 18. There are also no participants over 70 years old, whereas in VISTA 12% of the Melbourne participants are over 70. Since the

**Table 6.2** Household characteristics

| Category | Percentage |
|---|---|
| Household size | |
| 1 | 14% |
| 2 | 33% |
| 3 | 21% |
| 4 | 25% |
| 5+ | 7% |
| Number of vehicles in the household | |
| 0 | 19% |
| 1 | 40% |
| 2 | 27% |
| 3 | 9% |
| 4 | 4% |
| 5+ | 0% |

survey was predominantly advertised to the staff and students of the University of Melbourne, most participants are between 18 and 59 (91%) and have a tertiary degree in their education (67%). Eighty percent of the respondents have some type of employment (e.g., full-time, part-time, or self-employed), whereas the figure is 54% for VISTA respondents. High education and employment result in high income: 55% of all users have a yearly income more than AU$65000 (AU$1250 per week). There are no data for education or household income in VISTA for comparison. However, since VISTA surveys a valid sample of the population, other sources can be used to fill in. The Australian Bureau of Statistics reports an average equalized disposable household income in 2013–2014 of $998 per week (2017). It also reports from the 2011 census that 18.8% of the Australian population has a tertiary degree (2011).

More than 90% of the participants come from small households (four or fewer) and 86% of them have two or fewer cars in their households. The household structure proves to be highly similar to that of VISTA, with 91% of the respondents being from small households and 92% of the households having two or fewer vehicles.

In total, 1733 valid responses were recorded from the 114 users who answered the happiness questions for 1213 different activities. Table 6.3 presents a summary of the activity purposes for which happiness was reported and how they were grouped for analysis. They are further divided to indicate if the response was collected through the mobile phone or the web interface. Most of the responses were recorded at home (39%) or at work (29%). This confirms that many of the respondents were among the staff of the university, in comparison to students, since high income level and high education level were also observed in the sample.

Figure 6.1 shows the breakdown of reported happiness for each activity type. In general, the majority (71%) of the responses were in happy levels, regardless of activity purpose. Discretionary and other activity purposes had the highest level of happiness, with only 4% of the responses in unhappy levels. Meanwhile, education

**Table 6.3** Activity purpose breakdown

| | Phone | | Web | | Total | |
|---|---|---|---|---|---|---|
| Activity purpose | Count | Percent | Count | Percent | Count | Percent |
| Home | 356 | 35% | 328 | 46% | 684 | 39% |
| Home | 347 | 34% | 323 | 45% | 670 | 39% |
| Other home | 9 | 1% | 5 | 1% | 14 | 1% |
| Work | 302 | 30% | 209 | 29% | 511 | 29% |
| Work | 276 | 27% | 187 | 26% | 463 | 27% |
| Work-related business | 26 | 3% | 22 | 3% | 48 | 3% |
| Education | 91 | 9% | 40 | 6% | 131 | 8% |
| Education | 91 | 9% | 40 | 6% | 131 | 8% |
| Discretionary | 160 | 16% | 81 | 11% | 241 | 14% |
| Meal/eating break | 32 | 3% | 18 | 3% | 50 | 3% |
| Social | 66 | 6% | 43 | 6% | 109 | 6% |
| Entertainment | 8 | 1% | 2 | 0% | 10 | 1% |
| Recreation | 40 | 4% | 7 | 1% | 47 | 3% |
| Sports/exercise | 14 | 1% | 11 | 2% | 25 | 1% |
| Personal | 34 | 3% | 27 | 4% | 61 | 4% |
| Personal errand/task | 11 | 1% | 6 | 1% | 17 | 1% |
| Shopping | 21 | 2% | 21 | 3% | 42 | 2% |
| Medical/dental (self) | 2 | 0% | 0 | 0% | 2 | 0% |
| Travel | 53 | 5% | 18 | 3% | 71 | 4% |
| Travelling | 40 | 4% | 0 | 0% | 40 | 2% |
| Change mode/transfer | 13 | 1% | 18 | 3% | 31 | 2% |
| Other | 23 | 2% | 11 | 2% | 16 | 1% |
| To accompany someone | 7 | 1% | 2 | 0% | 9 | 1% |
| Pick up/drop off | 3 | 0% | 4 | 1% | 7 | 0% |
| Other | 13 | 1% | 5 | 1% | 18 | 1% |
| Total | 1019 | | 714 | | 1733 | |

had the highest level of unhappiness, with 38% of the answers in unhappy levels. Participants reported being unhappy at work only 12% of the time. Overall, the response distribution follows the trend highlighted by Diener (1984): single-item scales of well-being responses are often concentrated in *happy* categories.

This high level of happiness is fascinating compared to previous studies (Raveau et al. 2015). This can be explained by the context in which data was collected. Melbourne has been reported the most livable city in the world for seven consecutive years by the Economist Intelligence Unit (2017). This ranking considers factors such as safety, health care, educational resources, infrastructure, and the environment, meaning that people in Melbourne have a high standard of living. Thus, it can be assumed to be generally happier than other countries in which the same Happiness Survey has taken place before, such as Chile, China, Singapore, and United States (Raveau et al. 2015)—although others have shown that the economic impact on happiness is marginal (Oswald 1997). The same study also showed that the average

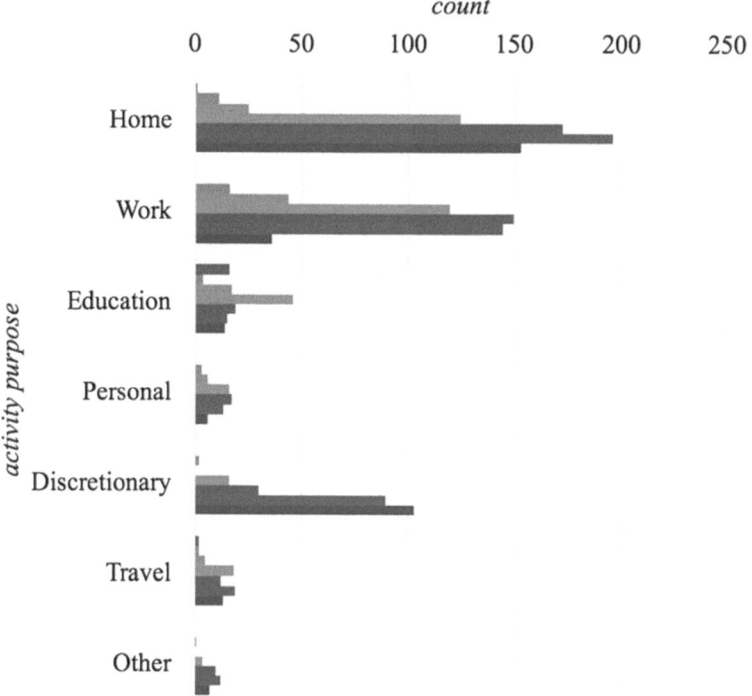

Fig. 6.1 Reported happiness by activity purpose

reported happiness between countries is significantly different, which points to cultural reasons as well. Moreover, according to the World Happiness Report 2017 (Helliwell et al. 2017), Australians are the ninth happiest nation of the world. Therefore, observing a high level of happiness is not surprising in Melbourne.

Figure 6.2 shows the distribution of the duration for the reported activities. Seventy-five percent of all activities are less than 12.6 h long, and 90% are less than 21.5 h long. Longer activities tended to be home-based. Figure 6.3 shows the distribution of time before the different reports for the activities. Seventy-five percent and 90% of all responses occurred within 9.5 h and 24.2 h of the end of the activity respectively, while 43% occurred within 1 h of the activity itself. Responses occurring after 24 h were mostly done through the web-based interface.

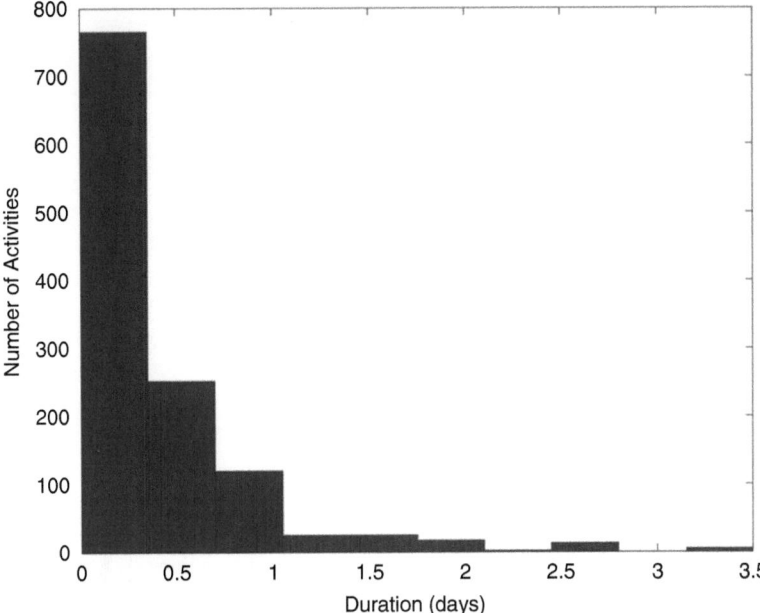

**Fig. 6.2** Distribution of activity duration

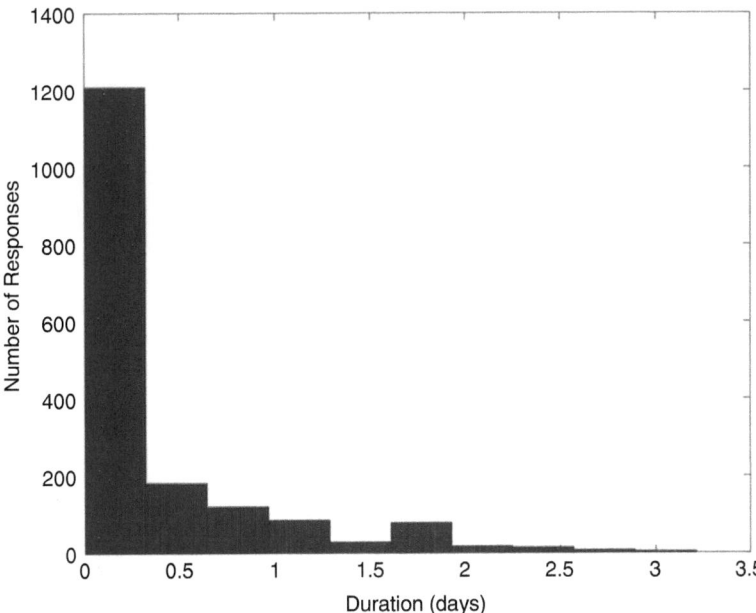

**Fig. 6.3** Distribution of elapsed time before response

**Table 6.4** Hedonic states counts

| Differences | Phone | | Web | | Total | |
|---|---|---|---|---|---|---|
| | Count | Percent | Count | Percent | Count | Percent |
| −4 | 14 | 1% | 1 | 0% | 15 | 1% |
| −3 | 28 | 3% | 18 | 3% | 46 | 3% |
| −2 | 68 | 7% | 25 | 4% | 93 | 5% |
| −1 | 213 | 21% | 136 | 19% | 349 | 20% |
| 0 | 414 | 41% | 352 | 49% | 766 | 44% |
| 1 | 238 | 23% | 162 | 23% | 400 | 23% |
| 2 | 35 | 3% | 19 | 3% | 54 | 3% |
| 3 | 9 | 1% | 1 | 0% | 10 | 1% |

## 6.3 Modeling Hedonic State

To account for potential inter-user discrepancy in the use of the happiness scale—a *Slightly Happy* to one person may have been comparable to another person's *Slightly Unhappy*—instead of modeling individuals' reported happiness, individuals' deviation from their own Set Point, or their Hedonic State, is modeled. To do so, two major assumptions are made. The first is that the study is conducted throughout a 2-week period that is quotidian, such that the activities selected for reporting happiness are representative of the users' day-to-day lives. Since all activities are recurring and the extent of the activities collected is insignificant compared to what has accumulated for an individual throughout a lifetime, a single activity does not significantly affect the Set Point. Therefore, instead of using a moving average or moving median, the Set Point is assumed to be the overall median across all activities. This is especially useful because of the limited number of sample points available for each user. The Set Point is rounded to the nearest integer to limit the available alternatives for the developed model. Note that the Set Point could have been activity purpose-specific, yet there are not enough observations of different activity purposes for each individual.

Secondly, since the individual's Set Point is stable for the period of time the data is collected, a user's Hedonic State is the difference between their reported happiness and their established Set Point. Table 6.4 shows the counts for the different Hedonic States across all users. Unlike the happiness responses, the Hedonic States are accumulated around the Set Point. Furthermore, 44% of the Hedonic States are actually 0, which translates to each individual's median.

To understand how different activity attributes and socio-demographic characteristics affect an individual's Hedonic State, a dynamic Ordinal Logit Model (OLM) was estimated. OLM models are a subset of Random Utility Maximization models. These models assume that individuals make choices that maximize their utility. While one's utility can be explained through a number of personal and situational characteristics, there is a part of the utility that is random, such that an individual's choice is probabilistic in nature. OLM models specifically recognize that there is an

**Table 6.5**  Model variables

| Variable name | Variable | Domain |
|---|---|---|
| Individual | $n$ | – |
| Activity | $a$ | – |
| Observation | $k$ | $\{1, 2\}$ |
| Real-time | $\delta_{realtime,\ na1}$ | Binary |
| Multiple observations | $\delta_{MultObs,\ na}$ | Binary |
| Time until observation | $ObsTime_{nak}$ | Continuous *days* |
| Duration of activity | $Dur_{na}$ | Continuous *day* |
| Activity purpose | $\delta_{i,\ na}$ *for* $i \in I$ | Binary |
|   Home | | |
|   Work | | |
|   Education | | |
|   Personal | | |
|   Discretionary | | |
|   Travel | | |
|   Other | | |
| Weekend | $\delta_{weekend,\ na}$ | Binary |
| Socioeconomic binaries | $\delta_{j,\ n}$ *for* $j \in J$ | Binary |
|   Female – *fixed* | | |
|   Male | | |
|   Full-time – *fixed* | | |
|   Part-time | | |
|   Retired | | |
|   Unemployed | | |
|   Self-employed | | |
| Single – *fixed* | | |
|   Married | | |
|   Divorced | | |
| Household income | $Income_{n}$ | Midpoint of income range AU$ *week*$^{-1}$ |
| Missing income | $\delta_{missingincome,\ n}$ | Binary |
| Hedonic state | $d_{nak}$ | |

underlying order to the discrete choices. Table 6.5 outlines the different variables used in the developed model.

Note that observation $k$, which refers to a happiness response for a specific activity instance, can take on the value of 1 if an individual answered the happiness question on their phone yet not on the web interface (during validation) or 2 if the individual answered both happiness questions for the same activity. $\delta_{MultObs,\ na}$ indicates if an activity $a$ for individual $n$ has multiple observations. While a phone-based response is judged to have been real-time if the individual responded before the end of the activity, the web-based response was always after the end of the activity because it was completed during validation. $ObsTime_{nak}$ is the time between the end of the activity and the response. It is set to zero if the response was real-time.

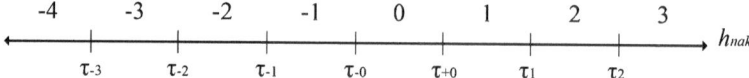

**Fig. 6.4** Hedonic state thresholds

**Fig. 6.5** Relationship between $h_{na1}$ and $h_{na2}$

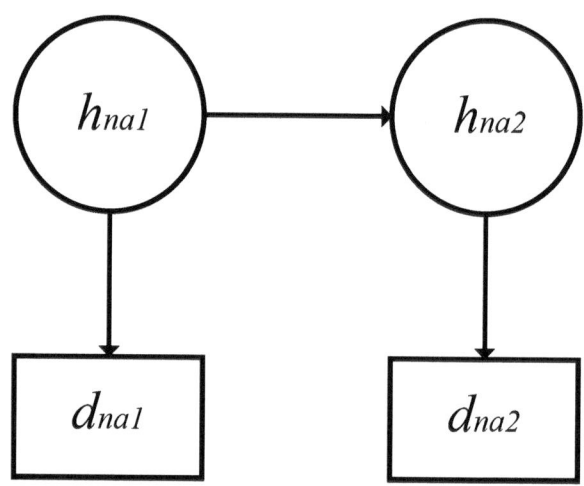

These attributes, along with the activity duration, $Dur_{na}$, were extracted from the user's activities from the FMS database.

As mentioned, the calculated Hedonic State, $d_{nak}$, reflects an individual's latent happiness, $h_{nak}$, such that

$$
d_{nak} = \begin{cases}
-4 & -\infty < h_{nak} \leq \tau_{-3} \\
-3 & \tau_{-3} < h_{nak} \leq \tau_{-2} \\
-2 & \tau_{-2} < h_{nak} \leq \tau_{-1} \\
-1 & \tau_{-1} < h_{nak} \leq \tau_{-0} \\
0 & \tau_{-0} < h_{nak} \leq \tau_{+0} \\
1 & \tau_{+0} < h_{nak} \leq \tau_{1} \\
2 & \tau_{1} < h_{nak} \leq \tau_{2} \\
3 & \tau_{2} < h_{nak} < +\infty
\end{cases}
\tag{6.1}
$$

where the $\tau$'s are the thresholds for the latent happiness. This is further described in Fig. 6.4. $d_{nak} = 0$ is centered between $\tau_{-0}$ and $\tau_{+0}$. Centering $d_{nak} = 0$ allows for clearer interpretation of variables.

Furthermore, the second happiness response $h_{na2}$ for the same activity $na$ is dependent on the first happiness response $h_{na1}$. Their causal relationship, together with the actualized Hedonic States $d_{na1}$ and $d_{na2}$, are described in Fig. 6.5.

$h_{na1}$ is specified as follows:

$$h_{na1} = \beta_{realtime} \cdot \delta_{realtime,na1} + \beta_{obstime} \cdot ObsTime_{na1}$$
$$+ \sum_{i \in I} \left( \beta_{i,dur} \cdot Dur_{na} + \beta_{i,dur2} \cdot Dur_{na}^2 \right) \cdot \delta_{i,na}$$
$$+ \sum_{i \in I} \beta_{i,weekend} \cdot \delta_{i,na} \cdot \delta_{weekend,na} + \sum_{i \in I} \beta_{i,weekday} \cdot \delta_{i,na} \qquad (6.2)$$
$$\cdot (1 - \delta_{weekend,na}) + \sum_{j \in J} \beta_j \cdot \delta_{j,n} \beta_{missingincome} \cdot \delta_{missingincomen,n}$$
$$+ \beta_{income,n} \cdot \left( 1 - \delta_{missingincomen,n} \right) \cdot Income_n + \eta_n + \omega_{na1} + \epsilon_{na1}$$
$$h_{na1} = \beta' X_{na1} + \eta_n + \omega_{na1} + \epsilon_{na1} \qquad (6.3)$$

where

$$\eta_n \sim \mathcal{N}\left(0, \sigma_\eta^2\right)$$
$$\omega_{na1} \sim \mathcal{N}\left(\mu, \sigma_\omega^2\right)$$
$$\epsilon_{na1} \sim logistic(0, 1).$$

The specification includes components for the response being real-time and for the time elapsed between the end of the activity and the response. For each activity purpose, a quadratic function of duration is included, as well as an intercept. The intercept distinguishes between the activity being performed during a weekday or the weekend. Socioeconomic variables are included linearly. $\eta_n$ is a panel effect to account for inter-individual heterogeneity and intra-individual unobserved correlation. $\omega_{na1}$, on the other hand, is an error term included in the phone-based happiness response equation to account for potential mistakes when selecting an answer on the screen. Including it also makes the estimation computationally easier. Finally, the model includes the random error, which is logistically distributed for OLM. Note that the $\beta$'s for weekday-home activities, full-time, and single are fixed to zero for estimation.

For simplicity, let $h_{na1}$ be decomposed as follows:

$$h_{na1} = \hbar_{na1} + \epsilon_{na1}. \qquad (6.4)$$

As previously mentioned, $h_{na2}$, the second happiness response for the activity $na$, is a function of $h_{na1}$ and is defined as

$$h_{na2} = \beta_{h1} \cdot \hbar_{na1} + \beta_{obstime} \cdot ObsTime_{na2} + \epsilon_{na2}. \qquad (6.5)$$

Since both happiness reports are made by the same individual $n$ about the same activity instance $a$, the only difference in activity attributes between the first and second reports are the time elapsed since the end of the activity. Therefore, $h_{na2}$ includes a scaled component of $h_{na1}$ and the observation time, as well as a random error $\epsilon_{na2}$, distributed similar to $\epsilon_{na1}$.

The error term for $k = 2$ is logistically distributed with position 0 and mean 1, such that the probability of the observed $d_{na2} = y_2$ for $y_2 \in \{-4, \ldots, 3\}$, conditional on the individual panel effect, $\eta_n$, and the phone-based error, $\omega_{na1}$, is the difference of logistics.

$$P(d_{na2} = y_2 | \eta_n, \omega_{na1}) = \left( F_{\epsilon_2} \left( \hbar_{na2} - \tau_{y_2-1} \right) - F_{\epsilon_2} \left( \hbar_{na2} - \tau_{y_2} \right) \right)^{\delta_{MultObs, na}} \quad (6.6)$$

where

$$\hbar_{na2} = \beta_{h1} \cdot \hbar_{na1} + \beta_{obstime} \cdot ObsTime_{na2} \quad (6.7)$$

is the systematic component of $h_{na2}$.

The conditional probability of $d_{na2} = y_2$ is raised to the power of $\delta_{MultObs, na}$, so that the term is expressed when there are multiple observations, but is 1 when there is only one observation for activity $a$ for individual $n$—that is, $d_{na2}$ does not exist.

Similarly, the conditional probability for $d_{na1} = y_1$, $y_1 \in \{-4, \dots, 3\}$, is

$$P(d_{na1} = y_1 | \eta_n, \omega_{na1}) = F_{\epsilon_1} \left( \hbar_{na1} - \tau_{y_1-1} \right) - F_{\epsilon_1} \left( \hbar_{na1} - \tau_{y_1} \right) \quad (6.8)$$

where

$$\hbar_{na1} = \beta' X_{na1} + \eta_n + \omega_{na1}. \quad (6.9)$$

The joint probability for individual $n$ and activity $a$, conditional on both $\eta_n$ and $\omega_{na1}$, is

$$P(d_{na1} = y_1 | \eta_n, \omega_{na1}) P(d_{na2} = y_2 | \eta_n, \omega_{na1}). \quad (6.10)$$

The joint probability must be integrated over the density of $\omega_{na1}$ to make the joint probability only conditional on the individual panel effect $\eta_n$, resulting in the probability of an activity $a$ for individual $n$.

$$\int_\omega P(d_{na1} = y_1 | \eta_n, \omega_{na1}) P(d_{na2} = y_2 | \eta_n, \omega_{na1}) f_\omega(\omega_{na1}) \, d\omega_{na1} \quad (6.11)$$

To account for the individual panel effect, the product of the above expression for all activities $a$ for individual $n$ must be integrated over the density of $\eta_n$.

$$\int_\eta \left( \prod_a \int_\omega P(d_{na1} = y_1 | \eta_n, \omega_{na1}) P(d_{na2} = y_2 | \eta_n, \omega_{na1}) f_\omega(\omega_{na1}) d\omega_{na1} \right) f_\eta(\eta_n) d\eta$$

$$(6.12)$$

This results in the joint probability for the sequence of activities for an individual $n$. The likelihood, $L$, is the product of the individual likelihood over all individuals.

$$L = \prod_n \int_\eta \left( \prod_a \int_\omega P(d_{na1} = y_1|\eta_n, \omega_{na1}) P(d_{na2} = y_2|\eta_n, \omega_{na1}) f_\omega(\omega_{na1}) d\omega_{na1} \right)$$
$$\times f_\eta(\eta_n) d\eta$$

$$(6.13)$$

And the log likelihood, $\mathcal{L}$, is the sum of the log of the joint probability for the sequence of activities for an individual $n$, over all individuals.

$$\mathcal{L} = \sum_n \log \left( \int_\eta \left( \prod_a \int_\omega P(d_{na1} = y_1|\eta_n, \omega_{na1}) \right. \right.$$
$$P(d_{na2} = y_2|\eta_n, \omega_{na1}) f_\omega(\omega_{na1}) d\omega_{na1}) f_\eta(\eta_n) d\eta) \qquad (6.14)$$

A number of other specifications were also estimated. These included models that repeated the variables from $h_{na1}$ in $h_{na2}$ and different inclusions of $ObsTime_{na2}$ in $h_{na2}$. The mentioned specification was chosen so that $\beta_{h1}$ could be treated as a scaling factor of $h_{na1}$, but $ObsTime_{na2}$ was still accounted for. The model was estimated using Python Biogeme (Bierlaire and Fetiarison 2009) with numerical integration. The resulting estimated model is presented in Table 6.6.

When comparing between activity purposes, a distinction between weekday and weekend is made. Figures 6.6 and 6.7 plot the effect of duration of each activity type on the latent happiness $h_{nak}$ for weekday and weekend activities, respectively, and use activity purpose-specific values as intercepts.

The weekday plot shows that discretionary and other activities have the highest positive effect on Hedonic State compared to staying at home on a weekday, and the effect is monotonically increasing for discretionary activities. This aligns with the category itself; it includes meals, socializing, recreation, entertainment, and exercise, all of which are activities that people typically do for pleasure. Similar results were found in Kahneman et al. (2004) for the positive effects of meals, exercising, and socializing. Education is the only other activity that has a positive weekday coefficient, yet it is considerably small in scale. While the coefficient for staying at home is fixed at zero, travel, personal, and work all have negative coefficients, with work being the most negative. This can be interpreted as work having the most negative effect on an individual's Hedonic State. These findings also agree with those of Kahneman et al. (2004), which associate work with one of the worst net effects, second only to individuals' morning commute.

The weekend plot, on the other hand, shows a bigger spread. While discretionary activities still contribute significantly more to a more positive Hedonic State, staying at home on weekends has a positive effect compared to staying at home on weekdays. Education has half of the positive effect, yet remains similar in magnitude compared to other activities. Curiously, work on weekends is less negative than work on weekdays. On weekends, however, personal activities contribute the most

**Table 6.6** OLM estimates

| Variable | Estimate | Standard error |
|---|---|---|
| Activity purpose | | |
| Weekday | | |
| Home | 0 | Fixed |
| Work | −0.816 | 0.581 |
| Education | 0.111 | 0.0729 |
| Discretionary | 1.77 | 0.505 |
| Personal | −0.626 | 0.796 |
| Travel | −0.638 | 0.796 |
| Other | 2.70 | 1.85 |
| Weekend | | |
| Home | 0.349 | 0.295 |
| Work | −0.553 | 0.502 |
| Education | 0.0512 | 0.0737 |
| Discretionary | 0.623 | 0.668 |
| Personal | −1.14 | 0.514 |
| Travel | −0.605 | 0.725 |
| Other | −0.0388 | 1.32 |
| Duration of activity | | |
| Duration (days) | | |
| Home | 2.61 | 0.678 |
| Work | −0.972 | 0.973 |
| Education | −0.667 | 0.155 |
| Discretionary | 5.53 | 1.04 |
| Personal | 4.98 | 3.03 |
| Travel | 3.77 | 1.77 |
| Other | −1.62 | 5.68 |
| Duration$^2$ (days$^2$) | | |
| Home | −1.08 | 0.298 |
| Work | 0.657 | 0.494 |
| Education | 0.261 | 0.0561 |
| Discretionary | −2.39 | 0.489 |
| Personal | −2.63 | 2.38 |
| Travel | −1.26 | 1.33 |
| Other | 7.70 | 6.98 |
| Time of response | | |
| Real-time | 0.314 | 0.163 |
| Time until observation (days) | 0.0156 | 0.0791 |
| Personal characteristics | | |
| Gender | | |
| Female | 0 | Fixed |
| Male | −0.211 | 0.189 |
| Household income | | |

(continued)

**Table 6.6** (continued)

| Variable | Estimate | Standard error |
|---|---|---|
| Income (AU$1000/week) | −0.133 | 0.113 |
| Missing income | −0.542 | 0.351 |
| Marital status | | |
| Single | 0 | Fixed |
| Married | −0.136 | 0.223 |
| Divorced | −0.124 | 0.489 |
| Employment | | |
| Full-time | 0 | Fixed |
| Part-time | −0.286 | 0.250 |
| Self-employed | 0.0904 | 0.432 |
| Unemployed | −0.224 | 0.291 |
| Retired | −0.509 | 0.889 |
| Panel effects | | |
| Individual error standard deviation ($\sigma_\eta$) | 0.471 | 0.118 |
| Phone-based error mean ($\mu$) | −0.241 | 0.349 |
| Phone-based error standard deviation ($\sigma_\omega$) | 1.77 | 0.140 |
| Effect of first observation on second response | | |
| $\theta_{na1}$ | 0.739 | 0.0675 |
| Thresholds | | |
| $\tau_{-3}$ | −6.66 | 0.270 |
| $\tau_{-2}$ | −4.89 | 0.134 |
| $\tau_{-1}$ | −3.52 | 0.119 |
| $\tau_{-0}$ | −1.47 | 0.0665 |
| $\tau_{+0}$ | 1.47 | 0.0665 |
| $\tau_1$ | 4.53 | 0.175 |
| $\tau_2$ | 6.96 | 0.346 |
| Number of happiness observations | 1733 | |
| Log likelihood | −2494.231 | |
| $\bar{\rho}^2$ | 0.259 | |

negatively to Hedonic State. This can be attributed to the nature of the category, which includes running errands, shopping, and medical and dental appointments.

The shape of the curves in both plots tells a lot about the value of the activities. Discretionary activities have the most rapidly increasing value, which means performing discretionary activities for longer periods of time contributes positively to one's Hedonic State. The value of staying at home increases with time, yet flattens out faster than the other monotonically increasing curves, which represents the diminishing returns of spending too much time at home. Travel activities have a significant increase in positive contribution with time. This can be attributed to people enjoying longer commutes because of pleasure derived from driving on for longer, or the free time that is made available to perform other activities during the commute, such as reading on public transport. However, the positive trend is still

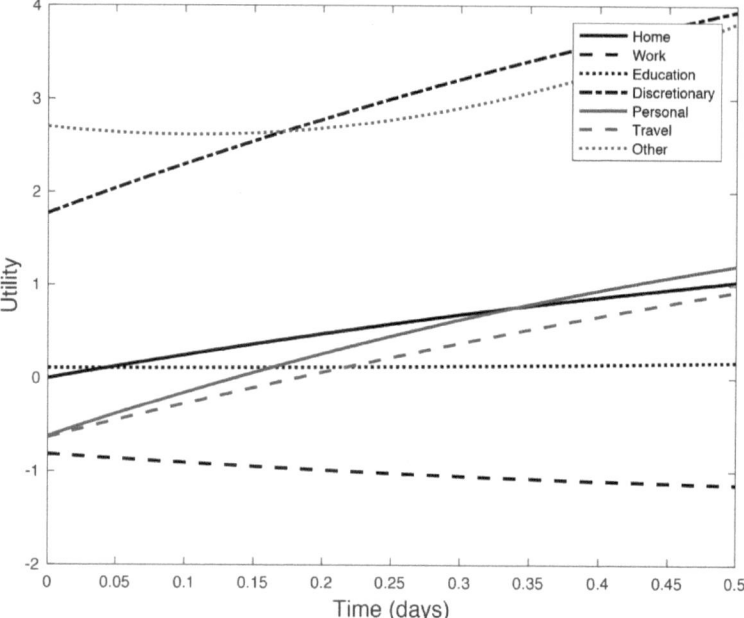

**Fig. 6.6** Effect of duration on utility by activity purpose for weekday activities

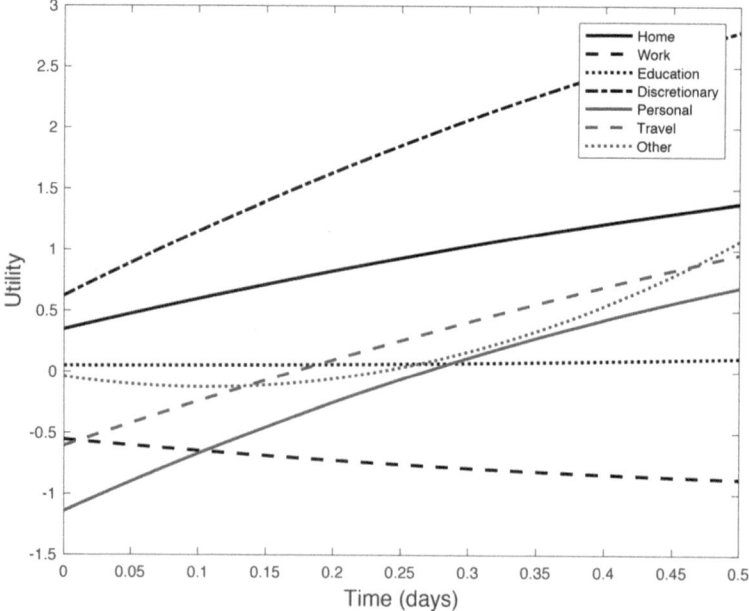

**Fig. 6.7** Effect of duration on utility by activity purpose for weekend activities

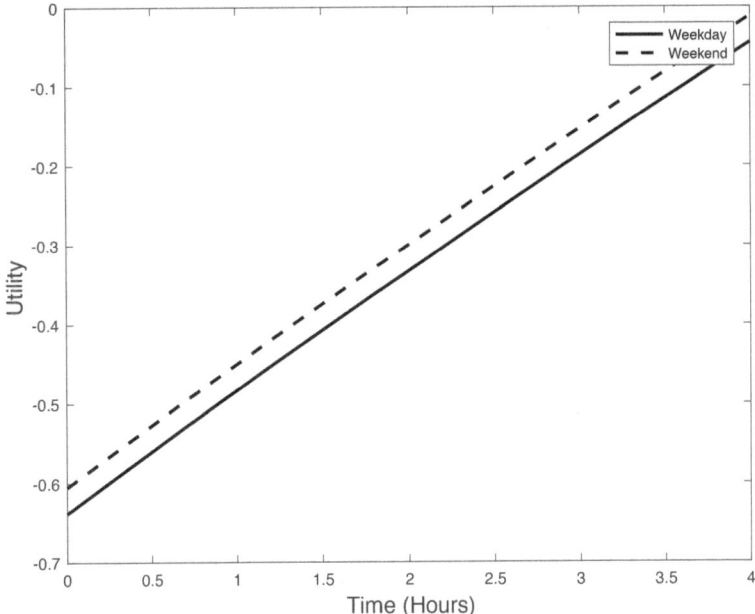

**Fig. 6.8** Effect of duration of travel activity on utility for weekday and weekend

significant for shorter travel activities, as shown in Fig. 6.8. Reasons for enjoying travel activities, discussed by and modeled by Ory and Mokhtarian (2005), include independence, exposure to environment, buffer between activities, conquest, and physical exercise—all which may have contributed to the observed curve. However, since literature (Kahneman et al. 2004; Kahneman and Krueger 2006) has shown that people do not enjoy commuting, it may also indicate the value of taking longer trips, such as a day trip out of the city. Activities labeled as other have the most distinct curve, yet it is not possible to exactly know why. With regards to accompanying people and escorting people—activities which tend to take a short amount of time—duration does not seem to have a very significant effect. Finally, education and work activities have the flattest curves. This indicates that duration has little effect on the added utility of work and educational activities. Overall, since 75% of activities are performed under 12.6 h, the activity purpose itself has a greater effect on happiness than the duration, which aligns with the developed theories of Duration Neglect.

The personal characteristics give insight into the skewness of the distribution of individuals' Hedonic States. Men's average Hedonic State tends to be below their median—or their Set Point—compared to women's. Furthermore, married and divorced individuals have an average Hedonic State that is below their Set Point compared to single individuals. In terms of employment, part-time, unemployed, and retired persons reported lower average Hedonic States compared to full-time employed people. On the other hand, self-employed individuals have an average that is slightly more positive than employed people—however, the difference is an order of magnitude smaller. Income appears to contribute negatively to average Hedonic State. However, this may be attributed to the non-representative number of high income individuals in the sample. It is worth noting that all of the personal characteristics have very high standard errors of their parameter estimates. This means that they are not as significant towards explaining Hedonic State. This makes sense because the Hedonic State was calculated around personal medians, such that it is expected that there be less variation across individuals and the sample, as previously shown in Table 6.4.

With regards to the response time, activities reported in real-time tend to have a more positive Hedonic State. The fact that the constant is significant and has a considerable parameter magnitude compared to activity purpose variables and socioeconomic variables may be a demonstration of the distinction between moment utility and remembered utility. Since the end of the activity has not happened, a happiness response reported in real-time is considered a single measurement of moment utility, which by itself is not necessarily predictive of how people remember the activity (Kahneman 1999). Similar positive effects of real-time measurements have been seen in Pedersen et al. (2011), who found that private vehicle users report higher satisfaction when riding public transport than they later remember. The time until observation is also significant, however, the magnitude of its effect is considerably smaller. Since approximately 90% of the activities are under one full day, the time before reporting has a small effect on the Hedonic State itself.

The individual and the phone-based panel effects both have significant standard deviations, yet the mean for $\omega_{na1}$ has a high standard error. This means that the added utility, in this case negative, to responding on the phone is not significant.

Finally, the coefficient of the systematic part of the $h_{na1}$, $\beta_{h1}$, is positive and less than one. A $t$-test can be performed to compare the estimate to one. The standard error, adjusted for the sample size of 714 activity instances with a second happiness report, is 0.0647, leading to a $t$-score of $-3.87$. For such sufficiently large sample size, the $t$ distribution approaches the standard normal distribution, such that the p-value is $5.4 \times 10^{-5}$, or 0.00. Therefore, $\beta_{h1}$ is significantly different than one for our sample size. This result for $\beta_{h1}$ indicates that the second happiness response for a given activity $a$ for an individual $n$ is closer to the Set Point. $\beta_{h1}$ is, therefore, a damping effect of $h_{na1}$. Recall that $h_{na1}$ is the first happiness response for a specific activity $a$ for an individual $n$ collected over the mobile phone, and that $h_{na2}$ is the second response collected during the web-based validation. This may be interpreted as an intra-activity Hedonic Treadmill, where the individual's perception of the happiness towards an activity instance is likely to be more neutral as time goes by. Like the Hedonic Treadmill described in Frederick and Loewenstein (1999), an intra-activity Hedonic Treadmill shows that remembered happiness also tends to become less accentuated, such that individuals' memories of their activity become more neutral in later reports. This would show that one's memory of their happiness is not objective; instead, it is susceptible to changes. This finding is in accordance with a number of studies which highlight that one's remembered well-being becomes more neutral, such as Abou-Zeid and Ben-Akiva (2012) and Pedersen et al. (2011), who found that car users' positive real-time report of satisfaction in public transport becomes less positive in memory. Furthermore, the finding that the second report of happiness is a moderated version of the first report aligns with Ariely's (1998) conclusions that self-reporting throughout an experience moderates the evaluations made retrospectively.

## 6.4  Conclusion

### 6.4.1  Summary

Overall, the conducted study contributes to the literature of applied models of happiness by analyzing an individual's Hedonic State using a dynamic Ordinal Logit Model, and by testing an intra-activity Hedonic Treadmill for a variety of day-to-day activities. Through the data collection platform, FMS, happiness data was collected over a varying period of time through phone- and web-based interfaces. The provided data was processed such that each individual was given a Set Point and the Hedonic State was calculated for each happiness observation. The dynamic OLM model showed that, while socioeconomic characteristics were less significant in modifying individuals' average happiness compared to their median, activity attributes—such as purpose, duration, and if it was performed during the weekend or a weekday—were more significant in explaining Hedonic State. Furthermore, the model demonstrated that the second report of happiness is a dampened version of the first report, implying that there exists an intra-activity Hedonic Treadmill.

### 6.4.2  Happiness Measurement Implications

The developed understanding of an intra-activity Hedonic Treadmill leads to a number of implications on how well-being is measured. Satisfaction surveys for an event, for example, could be significantly different if conducted directly after or a week after said event. If one's memory of their happiness with an activity becomes more neutral with time, data collection efforts can be planned to attain information that is relevant to the purpose of analysis. Real-time measurements of well-being when driving or in public transport can be used to improve the actual user experience. On the other hand, knowing that the remembered utility of an activity dampens with time may lead to better measurements for predictive purposes. Since people rely mostly on their memories of activities to decide whether to engage in the activity again (Wirtz et al. 2003), it becomes more relevant to understand people's remembered utility instead of their moment utility to predict future behavior. Further understanding how the intra-activity Hedonic Treadmill varies for different types of activities could give researchers even more insight as to when to conduct happiness measurements.

### 6.4.3   Limitations and Further Work

The major limitation of the model provided is the small number of happiness observations for each individual. On average, each individual had 15.2 happiness recordings on 10.6 activities. Since these were not enough to establish a proper moving Set Point, assumptions were made in order to determine individuals' Hedonic States. Ideally, if individuals had collected data for longer periods of time, the Set Point could have been a moving average or median. Furthermore, more data points could have resulted in more elaborate calculations of a Set Point, such as those described in Parducci (1984). One example would have been to create activity purpose-specific Set Points for each individual. Another approach that could have been used, independent of data size, is to model the Set Point itself as a latent variable. Finally, given more data, the Hedonic Treadmill Effect, as described in Frederick and Loewenstein (1999) among a progression of activities, could be tested.

With more available data, it would have been possible to test more elaborate specifications of activity duration. They could, for example, have been specific to weekdays or weekends, or be interacted with socioeconomic variables. This would lead to more understanding of what affects different users' Hedonic State. Moreover, other specifications may be tested to account for non-linear effects of the duration.

Data collection can also be improved with better inference from sensors. As an emerging methodology for collecting daily activity behavior, FMS still requires user input in fixing inferred activities and validating one's day. Despite eliminating a number of biases from traditional activity reporting, the methodology may still affect data quality, such as activity duration (Ghorpade et al. 2015). As reported, activity durations tended to be very large, especially with regards to travel activities. These may have been the result of incorrect reporting of activities between travel. Improvements in the data collection methodology should be investigated in further research.

Additionally, the model could be elaborated by including variables that take into account sequences of activities. This can be done with solely the reported activities, where the previous activity, $n(a - 1)k$, and the current activity, $nak$, are interacted. However, since FMS provides information on all of the user's activities throughout the day, the interaction can be based on the previous activity or activity pattern, even if an individual did not report on the happiness of said activity. Information on activities preceding and following the activity reported on could have also informed a distinction between commuting and other types of travel. This would allow for a difference in the categorization of travel and possibly eliminate the multiple interpretations of the travel curve. Furthermore, given information on what activity the user is performing while answering the happiness question retrospectively, the damping effect could be modified to understand the how different activities affect how an individual remembers happiness during a previous activity. This could illuminate mechanisms of the proposed intra-activity Hedonic Treadmill.

# References

Abou-Zeid, M., & Ben-Akiva, M. (2012). Well-being and activity-based models. *Transportation, 39*, 1189–1207.

Andrews, F., & Withey, S. B. (1976). Developing measures of perceived life quality: Results from several national surveys. *Social Indicators Research, 1*, 1–26.

Ariely, D. (1998). Combining experiences over time: The effects of duration, intensity changes and on-line measurements on retrospective pain evaluations. *Journal of Behavioral Decision Making, 11*, 19–45.

Ariely, D., & Zauberman, G. (2000). On the making of an experience: The effects of breaking and combining experiences on their overall evaluation. *Journal of Behavioral Decision Making, 13*, 219–232.

Australian Bureau of Statistics. (2011). Highest level of education (all persons aged 15 years and over). http://www.abs.gov.au/websitedbs/censushome.nsf/home/mediafactsheets2nd/$file/Topic%20-%20Highest%20Level%20of%20Education.pdf. Accessed 23 June 2017.

Australian Bureau of Statistics. (2017). Household income and wealth, Australia 2015–16. http://www.abs.gov.au/ausstats/abs@.nsf/mf/6523.0. Accessed 23 June 2017.

Baumeister, R. F., Vohs, K. D., & Oettingen, G. (2016). Pragmatic prospection: How and why people think about the future. *Review of General Psychology, 20*(1), 3–16.

Bergstad, C. J., Gamble, A., Hagman, O., Polk, M., Gärling, T., Ettema, D., Friman, M., & Olson, L. E. (2012). Influences of affect associated with routine out-of-house activities on subjective well-being. *Applied Research in Quality of Life, 7*, 49–62.

Bierlaire, M., & Fetiarison, M. (2009). Estimation of discrete choice models: Extending BIOGEME. Proceedings of the 9th Swiss Transport Research Conference (STRC), Monte Verità.

Cottrill, C., Pereira, F., Zhao, F., Dias, I., Lim, H., Ben-Akiva, M., & Zegras, P. C. (2013). Future mobility survey. *Transportation Research Record: Journal of the Transportation Research Board, 2354*, 59–67.

Diener, E. (1984). Subjective well-being. *Psychological Bulletin, 95*(3), 542–575.

Duarte, A., Garcia, C., Limão, S., & Polydropoulou, A. (2008). Happiness in transport decision making: The Swiss sample. 8th Swiss Transport Research Conference, Ascona, Switzerland.

Ettema, D., Gärling, T., Eriksson, L., Friman, M., Olsson, L. E., & Fujii, S. (2011). Satisfaction with travel and subjective well-being: Development and test of a measurement tool. *Transportation Research Part F, 14*, 167–175.

Frederick, S., & Loewenstein, G. (1999). Hedonic adaptation. In D. Kahneman, E. Diener, & N. Schwarz (Eds.), *Well-being: The foundations of hedonic psychology* (pp. 302–329). New York: Russell Sage.

Fujita, F., & Diener, E. (2005). Life satisfaction set point: Stability and change. *Journal of Personality and Social Psychology, 88*(1), 158–164.

Ghorpade, A., Pereira, F. C., Zhao, F., Zegras, C., Ben-Akiva, M. (2015). An integrated stop-mode detection algorithm for real world smartphone-based travel survey. 94th Annual Meeting of the Transportation Research Board, Washington, DC.

Giachanou, A., & Crestani, F. (2016) Like it or not: A survey of Twitter sentiment analysis methods. *ACM Computing Surveys, 49*(2), 28–28:41.

Hardie, B. G. S., Johnson, E. J., & Fader, P. S. (1993). Modeling loss aversion and brand dependence effects on brand choice. *Marketing Science, 12*, 378–394.

Helliwell, J., Layard, R., & Sachs, J. (2017). *World happiness report 2017*. New York: Sustainable Development Solutions Network.

Helson, H. (1964). *Adaptation-level theory: An experimental and systematic approach to behavior*. New York: Harper and Row.

Jariyasunan, J., Carrel, A., Ekambaram, V., Gaker, D. J., Kote, T., Sengupta, R., Walker, J. L. (2012). The quantified traveler: Using personal travel data to promote sustainable transport behavior. 91st Annual Meeting of the Transportation Research Board, Washington, DC.

Kahneman, D. (1999). Evaluation by moments: Past and future. In D. Kahneman & A. Tversky (Eds.), *Choices, values and frames*. New York: Cambridge University Press and Russell Sage.

Kahneman, D., & Krueger, A. B. (2006). Developments in the measurement of subjective well-being. *Journal of Economic Perspectives, 20*(1), 3–24.

Kahneman, D., Diener, N., & Schwarz, N. (1999). *Well-being: The foundations of hedonic psychology*. New York: Russell Sage.

Kahneman, D., Fredrickson, B., Schreiber, C., & Redelmeier, D. (1993). When more pain is preferred to less: Adding a better end. *Psychological Science, 4*(6), 401–405. Retrieved from http://www.jstor.org/stable/40062570

Kahneman, D., Krueger, A. B., Schkade, D. A., Schwarz, N., & Stone, A. A. (2004). A survey method for characterizing daily life experience: The day reconstruction method. *Science, 306* (5702), 1776–1780.

Killingsworth, M., & Gilbert, D. (2010). A wandering mind is an unhappy mind. *Science, 330* (6006), 932.

March, J. G. (1988). Variable risk preferences and adaptive aspirations. *Elsevier, 9*(1), 5–24.

Ory, D., & Mokhtarian, P. (2005). When is getting there half the fun? *Modeling the liking for travel. Transportation Research Part A, 39*, 97–123.

Oswald, A. J. (1997). Happiness and economic performance. *Economic Journal, 107*(445), 1815–1831.

Parducci, A. (1968). The Relativism of absolute judgments. *Scientific American, 219*, 84–90.

Parducci, A. (1984). *Value judgments: Toward a relational theory of happiness. Attitudinal judgement* (pp. 3–21). New York: Springer-Verlag.

Pedersen, T., Friman, M., & Kristensson, P. (2011). The role of predicted, on-line experienced and remembered satisfaction in current choice to use public transport services. *Journal of Retailing and Consumer Services, 18*, 471–475.

Raveau, S., Ghorpade, A., Zhao, F., Abou-Zeid, M., Zegras, C., & Ben-Akiva, M. (2015). Smartphone-based survey for real-time and retrospective happiness related to travel and activities. *Transportation Research Record: Journal of the Transportation Research Board, 2566*, 102–110.

Ravulaparthy, S., Yoon, S., & Goulias, K. (2013). Linking elderly transport mobility and subjective well-being: A multivariate latent modeling approach. *Transportation Research Record: Journal of the Transportation Research Board, 2382*, 28–36.

Roddis, S. (2016). *Victorian future mobility sensing (FMS) trial*. Project Report. Department of Infrastructure Engineering, The University of Melbourne.

Ryder, H. R., & Heal, G. M. (1973). Optimal growth with intertemporally dependent preferences. *Review of Economic Studies, 40*, 1–33.

Sinnott, R. O., & Cui, S. (2016). Benchmarking sentiment analysis approaches on the cloud. In *IEEE 22nd International Conference on Parallel and Distributed Systems (ICPADS)* (pp. 695–704). Wuhan: IEEE.

The Economist Intelligence Unit. (2017). The global liveability report 2017. The Economist Intelligence Unit Limited 2017. http://www.eiu.com/Handlers/WhitepaperHandler.ashx?fi=Liveability-Ranking-Free-Summary-Report-August-2017.pdf

The Victorian Department of Transport. (2011). *Victorian integrated survey of travel & activity 2009–10*. Survey Procedures and Documentation. Final Data Release v1.0.

Wirtz, D., Kruger, J., Scollon, C. N., & Diener, E. (2003). Research report: What to do on spring break? The role of predicted, on-line, and remembered experience in future choice. *Psychological Science, 14*(5), 520–524.

# Chapter 7
# Measuring Door-to-Door Journey Travel Satisfaction with a Mobile Phone App

Yusak O. Susilo and Fotis K. Liotopoulos

**Abstract** This chapter describes the lessons learned from designing, deploying and analysing the results from a smartphone applications, sbNavi™, in measuring door-to-door, multi-modal, travel satisfaction across eight different European cities. In this chapter, the process, the architecture design and the pros and cons of deploying such app are described. Challenges from technical and practical point of views are then discussed and the comparability of the results, compared to other survey methods, is presented.

**Keywords** App architectural design · Pros and cons of app deployments · Multimodal travel satisfaction · On-board measurement · Door-to-door journey

## 7.1 Introduction

In the last decade, there have been a surge of studies, investigating various aspects of passenger travel experience and the complexity underlie such evaluations (e.g. Friman and Gärling 2001; Stradling et al. 2007; Diana 2008; Páez and Whalen 2010; Susilo et al. 2012; Ettema et al. 2012; Friman et al. 2013). For example, previous studies (e.g. Pedersen et al. 2011; Susilo and Cats 2014) suggest that there is a systematic tendency to report higher satisfaction levels immediately after the completion of a public transport or cycling trip stage when compared with a retrospective satisfaction report. In contrast, private car travellers reported significantly lower travel satisfaction levels in retrospective reports. This opposing-behaviour highlights the importance to understand the implication on how such travel satisfaction were measured and interpreted, and how it is changing overtime

Y. O. Susilo (✉)
KTH Royal Institute of Technology, Stockholm, Sweden
e-mail: yusak.susilo@abe.kth.se

F. K. Liotopoulos
SBOING.net, Thessaloniki, Greece
e-mail: liotop@sboing.net

© Springer International Publishing AG, part of Springer Nature 2018
M. Friman et al. (eds.), *Quality of Life and Daily Travel*, Applying Quality of Life Research, https://doi.org/10.1007/978-3-319-76623-2_7

and influenced by its internal and external contexts. Travel satisfaction is a continuous self-learning and self-appreciation processes. Thus, individual specific contexts, such as different travel patterns and modes specific spots, events, and locations, would produce different outputs. These complexities, however, are largely ignored in most of today travel satisfaction surveys that are regularly deployed in measuring the public transport operators' performances in various metropolitans in the world.

One of the main reasons that such complexities have been overlooked in the past is because it is considered too complicated and demanding to ask respondents to provide such complex information in a traditional travel satisfaction survey. Many of travel satisfaction surveys (such as Passenger Focus 2011; SKT 2016) were organized by public transport operators which mainly interested to improve their particular service provision, periodically evaluating the operators' performance, and not about whole journey trip experience and not about how the satisfaction would be different in different context compositions. With the increased importance of providing inclusive transport services by the local and national authorities as well as with the emerging mobile and GPS technologies, measuring the whole (door-to-door) journeys in a cheaper and reliable way, without providing too much workload and burden to the respondents, seems now to be within a reaching distance. The current mobile positioning technology, however, is not without problems (Anderson et al. 2009; Cottrill et al. 2013; NCHRP 2014; Susilo et al. 2016). In many cases, although positioning technology can be used to directly record accurate time and geographic information of travel (e.g., Chung and Shalaby 2005; Gong and Chen 2012; Feng and Timmermans 2013; Rasouli and Timmermans 2014), the participants are still needed to be heavily involved by providing/verifying the entities and their attributes, especially when we are collecting information that cannot be derived from GPS data alone such as travel satisfaction.

This chapter describes the lessons learned from designing, deploying and analysing the results from a smartphone application, sbNavi™, in measuring door-to-door travel satisfaction. In this chapter, the pros and cons of deploying such app are discussed. Challenges from technical and practical point of views are discussed and the comparability of the results, compared to other survey methods, is presented.

## 7.2   The Survey and Tool Design

The smartphone application, sbNavi™, that is used to measure door-to-door travel satisfaction discussed in this paper is one of the outcomes of the METPEX FP7 EU project (www.metpex.eu, METPEX 2012–2015 (Susilo et al. 2015). The METPEX project aims to develop a Pan-European standardised measurement tool to measure passenger experience across whole journeys, whilst taking into account wider human socio-economic, cultural, geographic and environmental factors. In doing so, the project utilises five different survey methods, i.e.: (1) Paper-and-pencil, (2) Online (web-based) questionnaire, (3) Real-time questionnaire, embedded in the satellite navigation (sbNavi™) app for IOS and Android, (4) Real-time questionnaire, embedded in a specially developed Android Game app, and (5) Focused group interviewing. The data collection was then carried out in eight different European cities – Bucharest, Coventry, Dublin, Grevena, Rome, Stockholm, Valencia and Vilnius, and five FIA motorist networks (Germany, Poland, France, Spain and the United Kingdom), between September and November 2014. In total, 6360 completed responses were collected during the survey period. After the data had been cleaned and double checked for consistency and reliability across different sections, the total number of valid samples was 5275. The results were 984 responses from the paper-and-pencil survey, 3395 responses from the online web survey, 231 responses from the sbNavi™ app, 414 responses from the game app and 251 responses from the focus group method. Detailed comparison analysis on the survey results across different survey methods can be seen at (Susilo et al. 2017a) and the overview of the questionnaire design and survey deployment can be seen at (Susilo et al. 2017b). Further discussion on the METPEX project results, including the business case of the tool can be seen on (Tovey et al. 2017). The further focus of this chapter discussion is the development and the evaluation of the third tool, i.e. measurement of door-to-door travel satisfaction via a real-time questionnaire which is embedded in a personal route navigation app (SBOING GPS navigator, sbNavi™) for IOS and Android.

## 7.2.1  The Selection of a Personal Navigation Assistant (PNA) Platform in Deploying the Survey

A mobile navigation system or personal navigation assistant (PNA) is a satellite-based navigation system designed for use in mobile devices; car navigators or smartphones. It typically uses a GNSS (mostly GPS) receiver to acquire position data from a set of satellites, in order to locate the user on a road, on the device's map database. Using the map database, the unit can give routing directions to other locations, effectively providing guidance to the user of the device. The use of a mobile phone app in measuring travel satisfaction does not only provide us the travel satisfaction evaluation of that specific trip leg, but also offers opportunities to capture the actual route taken, the exact travel time, background context of the travel and individual relationship with the given trip leg (e.g., the frequency/familiarity of the individual with this particular trip leg). The use of an app that is not purposely built solely to capture the individual travel satisfaction, but also provides other functionality as well, (e.g., useful services and information, such as route navigation, and other incentivation, such as promotional offers, digital virtual currency, etc.) is expected to help the users appreciate more the usefulness of the app in their daily travel, as a return of their participation in the survey.

Limitations of PNAs include the requirement of visibility of at least four satellites (the more the better) for determining the position of the user, as well as the relatively low accuracy in determining this position (at least in the current commercial GPS system). The new Galileo GNSS promises higher (even sub-meter) accuracies with proper satellite receivers/sensors, especially combined with other GNSS. More accurate PNAs with wider applicability will increase their penetration in the society, thus broadening the user community exposed to measurement tools.

The add-on travel satisfaction tool that is embedded at sbNavi™, called sbSirVVays®, enables the respondents to submit a survey (response to a questionnaire) over their smartphone.

With this app tool:

- The responder can manage (add/delete/edit) whole Journeys, with each journey consisting of an arbitrary number of legs (stages).
- For each journey leg the responder may fill in a different questionnaire related with the given leg.
- The journey legs can also be re-ordered at any given time.
- The app calls a web-service to dynamically retrieve an appropriate questionnaire based on his/her profile information. The selection criteria during the survey were: random, travel mode, gender/age-group/income, disability, additional transport needs (generated based on the expected distribution of socio-demographic and/or travel modes of respondents).
- The users can fill in/edit any questionnaire at any time (during/after the journey).
- GPS coordinates and Date-Time info are recorded at various points (where/if available).
- The users may also use the current system/GPS time and date, or enter it manually.
- Source and Destination places can also be entered manually.
- Within each questionnaire, the user may record (pause/restart/stop) the route of his/her journey. The recorded route is attached to (linked with) the questionnaire.
- The questionnaire responses are securely uploaded to the METPEX servers (encrypted with strong encryption, use of digital certificates, etc.) as required.
- In response to the submission of a questionnaire, the participant is rewarded with a number of SCU (SBOING credit units) which can be used in their application and unlock new features (i.e. download the latest maps).

The SBOING navigator, sbNavi™, implements a collaborative, crowdsourcing methodology for advanced navigation and routing.

1. Instead of the static speed limit of a road used by today's navigators, the sbNavi™ technology is based on a collaborative methodology, which consists, for each road section, of the statistical recording of the average travelling time for every vehicle type, weather conditions, road conditions, season, day-of-the-week and time-of-day. Thus, for example, for a 100 m section of road XYZ average travel time may be 40 s., on Tuesday afternoon, or 15 s., on Sunday morning, etc.
2. While driving, the GPS navigator records and stores a number of parameters, including the vehicle's GPS position (GPS coordinates), velocity, altimeter and

timestamp. In addition, the user may also add extra map information, such as road hazards, traffic cameras, points-of-interest (POIs), map corrections, etc.

3. The users subsequently securely upload their collected traces to the SBOING/sbNavi™'s host web-site and in return they get updated maps for their PNAs, through a "credit-debit" system (based on credit units, which are called "SBOING Credit Units", or SCUs). SCUs can then be bought/exchanged/traded as any virtual currency, i.e. with other virtual currencies (Farmville gold or Facebook currency), or for products and services at reduced prices (with targeted and location-based push advertising).

4. The uploaded data undergoes certain statistical validity checks, carried out by the server backend, (to filter out any malicious or invalid data) and it is statistically integrated inside the SBOING's database and world maps. Uncharted areas are updated and new roads and pathways are added to the existing maps, just by users' driving around and recording GPS traces.

5. Based on their collected SCUs, the users can download at will maps and SBOING/sbNavi™ traffic data for any region of the world, through SBOING's web-site, which will enable them to enjoy better routing and faster map updates.

More detailed description on other services that are provided by sbNavi™ can be found at www.sboing.net.

## 7.2.2 Integrating Travel Satisfaction Questionnaire to sbNavi™ App

Deploying door-to-door travel satisfaction questionnaires, as what sbSirVVays® add-on does, is not without a challenge. From the earlier desktop research, stakeholder consultation and a small size experiment, more than 1000 users groups, travel modes and more than 400 context-specific indicators were gathered (Susilo et al. 2017b). Apparently, it is impossible to ask the users to provide answers for all these indicators. Thus, several rounds of Multi Criteria Analysis among experts and stakeholders were carried out to set weights to the various indicators.

Based on this approach, 600 questions in total were formulated and distributed into five sections, differentiated according to the location of the survey (which was identified as a different campaign per test site), nature of the survey (retrospective vs real-time), user groups and travel modes used, with rules as shown on Fig. 7.1:

- Individual attributes (i.e. socio-demographic, mobility behaviour)
- Attitudes (i.e. travel preferences, mobility-related opinions)
- Contextual variables (i.e. temporal, weather conditions, trip purpose, subjective well-being indices)
- Specific user groups and travel modes specific questionnaires

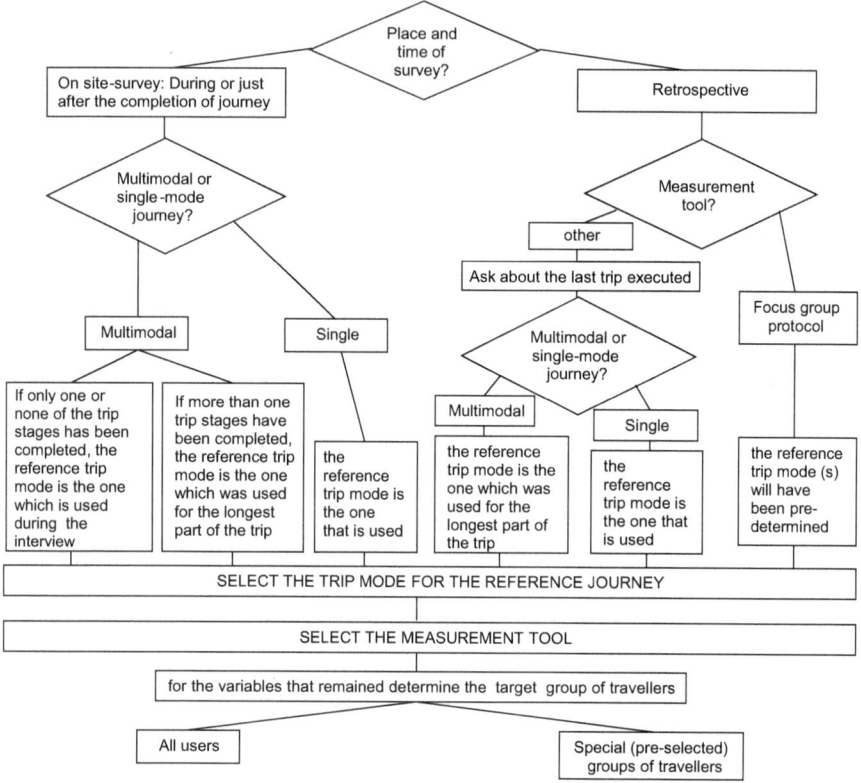

**Fig. 7.1** Flowchart of indicators deployment of questionnaire within METPEX system (Modified from: METPEX 2014; Susilo et al. 2017b)

- Travel experience factors (e.g. availability, travel time components, information provision, reliability, way-finding, comfort, appeal, safety and security, customer care, price, connectivity, etc.)

To limit the respondents' burden, it was decided that, for each specific user group and travel mode combination, each respondent was asked to answer 50–75 questions, maximum, which should only require the respondent to spend approximately 20–30 min, in total, to complete the entire questionnaire. In order to do this, the web-based survey and the sbNavi™ app survey tools have a capability to select and generate a questionnaire which is presented to the respondent dynamically.

The rules of the questions on deployment are shown in Fig. 7.2. The initial baseline questions cover, amongst other things, journey details and include control questions related to travel modes and user groups. This step provides detailed information on transport modes or on individuals with distinct travel needs and enables the PSS to overcome the challenge of acquiring both general travel experience information and information on specific individual groups. Tier 1 questions cover information at a high level on the satisfaction of each component of the

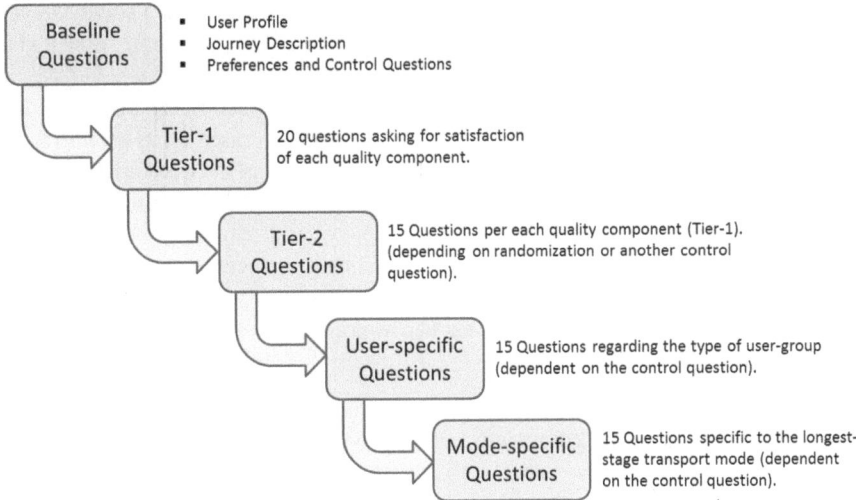

**Fig. 7.2** Flowchart of indicators deployment within METPEX system (Modified from: METPEX 2014)

transport experience. Tier 2 questions represent a focus on a particular sub-set of travel satisfaction selected at random. This structure is intended to enable the PSS to acquire both general information about the journey, as well as very detailed information about specific aspects whilst maintaining a practical limit on the number of questions a participant is asked – thereby responding to the concern about developing an overlong tool.

In order to deploy the planned questions as shown in Fig. 7.2, a dynamic survey concept is implemented. In technical and survey design terms, this means that there is one integrated main platform (server) where:

- The survey is described using XML. This description specifies each question's type (e.g. multiple choice, text, integer value, etc.), the visual components to be used in the questionnaire (e.g., checkbox, radio button, combo-box, slider, etc.) or the default response, amongst other things.
- A campaign, being a collection of surveys, is also described using XML. The description identifies its name, type and the set of surveys it contains.
- The surveys can be generated either statically (manually), or dynamically (e.g., with a query followed by an SQL-to-XML script-based conversion). Alternatively, the XML may be replaced with JSON format messaging (more Java friendly, for Android platforms).
- The passenger's response is also in XML and uploaded with strong encryption to the central servers.

Then, the app-server and back-end communication protocol, used to provide a questionnaire to the app user (survey responder) from the application's point of view, is as follows:

- Step 1: Upon the user's request, the survey tool places a query to a survey server. Based on the user's demographics and profile the user is subsequently assigned to one of the available active campaigns.
- Step 2: A survey is randomly chosen, out of the list defined in the campaign, and it is loaded (in XML/JSON). Note here that, if the user (based on its profile) is not compatible with the particular campaign, i.e., if he is a Greek male and the campaign is for French females, then the application should not launch the questionnaire.
- Step 3: The questionnaire form is dynamically generated from the survey description.
- Step 4: When the user completes his/her response, the application uploads/posts the response (in XML/JSON).

This integrated dynamic back-end system acts as the "central hub", the registry point of all organisations, campaigns and surveys. All surveys will be accessed by the survey app through that central hub. Organizations (i.e., transport stakeholders, policy makers, consultants, etc., the company's customers, in general) will register in this hub and may define and enable (launch) their individual campaigns and surveys (questionnaires) at will. The local survey organiser also would be able to identify the participant who has completed the survey and provide the reward as what they have been promised, if any. The snapshots of sbNavi™ and sbSirVVays®'s interfaces and also of the back-end system can be seen in Fig. 7.3.

### 7.2.3 Support Infrastructures Needed

The primary infrastructure that received the user data from the users' devices and host the data management services was located on the Internet Cloud. All services involving the communication and handling of sensitive user data, such as passwords, user response, etc. were secured through SSL-based access. A website scanner was installed to look for malware in the website and regularly (e.g. daily) crawl the website for security gaps and vulnerabilities that a hacker could exploit to steal sensitive customer information or infect visitors with spyware and viruses.

The secondary infrastructure that hosted the data collection and processing were at the backend computing facilities, hosted by SBOING. The backend infrastructure used also served as a backup facility centre, that would be enabled in case of failure of the primary (cloud) infrastructure. In addition, it was used for independent data backup and for specialized data processing purposes that required a "dedicated server" infrastructure. In particular, this backend infrastructure provided: (1) daily (or regular) automated backups of the data hosted at the primary infrastructure, (2) a mirror environment (software and services) of the primary infrastructure, and (3) an ability to take over within a few hours after a failure of the primary infrastructure.

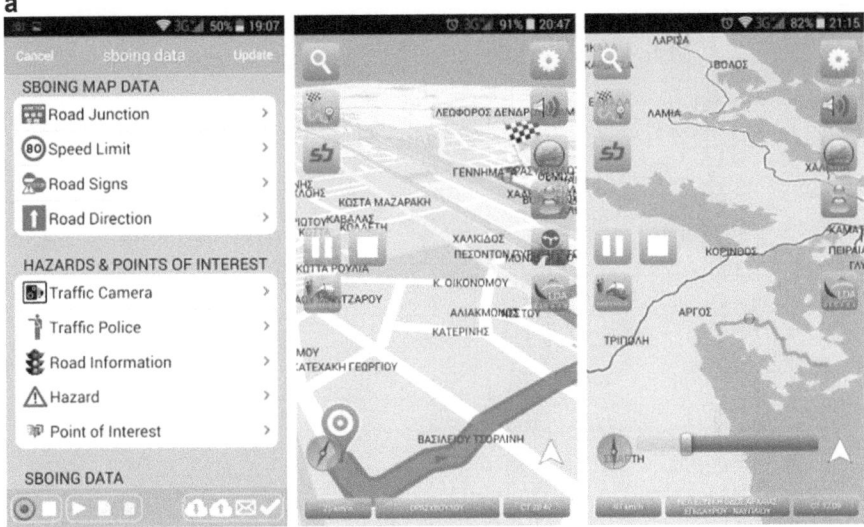

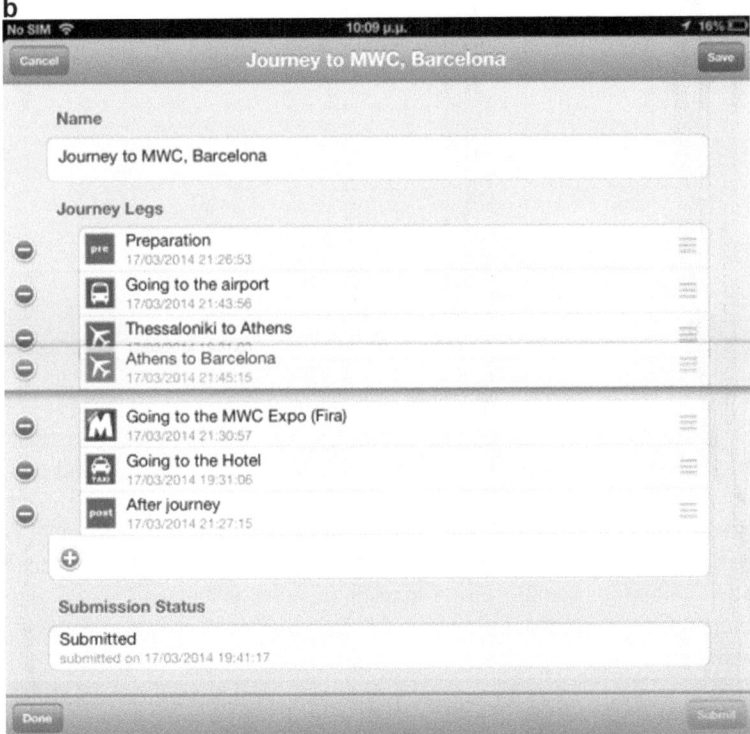

**Fig. 7.3** The snapshots of sbNavi™ and sbSirVVays®'s interfaces and also of the back-end system. (**a**) sbNavi™ app (Android version). (**b**) sbSirVVays® add-on to sbNavi™ app (for a multi-legged journey). (**c**) questionnaires management for a Campaign in the backend system

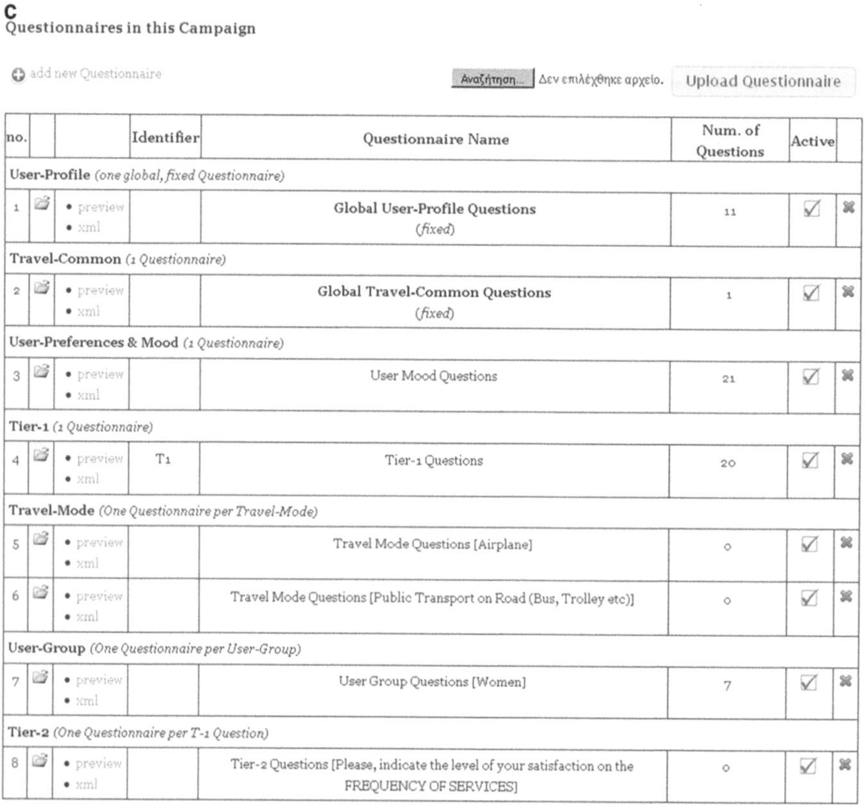

**C**
Questionnaires in this Campaign

⊕ add new Questionnaire                    Αναζήτηση... | Δεν επιλέχθηκε αρχείο.   Upload Questionnaire

| no. | | Identifier | Questionnaire Name | Num. of Questions | Active | |
|---|---|---|---|---|---|---|
| **User-Profile** *(one global, fixed Questionnaire)* | | | | | | |
| 1 | 📝 | • preview<br>• xml | Global User-Profile Questions<br>*(fixed)* | 11 | ✓ | ✖ |
| **Travel-Common** *(1 Questionnaire)* | | | | | | |
| 2 | 📝 | • preview<br>• xml | Global Travel-Common Questions<br>*(fixed)* | 1 | ✓ | ✖ |
| **User-Preferences & Mood** *(1 Questionnaire)* | | | | | | |
| 3 | 📝 | • preview<br>• xml | User Mood Questions | 21 | ✓ | ✖ |
| **Tier-1** *(1 Questionnaire)* | | | | | | |
| 4 | 📝 | • preview<br>• xml | T1 | Tier-1 Questions | 20 | ✓ | ✖ |
| **Travel-Mode** *(One Questionnaire per Travel-Mode)* | | | | | | |
| 5 | 📝 | • preview<br>• xml | Travel Mode Questions [Airplane] | 0 | ✓ | ✖ |
| 6 | 📝 | • preview<br>• xml | Travel Mode Questions [Public Transport on Road (Bus, Trolley etc)] | 0 | ✓ | ✖ |
| **User-Group** *(One Questionnaire per User-Group)* | | | | | | |
| 7 | 📝 | • preview<br>• xml | User Group Questions [Women] | 7 | ✓ | ✖ |
| **Tier-2** *(One Questionnaire per T-1 Question)* | | | | | | |
| 8 | 📝 | • preview<br>• xml | Tier-2 Questions [Please, indicate the level of your satisfaction on the FREQUENCY OF SERVICES] | 0 | ✓ | ✖ |

**Fig. 7.3**  (continued)

## 7.3  The Survey Field Preparation and Deployment

Prior the development, the surveyor coordinators that involve in the data collection were required to: (1) familiarise themselves with the tool, (2) translating the tool and the advertisement and dissemination materials (e.g. flyers, websites and newsletter) into local languages, (3) ensuring that local ethical procedures are met and all ethical and practical permissions that are required to test the tools are considered, (4) developing of a common survey plan, based on interface guideline (questionnaire) and expected minimum sample size for each traveller group and mode share, and (5) preparing a recruitment strategy, for each survey location and target group, including potential challenges and the plan to mitigate these.

### 7.3.1 Familiarisation with the Tools

All survey coordinators involved in the surveys needed to try-and-test the tool in advance and to learn how to use the backend system. In order to facilitate the familiarization process with the tool a manual was made available to all survey coordinators with instructions and details about the functioning of each tool. This familiarization stage was also meant to detect malfunctions and errors, so that tool developers could fix them before they were used in the real survey. At that stage the tool was also tested with a limited number of combinations of different user and transport mode groups to check the understandability of the questionnaire for different groups of respondents. As for the back-end system, the familiarization came with the navigation of its menus, testing the data entry system, checking the responses statistics and the export of test data.

### 7.3.2 Translation Process

The satisfaction survey in the sbNavi™ app was deployed in 10 different languages, i.e.: English, French, German, Spanish, Italian, Greek, Swedish, Lithuanian, Polish and Romanian. Since the original questionnaires had to be translated from English into nine languages, it was decided that the translation be jargon free, unambiguous and as clear as possible. These rules were adopted to avoid the following potential problems:

(a) Lexical and syntactic ambiguity. This happens when a word has more than one meaning or when a sentence can have more than one structure.
(b) Lexical and structural mismatching. Words that in the local language do not exist and therefore the translator must choose between a borrowing from another language, a neologism, or providing an explanation. For example, the a single word "*safety*" in English represents both "*safety from the danger*" and "*sense of security*", which in Swedish are usually represented by two different two words, either "*säkerhet*" or "*trygghet*", respectively.
(c) Another main problem was the quality of the whole sentence. Some of the sentences, although understandable and grammatically correct, did not sound natural when translated into other languages. This is a known problem of translations that may arise due to the paradox of having to choose between a grammatically correct translation, with the risk of changing the original meaning of the statements/questions, or rephrasing the questions to a more locally-acceptable one with the peril of changing the interpretation of the original one.

To reduce the impact of this problem, a reverse translation check was implemented. At the final checking stage, at least 20 randomly selected questions were reverse-translated back-and-forth into English and 9 other languages to ensure the quality and consistency of the translation process.

### 7.3.3  Respondents Recruitment

Since the survey deals with a multitude of different user types, of different transport modes, and within various sites, making sure that the sample size statistically reflected the structure of the population was of paramount importance. The stratification of travellers was decided to be based on two different characteristics: (1) the travel mode that respondents used on their main trip leg; and (2) the user group in which they belonged. With this approach, travellers with different needs and vulnerable travellers (elderly, people with mobility impairment, etc.) were included in the sampling. This approach ensured that a representative sample of travelers was chosen, for each travel mode and for each target user group, in every test site. It also facilitated testing whether the tool would be able to capture the individual door-to-door journey characteristics, regardless of the respondent's travel mode and user group. This information is crucial for Transport stakeholders and operators in improving their systems and services. The sampling process was based on the determination of several parameters that led to the computing of a statistically representative sample size. The survey campaigns were promoted via various channels and through the distribution of survey flyers.

During the survey period, the survey coordinators were able to periodically monitor statistics about the profiles of travellers that they were collecting. In case the yield of a particular user group were far from reaching their desired sample target, the survey coordinators could manage the quotas by properly prioritizing the targeted group. The prioritization of certain groups could be made by modifying at the back-end system the weights applied to a given user group.

### 7.3.4  Survey Deployment

The survey period began on September 15th, 2014 and ran until October 29th, 2014, with few exceptions, lasting a total of 45 days. The recruitment method varied depending on the trial site and the collection method. Some survey coordinators offered economic and other incentives to attract more respondents. For example, Stockholm offered a cinema ticket whilst Coventry offered a cup of coffee and lottery ticket to win an iPad. Some others used their stakeholders and membership networks (e.g. FIA, Bucharest, Dublin) to promote the survey. Some coordinators developed a strong media campaign to encourage online survey participation (e.g. in Valencia) and other deployed an efficient on-street survey campaign, distributing paper-based questionnaires and the online survey on their tablets and/or iPads. Some of the coordinators received strong support from their local stakeholders and were able to carry out surveys on board or at the stakeholders' premises. For example, Dublin carried out on-board surveys; and Dublin was allowed to set up a stand on a main railway station or at coffee shops (in Coventry).

In order to manage the quotas and reach the targets per user group and transport mode, the survey coordinators periodically checked their response statistics at the backend system querying the results and grouping them by user group, gender, age, etc., or by exporting the results on the given time. Therefore, the coordinators were able to check if their data collection process was progressing in the right direction, i.e., that they were collecting properly balanced number of samples per each targeted group. Thus, if a coordinator needed to collect more samples from a specific group, they could modify the weights given to each user group in real-time, in order to prioritize their favored groups.

## 7.4    The Results (and How This Different Than Other Survey Method)

Overall, the success of the trial was mixed. There are a number of sites and survey coordinators who managed to achieve the targeted number of the respondents, or even significantly more than was expected (see Table 7.1 below). However, at the same time, there were a few sites and survey coordinators who did not. Compared to other survey method that were simultaneously deployed during the survey period, the traditional online and the paper-and-pencil methods managed to attract the most respondents, whilst the more technological driven methods, sbNavi™ and game

**Table 7.1** Summary of collected vs. planned number of respondents, by the used survey methods

| City | Number of collected response | Paper and pencil | Web Online survey | sbNavi™ App | Game app | Focus group |
|------|------|------|------|------|------|------|
| Bucharest | 457 (600) | 59 (40) | 316 (440) | 13 (40) | 46 (40) | 23 (40) |
| Coventry | 479 (500) | 321 (100) | 104 (100) | 9 (100) | 33 (100) | 12 (100) |
| Dublin | 573 (600) | 231 (150) | 297 (150) | 11 (50) | 29 (50) | 5 (20) |
| Grevena | 320 (375) | 150 (100) | 65 (140) | 8 (20) | 2 (20) | 95 (95) |
| Rome | 832 (700) | 201 (280) | 532 (245) | 1 (55) | 22 (50) | 76 (70) |
| Stockholm | 996 (880) | 224 (200) | 252 (200) | 211 (200) | 228 (200) | 81 (80) |
| Valencia | 680 (600) | 22 (458) | 600 (20) | 17 (20) | 41 (20) | 0 (82) |
| Vilnius | 395 (600) | 291 (200) | 58 (200) | 22 (100) | 24 (100) | 0 (0) |
| FIA networks | 1611 (1500) | 0 (0) | 1611 (1460) | 0 (20) | 0 (20) | 0 (0) |
| Total | 6343 (6355) | 1791 (1528) | 3835 (2955) | 292 (605) | 425 (600) | 292 (487) |

Note: The ones in bracket are the target numbers that was stated on the survey plan

apps were found to be the most difficult. The acceptance level, however, was different in different countries.

Furthermore and overall, the game app had a higher acceptance rate than the sbNavi™ app. However, we cannot infer from this that sbNavi™ is less attractive than the game app, as that may have been the feeling of the responders because the Android game app contained fewer questions than the sbNavi™ app, which contained the full length of the questionnaire and provided more functionality, thus it was more complicated to handle, than the game app.

There was a consistent concern among respondents and surveyors that although the tools appeared *to be attractive,* the questionnaire was too long and too complicated. The disadvantages caused by this outweighed the attractiveness of the tools, thus many of the respondents did not manage to complete a whole questionnaire.

Furthermore, despite a surge in technology adoption and penetration of smartphones in Europe in the last several years, the acceptance of the smartphone app as a survey tool was still very low. There were significant privacy and data protection concerns among potential respondents (e.g., among FIA respondents) in installing an unknown app without being able to appreciate its benefits immediately. Indeed it is a common practice among smartphone users to download free game apps on a daily basis. But this may be because there was an expectation that the users would get a very professional and enjoyable game experience in exchange for their participation in the survey. Users' appetite to have a more entertaining app was also evidenced in our trial by having a higher participation rates for the Game app, even though it was launched much later than the sbNavi™ app.

It needs to be noted here that in some trial sites, Android smartphones have much wider and diverse market than the iOS (apple/sbNavi™) system. For instance, in the UK the Android market share is 61%, in Italy 76% and in Spain 84%.[1]

A similar tendency could also be seen in terms of the distribution of travel modes (see Table 7.2). Pedestrians and cyclists were more difficult to capture than rail-based travellers. This is probably because many of the recruitment processes focused on the main interchanges where the travellers' main travel modes were other than walking and cycling. Furthermore, it is very difficult, if not impossible, for pedestrians, cyclists and car drivers to participate in online based survey (e.g., filling the online questionnaire or app-based surveys) whilst travelling.

Another common concern among many trial sites was the requirement for a high-speed Internet connection to download and complete the apps and online questionnaires. At the trial sites where the speed and bandwidth of the Internet were rather limited, the apps and the online questionnaire required a very long time to download, respond, and move between pages. Sometimes, maybe because it took too much time to wait for a response from the server, the app may have a timed-out (delay in response) and/or the respondents gave up the survey and cancelled their participation. Although many of these connectivity/communications problems were due to

---

[1]http://www.smartcompany.com.au/technology/trends/43064-google-android-gains-ground-on-apple-iphone-in-australia-windows-phone-beating-ios-in-key-european-markets.html#

**Table 7.2** Summary of collected vs. planned number of respondents, by travel mode

| City | Private vehicle | PT road | PT Rail (Tram, Rail, Underground) | Pedestrian and bike | PT waterborne | Demand responsive transit | Mobility vehicles |
|---|---|---|---|---|---|---|---|
| Bucharest | 76 (182) | 111 (147) | 160 (141) | 46 (130) | 0 (0) | 20 (0) | 3 (0) |
| Coventry | 150 (100) | 98 (100) | 103 (100) | 77 (150) | 0 (0) | 15 (25) | 2 (25) |
| Dublin | 31 (100) | 390 (200) | 122 (200) | 20 (100) | 1 (0) | 1 (0) | 0 (0) |
| Grevena | 98 (150) | 154 (60) | 8 (0) | 62 (165) | 6 (0) | 1 (0) | 0 (0) |
| Rome | 232 (458) | 185 (95) | 362 (107) | 26 (40) | 1 (0) | 0 (0) | 5 (0) |
| Stockholm | 168 (230) | 161 (150) | 368 (190) | 109 (310) | 3 (0) | 20 (0) | 0 (0) |
| Valencia | 178 (191) | 110 (96) | 61 (44) | 291 (270) | 0 (0) | 0 (0) | 0 (0) |
| Vilnius | 121 (200) | 146 (200) | 5 (0) | 92 (200) | 0 (0) | 6 (0) | 4 (0) |
| FIA networks | 639 (1500) | 297 (0) | 427 (0) | 151 (0) | 21 (0) | 19 (0) | 57 (0) |
| Total | 1693 | 1652 | 1616 | 874 | 32 | 82 | 71 |

Note: The ones in brackets are the target numbers that were stated on the survey plan. The Game app tool recorded neither the respondents' travel mode nor any tier 2 questions. Thus, the responses that were collected via the Game app are not included in this Table. On the other hand, sbNavi™ allowed the respondent to record more than one trip leg, thus, if he/she did that, the respondent may have had their trip record with more than one travel modes

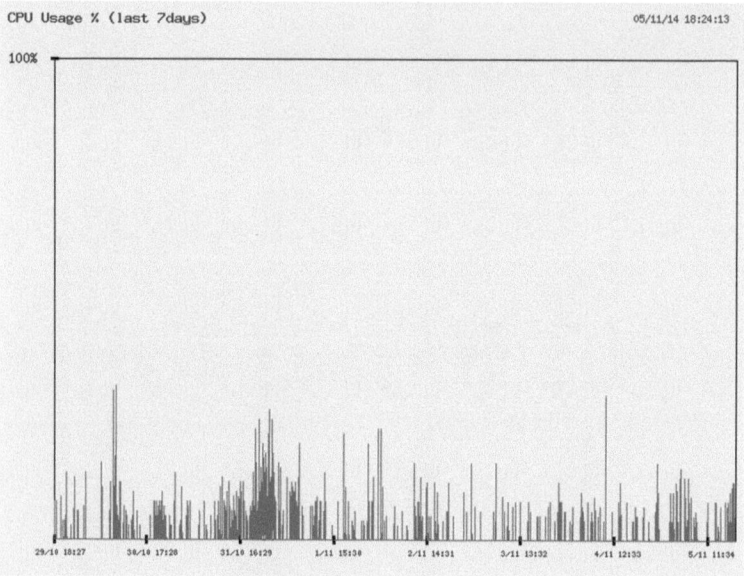

**Fig. 7.4** The backend server utilization during the survey period

the local Internet connection of the client, it is something that needs further analysis in future versions of the tools. Performance statistics from the backend server show that it only had 5% cpu utilization and 5.5 ms ping time to Google, throughout the trial period (see Fig. 7.4). To avoid this problem in the future, perhaps a lighter app and shorter questionnaire pages, that requires much lower Internet data transmission from the client may actually work better and have a higher acceptance among potential respondents, especially if we deployed the tool in a country where has a rather limited/slow access of internet.

From time to time, the communication between the game app and the server was also disrupted. This was noticed by the Valencia and Stockholm teams when some of their registered respondents' responses could not be found at the backend database.

Another concern was the quality of the language used. Despite several rounds of language checking and improvements, there were still some confusing terms and/or not-reader-friendly jargon found on the questionnaire. However, fortunately, this problem was relatively quick and easy to fix during the survey period since all tools were connected to a well-established and robust common questions generator system.

Based on the feedback from the trials, there were also a set of questions that was not really relevant to or they were misplaced in a given socio-demographic and travel mode combination group. For those questions, the respondents were still required to choose 'N/A' for the entire section (e.g., in the set of questions that was aimed for pedestrians there were still questions related to public transport quality, etc.). Such cases should be avoided in the next versions of the tools. As reported by teams from Bucharest, Grevena, Coventry and Stockholm, the questions which seemed irrelevant (and prompted for an 'N/A' answer) have deterred the respondents to complete the remaining questionnaire.

Furthermore, the trial feedback also highlighted several ways in which participation rates and the experience of the respondents could be improved. This included providing an incentive and/or a token to appreciate the respondents' efforts to complete the questionnaire. The Coventry team highlighted the effectiveness of attracting potential respondents with free coffee and an iPad lottery. The same evidence was also found in Stockholm, where the team was providing cinema tickets (worth about 10–15 Euro) for every completed response.

To support and urge potential respondents to participate in the app surveys, the Stockholm team also provided step-by-step input guidance in the local language and snapshots of the screen. As an addition to this, a full-time dedicated staff member was provided to answer any enquiries and complaints by the respondents, for the entire day, during the trial period.

Finally, extra time to plan the survey and to collect the data would have been very helpful and would have most likely enabled partners to achieve better survey throughputs. The survey campaign planning and its implementation was strongly dependent on the development of the tools. The current trial period started late due to the delayed delivery of the tools. Even when the trial period was opened, not all tools were ready to be deployed. Among those that were deployed, some still had bugs which needed to be fixed immediately. These events created difficulties among trial coordinators in planning their campaigns and have hindered the achievement of their campaign objectives. On the other hand, there will always be some bugs that cannot be detected before being tested widely by survey coordinators and users.

## 7.5   Reflection and Conclusion

Overall, although there was a consistent agreement among respondents and surveyors that the tools were attractive, the questionnaire was found to be too long and complicated. It is also apparent from the survey feedback that – despite a surge in technology adoption and smartphone penetration in Europe in the last few years – the acceptance of a smartphone app as a survey tool is still very low. There were also significant privacy and data protection concerns among potential respondents in terms of installing an unknown app.

The general summary of the common problems found and the potential solutions and improvements that will be followed up in other tasks can be seen in Table 7.3.

**Table 7.3** Common reported problems in using the sbNavi™ app in measuring travel satisfaction and plausible solutions to improve it

| Most common problems found | Plausible solutions |
|---|---|
| Irrelevant/misplaced questions (very often requires respondents to fill 'N/A') | Recheck the (Excel) macro generating the questions' assignment and revisit the set of questions that seem irrelevant |
| Slow internet connection | Make the download and upload size smaller, e.g. reduce the length of the questionnaire page and make the app size lighter |
| Typos and the use of unclear jargons | Recheck the wording of the questions again |
| Confusion about using the app | Provide training, user support and a user-friendly manual in the local language |
| | From the tool designer's point of view, making it more user-friendly would significantly increase the appeal of the tools |
| Too long and too complicated questionnaires | Try to reduce the number of questions |
| Lack of interest and participations among relevant respondents and stakeholders | Provide incentives and make the questionnaire look more attractive and less complicated |

It also was learned during the study period that once app is designed and deployed as a survey tool, it became not just a survey tool; but, it will be seen as a product. Delivering the survey tool as a complete useful product (for the users) would increase the project significantly since we would need a multidisciplinary team to design, cleaning bugs, developed support systems and communicating with always-connected users. Furthermore, as launching a product through somebody else's platform (e.g. Google Play or iTunes store), we need to understand the various platforms better and understand the requirements and limitations of them. That said, once we are able to establish a system and a methodology keep the users engaged, this methodology will not only allow us to collect a very informative cross-section observation, but multi-day observations that will open us a new perspective of understanding of how people behave and appreciate the public transport services over different time-frames and spatial distributions.

Despite the above, crowdsourcing seems to be a very powerful and scalable new means of conducting survey campaigns. Smartphone apps in particular, with satellite navigation functionality and gamification and incentivation principles can furthermore be very useful tools for location-based and transport related survey campaigns, in general.

**Acknowledgement** The trials of these tools were funded by the METPEX (MEasurement Tool to determine the quality of the Passenger EXperience) project (www.metpex.eu), which was funded by the European Union's Seventh Framework Programme for Research, Technological Development and Demonstration under grant agreement no. 314354.

# References

Anderson, T, Abeywardana, V, Wolf, J், & Lee, M. (2009). *National travel survey–GPS feasibility study: Final report*. National Centre for Social Research, UK.

Chung, E., & Shalaby, A. (2005). A trip reconstruction tool for GPS-based personal travel surveys. *Transportation Planning and Technology, 28*(5), 371–401.

Cottrill, C.D., Pereira, F.C., Zhao, F., Dias, I.F., Lim, H.B., Ben-Akiva, M.E., et al. (2013). The future mobility survey: Experiences in developing a smartphone based travel survey in Singapore, in Annual Meeting of the Transportation Research Board, Washington, DC.

Diana, M. (2008). Making the "primary utility of travel" concept operational: A measurement model for the assessment of the intrinsic utility of reported trips. *Transportation Research Part A, 42*, 455–474.

Ettema, D. F., Friman, M., Gärling, T., Olsson, L. E., & Fujii, S. (2012). How in-vehicle activities affect work commuters' satisfaction with public transport. *Journal of Transport Geography, 24*, 215–222.

Feng, T., & Timmermans, H. J. P. (2013). Transportation mode recognition using GPS and accelerometer data. *Transportation Research Part C, 37*, 118–130.

Friman, M., & Gärling, T. (2001). Frequency of negative critical incidents and satisfaction with public transport services. II. *Journal of Retailing and Consumer Services, 8*, 105–114.

Friman, M., Fujii, S., Ettema, D., Gärling, T., & Olsson, L. E. (2013). Psychometric analysis of the satisfaction with travel scale. *Transportation Research Part A, 48*, 132–145.

Gong, H., & Chen, C. (2012). *Automating web collection and validation of GPS data for longitudinal urban travel studies: Final report*. US DOT – Research and Innovative Technology Administration.

METPEX. (2014). Report on survey and data collection processes at each location (Deliverable 4.1 of the METPEX project), EU Commissions.

NCHRP. (2014). Applying GPS data to understand travel behaviour: Background, methods and tests, Report 775, Transportation Research Board.

Páez, A., & Whalen, K. (2010). Enjoyment of commute: A comparison of different modes. *Transportation Research: Part A, 44*, 537–549.

Passenger Focus. (2011). *National passenger survey: Autumn 2010 main report*. London: Passenger Focus.

Pedersen, T., Friman, M., & Kristensson, P. (2011). The role of predicted, on-line experienced and remembered satisfaction in current choice to use public transport services. *Journal of Retailing and Consumer Services, 18*, 471–475.

Rasouli, S., & Timmermans, H. J. P. (2014). *Mobile technologies for activity-travel data collection and analysis*. New York: IGI.

SKT – Swedish Public Transport Association. (2016). Annual public transport barometer for 2016 (in Swedish).

Stradling, S., Anable, J., & Carreno, M. (2007). Performance, importance and user disgruntlement: A six-step method for measuring satisfaction with travel modes. *Transportation Research Part A, 41*, 98–106.

Susilo, Y. O., & Cats, O. (2014). Exploring key determinants of travel satisfaction for multi-modal trips by different travellers' groups. *Transportation Research A, 67*, 366–380.

Susilo, Y. O., Lyons, G., Jain, J., & Atkins, S. (2012). Great Britain rail passengers' time use and journey satisfaction: 2010 findings with multivariate analysis. *Transportation Research Record, 2323*, 99–109.

Susilo, Y. O., Cats, O., Diana, M., Hrin, G. R., & Woodcock, A. (2015). Implementing a behavioural pilot survey for the stage-based study of the whole journey traveller experience. *Transportation Research Procedia, 11*, 172–184. https://doi.org/10.1016/j.trpro.2015.12.015.

Susilo, Y. O., Prelipcean, A. C., Gidófalvi, G., Allström, A., Kristoffersson, I., Widell, J. (2016). *Lessons from a trial of MEILI, a smartphone based semi-automatic activity-travel diary collector, in Stockholm city, Sweden.* World Conference on Transport Research 2016, Shanghai. China.

Susilo, Y. O., Abenoza, R. F., Woodcock, A., Liotopoulos, F., Duarte, A., Osmond, J., Georgiadis, A., Hrin, G. R., Bellver, P., Fornari, F., Tolio, V., O'Connell, E., Markucevičiūtė, I., & Diana, M. (2017a). Findings from measuring door-to-door travellers' travel satisfaction with traditional and smartphone app survey methods in eight European cities. *The European Journal of Transport and Infrastructure Research, Issue, 17*(3), 384–410. ISSN: 1567-7141.

Susilo, Y. O., Woodcock, A., Liotopoulos, F., Duarte, A., Osmond, J., Abenoza, R. F., Anghel, L. E., Herrero, D., Fornari, F., Tolio, V., O'Connell, E., Markucevičiūtė, I., Kritharioti, C., & Pirra, M. (2017b). Deploying traditional and smartphone app survey methods in measuring door-to-door travel satisfaction in eight European cities. *Transportation Research Procedia, 25,* 2262–2280.

Tovey, M., Woodcock, A., & Osmond, J. (2017). *Designing mobility and transport services: developing traveller experience tools.* Oxon: Routledge.

# Chapter 8
# Satisfaction with Leisure Trips: Findings from Ghent, Belgium

Jonas De Vos

**Abstract** Recently, studies have started analysing how people perceive their travel and how satisfied they are with it. This travel satisfaction – i.e., the mood during trips and the evaluation of these trips – can be affected by trip characteristics, such as the used travel mode and trip duration. In this study – analysing leisure trips of 1720 respondents living in the city of Ghent (Belgium) – we do not only look at the effect of trip characteristics on travel satisfaction, but also on the effects of travel-related attitudes and the residential location on travel satisfaction, both singly and each controlling for the other. The latter makes it possible to analyse whether people who live in their preferred neighbourhood based on travel preferences (e.g., car lovers living in suburban-type of neighbourhoods) are more satisfied than people who do not. Furthermore, this chapter also explores possible outcomes of travel satisfaction. It is possible that satisfying trips with a certain travel mode increase the chance of choosing that mode for future trips of the same kind, whether or not indirect through changes in attitudes. Repetitive positively or negatively perceived trips might also affect longer-term well-being, such as life satisfaction, both directly and indirectly through the performance of – and satisfaction with – activities at the destination of the trip. On the other hand, life satisfaction can also influence people's satisfaction with short-term activity episodes, such as satisfaction with leisure trips and activities.

**Keywords** Travel behaviour · Travel satisfaction · Attitudes · Well-being · Residential location

## 8.1 Introduction

Over the past decades there has been an increased attention towards subjective well-being across multiple disciplines. Although travel occupies a considerable share of our daily time budget and enables out-of-home activity participation, the

J. De Vos (✉)
Geography Department, Ghent University, Ghent, Belgium
e-mail: jonas.devos@ugent.be

© Springer International Publishing AG, part of Springer Nature 2018
M. Friman et al. (eds.), *Quality of Life and Daily Travel*, Applying Quality of Life
Research, https://doi.org/10.1007/978-3-319-76623-2_8

effect of travel on well-being has only been examined recently. Since approximately 2010, studies have started analysing how people perceive their trips, mostly focussing on the effect of trip characteristics (e.g., trip duration, travel mode) on trip satisfaction. Most of these studies found that long trip duration and public transport use are related with low levels of travel satisfaction, while short trips and active travel mostly result in high travel satisfaction (e.g., Mao et al. 2016; Morris and Guerra 2015a, b; Legrain et al. 2015; Olsson et al. 2013; Páez and Whalen 2010; St-Louis et al. 2014; Ye and Titheridge 2017). Although valuable insights have been gathered from these studies, the effects of the built environment and internal factors (such as travel-related preferences and attitudes) on trip satisfaction remain underexplored. Furthermore, most studies regard trip satisfaction as an outcome of certain travel-related choices and trip characteristics. However, satisfaction with travel could affect attitudes towards the used travel mode and could therefore affect future mode choices. Additionally, trip satisfaction might also affect the performance of − and satisfaction with − the activity at the destination of the trip. As a result, experiencing frequent positive emotions during travel and positively evaluating trips may not only affect long-term well-being − such as life satisfaction − directly, but also indirectly, through the experience of the activity at the destination (Bergstad et al. 2011; De Vos et al. 2013; Ettema et al. 2010). However, besides these bottom-up effects from short-term satisfaction (with travel and activities enabled by travel) to long-term life satisfaction, life satisfaction might also affect satisfaction with short-term activity episodes. A person who is satisfied with his/her life, might also be more satisfied with travel, compared to a person with low levels of life satisfaction. At present, however, our insights in the link between travel and well-being remain limited. We consequently raise three research questions which can help to fill the gaps in existing literature concerning travel satisfaction:

RQ1: What affects travel satisfaction?
RQ2: What are the possible outcomes of travel satisfaction?
RQ3: How is travel satisfaction related with long-term well-being?

This chapter will try to provide answers on the above mentioned research questions based on an Internet survey with 1720 respondents from the city of Ghent, Belgium. This survey contains information regarding respondents' satisfaction with the most recent leisure activity, satisfaction with the trip towards this activity and satisfaction with life in general. This chapter is organised as follows. Section 8.2 describes neighbourhood selection and sample recruitment. Section 8.3 explains the key variables used in this research. The main results are described in Sect. 8.4, while the discussion and conclusion are provided in Sect. 8.5.

## 8.2 Neighbourhood Selection and Sample Recruitment

In this study we use data from a 2012 Internet survey on residential location (choice), travel behaviour, travel satisfaction and well-being, which took place in the city of Ghent, Belgium (250,000 inhabitants). We stratified Ghent's total population based on residential neighbourhood in order to examine differences in travel behaviour and travel satisfaction between people living in urban neighbourhoods and those living in suburban neighbourhoods. In total 27,780 invitations with a link to the survey were distributed by hand in two internally homogeneous sets of five urban and seven suburban neighbourhoods within the city of Ghent. The five urban neighbourhoods, built before the Second World War, have a high density (average density: 7900 inhabitants per km$^2$), a high diversity, extensive public transport services and a design stimulating active travel. The seven suburban neighbourhoods, mainly built after the Second World War, are characterised by low densities (average density: 1700 inhabitants per km$^2$), low diversities, a street configuration stimulating car use (e.g., T-intersections and dead-end streets) and limited public transport services (Fig. 8.1). All households within the selected neighbourhoods received an invitation, covering about one fourth of all households in Ghent (see De Vos et al. 2016).

In socio-demographic terms, the urban neighbourhoods are characterised by lower household car possession, smaller household sizes and lower median incomes, compared to suburban neighbourhoods. Urban neighbourhoods are also inhabited by a relatively high share of citizens from outside the EU-15 area (9.5%), while this is not the case in suburban neighbourhoods (non-EU-15 citizens only account for 1.6%). Urban residents are in general younger than suburban residents, although age distributions can vary between the different urban and suburban neighbourhoods. While there are small variations within urban versus suburban neighbourhoods, physical characteristics of the neighbourhood and socio-demographics of the residents differ more considerably between urban versus suburban neighbourhoods (Table 8.1, see also City of Ghent 2012; De Vos et al. 2016).

The cover letter asked for an adult household member who participated in the residential location choice to complete the survey. Eventually, 1807 persons completed the survey, of which 1720 were retained after data cleaning. Table 8.1 indicates that urban and suburban respondents are approximately representative of the total population of the chosen urban and suburban neighbourhoods. The age distribution of urban and suburban respondents is comparable with the age distribution of the total population of the chosen neighbourhoods; on average, urban respondents are younger than suburban respondents. Similar to the total population of the neighbourhoods, the size, income and car ownership of households in our sample is considerably higher in suburban neighbourhoods than in urban neighbourhoods. Furthermore, in comparison with suburban respondents, more

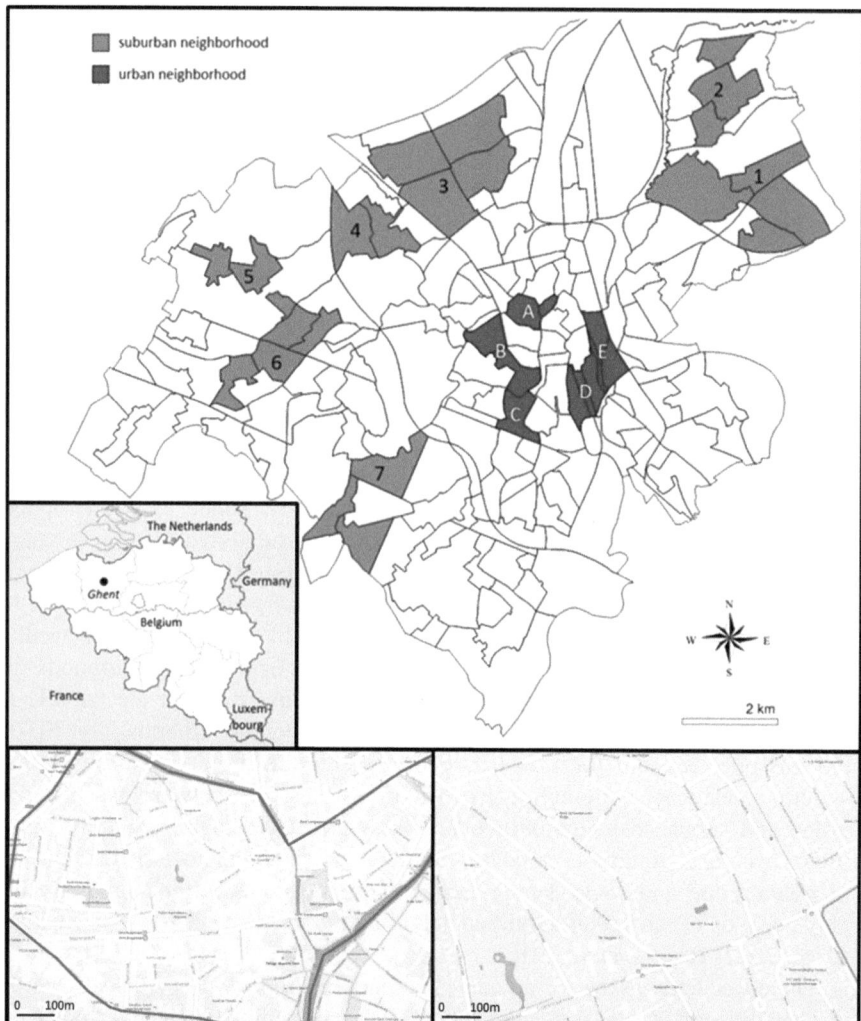

**Fig. 8.1** Distribution of neighbourhoods in Ghent Region (Suburban neighbourhoods: (1) Oostakker; (2) Oostakker-centre; (3) Mariakerke/Wondelgem; (4) Mariakerke-centre; (5) Drongen Luchteren/Campagne; (6) Drongen-centre; (7) Sint-Denijs-Westrem. Urban neighbourhoods: A: Patershol/Begijnhofdries; B: Ekkergem/Bijloke; C: Station; D: Zuid; E: Heernis/Sint-Macharius.) and street network of an urban (left) and suburban (right) neighbourhood (neighb. Patershol/Begijnhofdries (boundary indicated by *red line*) and neighb. Mariakerke/Wondelgem, respectively) (Source: City of Ghent 2012; Google maps)

women and highly educated people in our sample live in urban neighbourhoods (Table 8.1). Although the recruitment method results in a rather low response rate (i.e., 6.5%; which is comparable with other travel behaviour studies using the same

**Table 8.1** Socio-demographic statistics for urban and suburban participants (for more information, see De Vos et al. 2015, 2016)

| | Urban | | Suburban | | Total |
|---|---|---|---|---|---|
| | Sample | Population | Sample | Population | sample |
| Age (distribution) | | | | | |
| 18–34 (%) | 43.5 | 41.3 | 20.4 | 22.2 | 33.7 |
| 35–49 (%) | 23.2 | 22.7 | 27.3 | 26.2 | 24.9 |
| 50–64 (%) | 19.6 | 17.9 | 31.5 | 26.8 | 24.7 |
| 65 + (%) | 13.7 | 18.1 | 20.7 | 24.8 | 16.7 |
| Gender | | | | | |
| Female (%) | 48.8 | 49.5 | 41.4 | 51.0 | 45.7 |
| Education | | | | | |
| High educ. (university degree) (%) | 82.1 | N/A | 70.8 | N/A | 77.3 |
| Household composition | | | | | |
| Average household size | 2.0 | 1.8 | 2.7 | 2.5 | 2.3 |
| Household net income/month | | | | | |
| Low income (<1750 euro) (%) | 24.1 | N/A | 9.9 | N/A | 17.9 |
| Avg. income (1750–3499 euro) (%) | 49.3 | N/A | 49.4 | N/A | 49.4 |
| High income (3500+ euro) (%) | 26.5 | N/A | 40.7 | N/A | 32.7 |
| Household car possession | | | | | |
| 0 (%) | 32.4 | 35.9 | 7.7 | 9.7 | 21.9 |
| 1 (%) | 54.4 | 52.5 | 50.3 | 55.5 | 52.6 |
| >1 (%) | 13.2 | 11.6 | 42.3 | 34.8 | 25.5 |
| N | 991 | 23,279[a] | 729 | 23,440[a] | 1720 |
| % | 57.6 | 49.8 | 42.4 | 50.2 | 100 |

[a]Only adult inhabitants were taken into account

sampling method (e.g., Ben-Elia et al. 2014; Cao 2012)), the respondents are roughly comparable to the population of the selected neighbourhoods in socio-economic and demographic terms. Since the main goal of this study is to achieve an analytical representation of relationships among multiple variables, it is important to have a large and sufficiently diverse sample (Groves 1989). As our sample size is relatively large, this allows us to estimate relationships with ample confidence. The collected data for this study is cross-sectional. Although the used data provides us with a large amount of information, it does not capture possible changes over time in respondents' behaviour, attitudes and satisfaction concerning travel.

## 8.3   Key Variables

### 8.3.1   Satisfaction with the Trip to the Most Recent Leisure Activity

The survey asked respondents how they experienced the trip to their most recent out-of-home leisure activity. In order to measure people's travel satisfaction we used the Satisfaction with Travel Scale (STS) (De Vos et al. 2015; Ettema et al. 2011; Friman et al. 2013). This scale measures travellers' mood (i.e., experienced emotions) during a trip and travellers' evaluation of this trip. The affective emotions are measured by six items based on two dimensions, i.e., valence (ranging from unpleasant to pleasant) and activation (ranging from deactivation to activation), which are assessed by the Swedish Core Affect Scale (SCAS) (Västfjäll et al. 2002; Västfjäll and Gärling 2007). The endpoints of each item are combinations of the valence and activation dimensions. Three items range from negative activation to positive deactivation (i.e., stressed – calm; worried – confident; hurried – relaxed) and the other three from negative deactivation to positive activation (i.e., bored – enthusiastic; tired – alert; fed up – engaged). A cognitive evaluation of the trip being made is measured by three additional items that refer to the general quality and efficiency of the trip (i.e., *the trip was the worst – best I can think of; the trip was low – high standard; the trip did not go well – went well*). For all the nine scales, scores vary from −3 to 3 with a higher score implying higher satisfaction.

Since the internal consistency (i.e., the average correlation of a scale's items) of the six items measuring emotions during the trip and the three items measuring the cognitive evaluation of the trip are assessed as good (Cronbach's alpha is respectively 0.87 and 0.86), we created a positive emotions variable by averaging the scores of the six items measuring affective emotions and a positive evaluation variable by averaging the scores of the three items measuring cognitive evaluation.

### 8.3.2   Satisfaction with the Most Recent Leisure Activity

In order to measure how satisfied respondents were with their most recent out-of-home leisure activity (visiting family/friends; going out to restaurant, bar, club; going to forest, park, nature; participating in sports or cultural activity; recreational shopping) we used a similar scale as the STS, but applied on the activity instead of on the trip (see De Vos 2018). This Satisfaction with Activity Scale (SAS) therefore also contains six items analysing the experienced emotions during the (leisure) activity, ranging from negative to positive with varying levels of activation (i.e., stressed – calm; worried – confident; hurried – relaxed; bored – enthusiastic; tired – alert; fed up – engaged). A cognitive evaluation of the leisure activity made is measured by three additional items that refer to the general quality of the activity (i.e., *the activity was the worst – best I can think of; the activity was low – high standard; the activity did not go well – went well*). In analogy with the STS, the scores of the SAS vary from −3 to 3 with a higher score implying higher satisfaction.

Parallel to the STS, we separated the affective component of activity satisfaction (i.e., emotions during the leisure activity) from the cognitive component of activity satisfaction (i.e., evaluation of the leisure activity). Since the internal consistency of the six items measuring emotions during the activity and the three items measuring the cognitive evaluation of the activity are good (Cronbach's alpha is 0.82 and 0.79, respectively), we created a positive emotions variable by averaging the scores of the six items measuring affective emotions and a positive evaluation variable by averaging the scores of the three items measuring cognitive evaluation.

### 8.3.3 Life Satisfaction

Life satisfaction – a cognitive evaluation of how good one's life is over a longer period of time – has been measured using the Satisfaction With Life Scale (SWLS) (Diener et al. 1985; Pavot and Diener 1993). This scale asks respondents – on a five-point scale going from 1 (strongly disagree) to 5 (strongly agree) – to which extent they agree with five statements: i.e., *In most ways my life is close to my ideal; The conditions of my life are excellent; I am satisfied with my life; So far I have gotten the important things I want in life; If I could live my life over, I would change almost nothing.* Since the internal consistency (reliability) of this scale is high (Cronbach's Alpha = 0.88), one life satisfaction variable was created by averaging the scores on the five items.

### 8.3.4 Travel-Related Attitudes

In this study we make a distinction between mode-specfic attitudes and travel-liking attitudes. In order to measure respondents' attitudes and preferences towards different travel modes three types of variables were used. First, respondents were asked to which degree they like to travel with different travel modes (car; bus or tram; train; bicycle; on foot) on a five-point Likert scale. Second, the survey asked respondents which of the following 12 positive aspects they linked with the use of the five travel modes (yes/no): good for image; environmentally friendly; relaxing; comfortable; time saving; flexible; cheap; offering privacy; healthy; safe; reliable; possibility to perform activities during travel. For each travel mode we added up the number of positive aspects respondents indicated. Finally, ten questions asked respondents to indicate (on a scale from 1 to 10) what their ideal neighbourhood looks like, from a travel-related perspective (e.g., a neighbourhood with good car accessibility, a neighbourhood with good public transport facilities). Based on factor analyses we created factors which represent attitudes towards specific travel modes (for more information regarding these factor analyses, see De Vos et al. 2016, 2018).

Besides mode-specific attitudes, we also analysed travel-liking attitudes. In order to measure people's liking for travel – independent from elements such as mode choice and the type of trip – respondents were asked to indicate to which extent they agree with the following six statements on a scale from one (totally disagree) to five (totally agree): *I like to discover new and unfamiliar places; Reaching my destination is the only good thing about travel; Traffic makes me nervous; I like to travel; Travelling is boring; Travel time is wasted time.* After reversing the scores on the negative statements on travel liking (statement 2, 3, 5 and 6), Cronbach's alpha was measured. Although the value of Cronbach's alpha is satisfactory (i.e., 0.75), the value increases to 0.81 when deleting the first and third statements (i.e., *I like to discover new and unfamiliar places* and *Traffic makes me nervous*). We therefore created a travel-liking variable by averaging the scores on statements 4 and the reverse scores of statements 2, 5 and 6 (for more information, see De Vos and Witlox 2016).

### 8.3.5   Trip Characteristics, Residential Location, Household Car Ownership and Socio-demographics

Respondents were asked to indicate which travel mode (car; train; bus/tram; bicycle or on foot) they used to reach their most recent out-of-home leisure activity. If they used more than one travel mode to reach their destination, they were asked to indicate the travel mode covering the longest distance. Somewhat more than half of the respondents (i.e., 883; 51.8%) travelled by car, 165 respondents (9.6%) used public transport (117 bus/tram users and 48 train users), 337 respondents (19.8%) cycled and 319 (18.7%) respondents walked to their most recent out-of-home leisure activity. Sixteen respondents did not indicate which travel mode they used. The survey also asked for trip distance and trip duration of the most recent leisure trip. Almost half of the trips (48.8%) were shorter than 5 km, while slightly more than half of the trips (53.9%) had a duration of less than 15 min. It has to be noted that trip distance and trip duration are highly affected by respondents' residential location. Trip duration and especially trip distance of suburban residents are significantly higher compared to trip duration and distance of urban residents. Finally, respondents were also asked with whom they travelled (alone, or together with their partner, family, friends or colleagues/acquaintances).

Since survey invitations were distributed in two internally homogeneous sets of typical urban and suburban neighbourhoods in Ghent, we have information on the residential neighbourhood of respondents, i.e., suburban versus urban. Somewhat more than half of the respondents (i.e., 57.6%) live in urban neighbourhoods, while 42.4% of the respondents lives in suburban neighbourhoods.

The survey also asked respondents to indicate the number of cars their household owns. About half of the respondents (52.6%) lives in a household with one car, 21.9% of the respondents lives in a household without a car, while 25.5% of the respondents' households possesses two or more cars. Finally, we also asked for respondents' socio-demographics. Information on the following socio-demographic characteristics was collected: participants' age, gender, educational attainment, job status, the monthly net income of respondents' household, household size and household composition (see Table 8.1).

## 8.4    Results

In order to present the major results of this research, we provide answers to the three research questions separately.

*RQ1: What affects travel satisfaction?*

In this study, we analysed the effect of trip characteristics (i.e., trip duration, trip distance, travel mode and trip companionship), travel-related attitudes (i.e., mode-specific attitudes and travel-liking attitudes), and the residential location on satisfaction with leisure trips.

In line with previous studies (e.g., Mao et al. 2016; Morris and Guerra 2015b; Olsson et al. 2013; Páez and Whalen 2010; St-Louis et al. 2014; Ye and Titheridge 2017), results of our data indicate that people using public transport are least satisfied with their trips and that active travel – especially walking – results in the highest levels of travel satisfaction; intermediate levels are found for car users (De Vos et al. 2015, 2016). Consistent with other studies (e.g., Ettema et al. 2011; Morris and Guerra 2015a; Olsson et al. 2013; St-Louis et al. 2014), trip duration has a negative effect on trip satisfaction, although we only found significant negative effects for car and public transport users (De Vos et al. 2016). Travel time has no significant effect on trip satisfaction of active travellers – a result that has also been found by Mao et al. (2016) – possibly indicating people's enjoyment for walking and cycling itself. For car users we also found positive significant effects of trip distance on trip satisfaction (De Vos et al. 2016). This might be explained by possible confounding between the liking for the trip and the liking for the activity at the destination, together with the fact that out-of-home leisure activities located farther away are mostly performed less common and might therefore being perceived more rewarding. On the other hand, it can also indicate that people like, among other factors, to enjoy scenic beauty and explore new places. Finally, we also found that travelling alone results in significantly lower levels of trip satisfaction compared to when travelling with others. No significant differences were found between travelling with partner, friends, family and colleagues/acquaintances (De Vos 2018). To the best of our knowledge, this is the first study that analyses the effects of trip distance and travel companionship on trip satisfaction.

Although most studies indicate that travel satisfaction is affected by external trip characteristics, such as trip duration, congestion levels and travel mode, it is also possible that travel satisfaction is affected by internal factors such as travel-related preferences and attitudes (St-Louis et al. 2014; Ye and Titheridge 2017). We analysed the effect of both mode-specific attitudes and travel-liking attitudes on trip satisfaction. Mode-specific attitudes have a significant positive effect on trip satisfaction when using that particular mode. Trip satisfaction of car users, for instance, is positively affected by a positive stance towards car use (De Vos et al. 2016). Furthermore, travel-liking attitudes also have a significant impact on trip satisfaction. People with a negative stance towards travelling in general (e.g., people perceiving travel time as wasted time), have significantly lower levels of trip satisfaction compared to people who like – or at least do not dislike – travelling (De Vos and Witlox 2016).

We found higher levels of travel satisfaction for suburban respondents compared to urban respondents, and this for all travel modes. However, when controlling for other variables (such as socio-demographics, attitudes and trip characteristics), residing in an urban neighbourhood only has significant negative effects on trip satisfaction for car and public transport users, possibly due to congestion levels in urban areas. Higher levels of travel satisfaction of suburban respondents can partly be explained by the fact that elements like age, travel distance, household income and driver's license possession are all higher, on average, for suburban residents than for urban residents, and that satisfaction tends to be higher for those with higher values on those variables (De Vos et al. 2016).

Previous studies have indicated that both the residential location and travel-related attitudes have an important effect on travel mode choice. However, these attitudes can also affect mode choice indirectly, through the residential location choice (De Vos et al. 2012; Handy et al. 2005; Schwanen and Mokhtarian 2005). People with a preference for car use, for instance, will probably also have a preference for living in a suburban-style of neighbourhood, which are mostly designed to be well-accessible by car. As a result, it can also be argued that people try to select themselves in neighbourhoods enabling them to have satisfying trips (Cao and Ettema 2014; De Vos and Witlox 2016). However, due to elements such as income, distance to work and varying preferences within households, people might end up residing in a (non-preferred) neighbourhood which does not enable them to travel in a desired way. Consequently, these people might be less satisfied with their performed trips. Results of this study indicate that not living in the desired neighbourhood – based on travel-related attitudes – can reduce travel satisfaction levels. Urban residents with a preference for car use and suburban environments have significantly lower levels of travel satisfaction compared to urbanites with a preference for active travel, public transport and an urban setting. For suburban residents, however, travel satisfaction levels do not significantly differ according to travel-related attitudes and preferences (De Vos et al. 2016).

*RQ2: What are the possible outcomes of travel satisfaction?*

Travel satisfaction is often regarded as the outcome of certain trip characteristics (e.g., trip duration) and travel-related choices (e.g., travel mode choice). However, what is often neglected is that satisfaction with trips might also affect future travel behaviour. To the best of our knowledge, only the effect of travel satisfaction on travel mode choice has been analysed so far. The limited studies that have explored this relationship indicate that the frequency of choosing a certain mode is positively affected by satisfaction with previous trips using that particular mode (Abou-Zeid and Ben-Akiva 2012; Beirão and Cabral 2007; Reibstein et al. 1980). This is in line with studies from Kahneman et al. (1997) and Kahneman and Krueger (2006), indicating that a retrospective evaluation of a past episode can affect the prospective choice of an alternative in order to maximise happiness. Although not analysed before, it is also plausible that travel satisfaction influences travel-related attitudes. Satisfying trips with a certain mode might result in a more positive stance towards that specific mode. In this study we analysed a cyclical process between travel mode choice, travel satisfaction and travel-related attitudes using a structural equation modelling approach. Results of this study, focussing on walking and cycling, indicate that the cognitive evaluation of walking and cycling trips – itself being highly affected by the experienced emotions during the trip – has a positive effect on the attitudes towards the respective mode. In turn, these attitudes have a positive effect on choosing to walk or cycle, respectively (De Vos et al. 2018). If this process repeats itself multiple times, positive reinforcement might generate scripted choice and habitual mode use.

Although not emperically analysed, it is also possible that travel satisfaction affects the residential location (choice). People who are not satisfied with their daily travel might also not be satisfied with their residential location as their residential neighbourhood – setting the parameters within which many travel choices are made for a considerable amount of time – might force them to travel in an undesired way. Car travel in urban areas might be hampered by congestion, car-free zones and limited parking space, while people living in suburban or rural areas might have to travel longer distances than desired, possibly with an undesired mode (i.e., the car). Therefore, low satisfaction with daily travel might result in low residential satisfaction and an increased intention to change the residential location in favour of a neighbourhood enabling people to travel in a desired way (De Vos and Witlox 2017).

*RQ3: How is travel satisfaction related with long-term well-being?*

Travel satisfaction can be regarded as short-term satisfaction (i.e., in case of a person's mood during trips) or medium-term satisfaction (i.e., in case of overall satisfaction with daily travel), and is related with long-term life satisfaction (De Vos and Witlox 2017). Life satisfaction is directly affected by medium-term domain satisfaction and both directly and indirectly affected – through domain satisfaction – by short-term emotional well-being (i.e., the experience of positive emotions). As a result, travel can have an important impact on life satisfaction. However, besides direct effects of travel satisfaction on life satisfaction, it is also possible that travel influences life satisfaction indirectly. Since participating in out-of-home activities has a clear impact on life satisfaction (Abou-Zeid and Ben-Akiva 2012; Diener

2000; Lyubomirsky et al. 2005), travel has an important indirect effect on satisfaction with life. In case of social exclusion, for instance, where a lack of travel options makes it impossible to engage in rewarding activities, a person's well-being will be negatively affected (e.g., Currie et al. 2009; Lucas 2012). Furthermore, spill-over effects of the (perceived) quality of the trip on the performance and perception of the activity at the destination of the trip are possible (Bergstad et al. 2011; De Vos et al. 2013; Ettema et al. 2010). A stressful trip, for instance, might lower satisfaction with the upcoming activity and can therefore dampen the activity's well-being enhancing effect. On the other hand, travel time can give travellers the opportunity to mentally prepare for the activity ahead, facilitating the performance of that activity (Jain and Lyons 2008; Mokhtarian and Salomon 2001). Besides these bottom-up effects from short-term and medium-term satisfaction on long-term life satisfaction, it is also possible that top-down effects exist in which people with high levels of life satisfaction experience more frequent positive emotions compared to people with lower levels of life satisfaction. As a result, people evaluating their life positively would have a higher probability of being satisfied with their trips, compared to people with a lower life satisfaction.

In order to analyse the relationships between travel and well-being, we used a structural equation modelling approach. In this model, both top-down and bottom-up effects between long-term life satisfaction and short-term satisfaction with the most recent leisure activity and the foregoing trip were analysed, next to the effect of trip satisfaction on satisfaction with the leisure activity at the destination (De Vos 2018). Results indicate that spill-over effects exist from satisfaction with the trip preceding a leisure activity on satisfaction with that activity. The experienced emotions during the leisure activity are strongly affected by the mood during the foregoing trip, while the evaluation of this activity is affected by the evaluation of that trip.[1] Furthermore, results suggest that satisfaction with out-of-home leisure activities has an important effect on life satisfaction, while satisfaction with the trip towards this activity mainly has an indirect effect on life satisfaction, through leisure activity satisfaction. Although significant effects have been found from a positive mood during trips on life satisfaction, the effect of travel on life satisfaction is mainly indirect, by enabling activity participation and by spill-over effects on these activities. This might not come as a big surprise as leisure activities are often performed to satisfy certain needs and maintain or enhance well-being, while travel is mostly a derived demand; in this case to enable participation in leisure activities. Besides effects of satisfaction with short-term activity episodes on longer-term life satisfaction, results also indicate a strong positive effect of life satisfaction on both travel satisfaction and activity satisfaction (De Vos 2018).

---

[1]It has to be noted that our data does not make it possible to analyse how long spill-over effects last. As a result, we do not know, for instance, if a stressful trip towards a leisure activity negatively affects the perception of the rest of the leisure activity or if only the beginning of the activity will be negatively affected.

## 8.5   Discussion and Conclusion

Based on the results found from the 2012 data sample from Ghent, Belgium, it can be argued that travel satisfaction is both influenced by – and in itself affects – multiple travel-related elements. As a result, it is possible that travel satisfaction plays a central role in a continuous cyclical travel process (Fig. 8.2). Travel satisfaction is affected by life satisfaction, the residential location, travel-related attitudes and trip characteristics, while on the other hand it also affects these four elements (De Vos and Witlox 2017).[2] Furthermore, satisfaction with the activity at the destination of the trip – which is related with life satisfaction – is also influenced by travel satisfaction. In this continuous cyclical process, the perception of every trip can slightly affect life satisfaction, residential location preferences, travel attitudes and

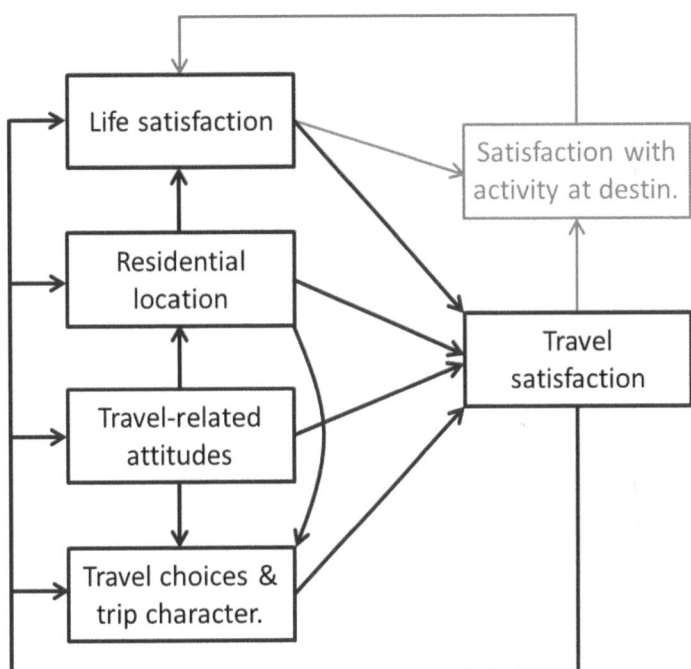

**Fig. 8.2** The central role of travel satisfaction in a travel behaviour process (Based on De Vos and Witlox 2017)

[2]Life satisfaction, residential location, travel-related attitudes and travel choices/outcomes are also related with each other (for more information, see De Vos and Witlox 2017). Travel-related attitudes have an impact on travel choices (e.g., travel mode choice), both direct and indirect through the residential location (choice) (i.e., residential self-selection). Furthermore, it is also possible that the residential location (directly) affects life satisfaction.

(future) travel-related choices/outcomes (e.g., travel mode (choice)), four elements which play a role in the perception of future trips. The process shown in Fig. 8.2 is therefore not an isolated process, but a process repeated every time a trip is made (De Vos and Witlox 2017).

The process described above and shown in Fig. 8.2 may play a crucial role in possible habit formation. Travel-related choices, such as destination choice, route choice and especially travel mode choice, often have a repetitive character. For instance, if people choose the same mode over and over again it is possible that behaviour has become habitual and that people choose the same alternative − that satisfied their needs in previous decision making − without a deliberate decision process (i.e., a decision based on attitudes and intentions) (Aarts et al. 1998; Verplanken et al. 1997). However, always choosing the same travel mode for a certain type of trip may not always be the results of habits, but can be the outcome of repeated decision-making processes. According to Triandis (1977), the relationship between habits and deliberate choice making (based on behavioural intentions) is reciprocal: the stronger the determinant habit is, the weaker the determinant intention is, and vice versa. As a result, the role of attitudes in our proposed process (Fig. 8.2) will depend on how habitual travel decisions are. In case, for instance, travel mode choice is a deliberate choice, attitudes play an important role in the process between attitudes, mode choice, residential location and travel satisfaction. In case mode choice has become habitual, the role of attitudes in this process becomes limited and people will most likely repeat past satisfying behaviour (De Vos and Witlox 2017).

Although the used data and found results from this study have provided valuable insights in the research domain of travel and well-being, we feel that this research can benefit from (i) longitudinal data, (ii) qualitative data, (iii) real-time measures, (iv) data from other regions, (v) a focus on satisfaction with travel in general, and (vi) a focus on other trip purposes. First, using longitudinal data makes it possible to capture changes in people's attitudes, behaviour and satisfaction levels, and can consequently provide new insights in the (possible) formation of travel habits. Furthermore, longitudinal data also improves the identification of causal relationships. Second, qualitative research can help explain findings from quantitative studies. Applying in-depth interviews can tell us, for instance, why public transport users perceive trips so negatively or why the effect of travel time and trip distance is different for varying travel modes, which is rather unfeasible with quantitative data. Third, repetitive real-time measures of people's emotions before, during and after a trip − e.g., a few times during the activity at the destination − might provide researchers with detailed information on how emotions developed during a trip flatten out afterwards. Real-time information − possibly gathered by smartphone surveys (Ettema and Smajic 2015; Friman et al. 2017) − also has the benefit that (potential) memory distortions will be avoided and people will not as much relate or confound trip satisfaction with the liking for the activity at the destination of the trip, as might happen when applying a single retrospective method asking information about travel satisfaction (and activity satisfaction) after the activity episode(s) have taken place. Fourth, although the insights from this study are not only of interest for the city of Ghent (as our rather large data set makes it possible to estimate specific relationships among multiple variables with ample confidence), it might be interesting to conduct a similar study in regions with other mobility cultures, where general attitudes towards certain modes might be different and where certain amenities (e.g., cycling infrastructure) might be lacking. Fifth, analysing satisfaction with daily travel − instead of satisfaction with one specific trip − might result in a stronger and perhaps more realistic link between travel satisfaction and travel behaviour as people's attitudes towards a specific mode, for instance, are formed by the perception of multiple previous trips and not only the most recent one. Finally, focusing on trips and succeeding activities other than leisure might result in different outcomes as they might have different characters. For instance, commute trips and work activities − mostly having a rather mandatory and invariable character − might have different satisfaction levels with trip and activity and different spill-over effects from the commute trip on the work activity.

**Acknowledgements** This research has been funded by the Research Foundation − Flanders (FWO), grant 12F2516N. The author would like to thank dr. Tim Schwanen, prof. Patricia L. Mokhtarian, dr. Veronique Van Acker and prof. Frank Witlox for their supervising role in the author's doctoral research (De Vos 2015), on which this chapter is partly based.

# References

Aarts, H., Verplanken, B., & Van Knippenberg, A. (1998). Predicting behaviour from actions in the past: Repeated decision making or a matter of habit? *Journal of Applied Social Psychology, 28* (15), 1355–1374.

Abou-Zeid, M., & Ben-Akiva, M. (2012). Well-being and activity-based models. *Transportation, 39*(6), 1189–1207.

Beirão, G., & Cabral, J. A. S. (2007). Understanding attitudes towards public transport and private car: A qualitative study. *Transport Policy, 14*(6), 478–489.

Ben-Elia, E., Alexander, B., Hubers, C., & Ettema, D. (2014). Activity fragmentation, ICT and travel: An exploratory path analysis of spatiotemporal interrelationships. *Transportation Research Part A, 68,* 56–74.

Bergstad, C. J., Gamble, A., Gärling, T., Hagman, O., Polk, M., Ettema, D., Friman, M., & Olsson, L. E. (2011). Subjective well-being related to satisfaction with daily travel. *Transportation, 38* (1), 1–15.

Cao, X. (2012). The relationships between e-shopping and store shopping in the shopping process of search goods. *Transportation Research Part A, 46*(7), 993–1002.

Cao, X., & Ettema, D. (2014). Satisfaction with travel and residential self-selection: How do preferences moderate the impact of the Hiawatha Light Rail Transit line? *Journal of Transport and Land Use, 7*(3), 93–108.

City of Ghent. (2012). Buurtmonitor Gent. http://gent.buurtmonitor.be. Last accessed August 2013.

Currie, G., Richardson, T., Smyth, P., Vella-Brodrick, D., Hine, J., Lucas, K., Stanley, J. R., Morris, J., Kinnear, R., & Stanley, J. K. (2009). Investigating links between transport disadvantage, social exclusion and well-being in Melbourne − Preliminary results. *Transport Policy, 16*(3), 97–105.

De Vos, J. (2015). *Travel satisfaction: Analysing the link between travel behaviour, residential location choice and well-being* (Doctoral dissertation). Ghent University, Ghent.

De Vos, J. (2018). Analysing the effect of trip satisfaction on satisfaction with the leisure activity at the destination of the trip, in relationship with life satisfaction. *Transportation*. https://doi.org/10.1007/s11116-017-9812-0.

De Vos, J., & Witlox, F. (2016). Do people live in urban neighbourhoods because they do not like to travel? Analysing an alternative residential self-selection hypothesis. *Travel Behaviour and Society, 4*, 29–39.

De Vos, J., & Witlox, F. (2017). Travel satisfaction revisited. On the pivotal role of travel satisfaction in conceptualising a travel behaviour process. *Transportation Research Part A, 106*, 364–373.

De Vos, J., Derudder, B., Van Acker, V., & Witlox, F. (2012). Reducing car use: changing attitudes or relocating? The influence of residential dissonance on travel behavior. *Journal of Transport Geography, 22*, 1–9.

De Vos, J., Schwanen, T., Van Acker, V., & Witlox, F. (2013). Travel and subjective well-being: A focus on findings, methods and future research needs. *Transport Reviews, 33*(4), 421–442.

De Vos, J., Schwanen, T., Van Acker, V., & Witlox, F. (2015). How satisfying is the scale for travel satisfaction. *Transportation Research Part F, 29*, 121–130.

De Vos, J., Mokhtarian, P. L., Schwanen, T., Van Acker, V., & Witlox, F. (2016). Travel mode choice and travel satisfaction: bridging the gap between decision utility and experienced utility. *Transportation, 43*(5), 771–796.

De Vos, J., Schwanen, T., Van Acker, V., & Witlox, F. (2018). *Do satisfying walking and cycling trips result in more future trips with active travel modes? An exploratory study*. Manuscript submitted for publication.

Diener, E. (2000). Subjective well-being: The science of happiness and a proposal for a national index. *American Psychologist, 55*(1), 34–43.

Diener, E., Emmons, R. A., Larsen, R. J., & Griffen, S. (1985). The satisfaction with life scale. *Journal of Personality Assessment, 49*(1), 71–75.

Ettema, D., & Smajic, I. (2015). Walking, places and wellbeing. *The Geographical Journal, 181*(2), 102–109.

Ettema, D., Gärling, T., Olsson, L. E., & Friman, M. (2010). Out-of-home activities, daily travel, and subjective well-being. *Transportation Research Part A, 44*(9), 723–732.

Ettema, D., Gärling, T., Eriksson, L., Friman, M., Olsson, L. E., & Fujii, S. (2011). Satisfaction with travel and subjective well-being: Development and test of a measurement tool. *Transportation Research Part F, 14*(3), 167–175.

Friman, M., Fujii, S., Ettema, D., Gärling, T., & Olsson, L. E. (2013). Psychometric analysis of the satisfaction with travel scale. *Transportation Research Part A, 48*, 132–145.

Friman, M., Olsson, L. E., Ståhl, M., Ettema, D., & Gärling, T. (2017). Travel and residual emotional well-being. *Transportation Research Part F, 49*, 159–176.

Groves, R. M. (1989). *Survey errors and survey costs*. New York: Wiley.

Handy, S. L., Cao, X., & Mokhtarian, P. L. (2005). Correlation or causality between the built environment and travel behavior? Evidence from Northern California. *Transportation Research Part D, 10*(6), 427–444.

Jain, J., & Lyons, G. (2008). The gift of travel time. *Journal of Transport Geography, 16*, 81–89.

Kahneman, D., & Krueger, A. B. (2006). Developments in the measurement of subjective well-being. *Journal of Economic Perspectives, 20*(1), 3–24.

Kahneman, D., Wakker, P. P., & Sarin, R. (1997). Back to Bentham? Explorations of experienced utility. *Quarterly Journal of Economics, 112*(2), 375–405.

Legrain, A., Eluru, N., & El-Geneidy, A. (2015). Am stressed, must travel: The relationship between mode choice and commuting stress. *Transportation Research Part F, 34*, 141–151.

Lucas, K. (2012). Transport and social exclusion: Where are we now? *Transport Policy, 20*, 105–113.

Lyubomirsky, S., King, L., & Diener, E. (2005). The benefits of frequent positive affect: Does happiness lead to success? *Psychological Bulletin, 131*(6), 803–855.

Mao, Z., Ettema, D., & Dijst, M. (2016). Commuting trip satisfaction in Beijing: Exploring the influence of multimodal behavior and modal flexibility. *Transportation Research Part A, 94*, 592–603.

Mokhtarian, P. L., & Salomon, I. (2001). How derived is the demand for travel? Some conceptual and measurement considerations. *Transportation Research Part A, 35*(8), 695–719.

Morris, E. A., & Guerra, E. (2015a). Are we there yet? Trip duration and mood during travel. *Transportation Research Part F, 33*, 38–47.

Morris, E. A., & Guerra, E. (2015b). Mood and mode: Does how we travel affect how we feel? *Transportation, 42*(1), 25–43.

Olsson, L. E., Gärling, T., Ettema, D., Friman, M., & Fujii, S. (2013). Happiness and satisfaction with work commute. *Social Indicators Research, 111*(1), 255–263.

Páez, A., & Whalen, K. (2010). Enjoyment of commute: A comparison of different transportation modes. *Transportation Research Part A, 44*(7), 537–549.

Pavot, W., & Diener, E. (1993). Review of the satisfaction with life scale. *Psychological Assessment, 5*(2), 164–172.

Reibstein, D. J., Lovelock, C. H., & Dobson, R. P. (1980). The direction of causality between perceptions, affect, and behavior: An application to travel behavior. *Journal of Consumer Research, 6*(4), 370–376.

Schwanen, T., & Mokhtarian, P. L. (2005). What affects commute mode choice, neighbourhood physical structure or preferences toward neighborhoods? *Journal of Transport Geography, 13*(1), 83–99.

St-Louis, E., Manaugh, K., Van Lierop, D., & El-Geneidy, A. (2014). The happy commuter: A comparison of commuter satisfaction across modes. *Transportation Research Part F, 26*, 160–170.

Triandis, H. C. (1977). *Interpersonal behaviour*. Monterey: Brooks/Cole.

Västfjäll, D., & Gärling, T. (2007). Validation of a Swedish short self-report measure. *Scandinavian Journal of Psychology, 48*(3), 233–238.

Västfjäll, D., Friman, M., Gärling, T., & Kleiner, M. (2002). The measurement of core affect: A Swedish selfreport measure. *Scandinavian Journal of Psychology, 43*(1), 19–31.

Verplanken, B., Aarts, H., & Van Knippenberg, A. (1997). Habit, information acquisition, and the process of making travel mode choices. *European Journal of Social Psychology, 27*(5), 539–560.

Ye, R., & Titheridge, H. (2017). Satisfaction with the commute: The role of travel mode choice, built environment and attitudes. *Transportation Research Part D, 52B*, 535–547.

# Chapter 9
# Examining the Relationship Between Commuting and it's Impact on Overall Life Satisfaction

**Lesley Fordham, Dea van Lierop, and Ahmed El-Geneidy**

**Abstract** Commuting to work and school can be viewed as an unpleasant and necessary task. However, some people enjoy their commutes and be satisfied with it. Trip satisfaction can have a positive impact on overall life satisfaction of individual. The purpose of this study is to analyze the relationship between individuals' satisfaction with their commuting trips and its impact on overall life satisfaction. This study is based on the results of the 2015/2016 McGill Commuter Survey, a university-wide travel survey in which students, staff and faculty described their commuting experiences to McGill University, located in Montreal, Canada. Using a Factor-Cluster analysis, the study reveals that there is a relationship between trip satisfaction and the impact of commuting on overall life satisfaction. One result of the study shows that cyclists and pedestrians who have the highest overall trip satisfaction, report that their life satisfaction is most impacted by their commute, and have the highest overall life satisfaction. Also, for all mode users, one or two clusters exhibit lower trip satisfaction, report that satisfaction with their commute does not greatly influence their life satisfaction, and claim having access to and using fewer modes relative to other users of the same mode. These results, in addition to the results that active mode users have high life and trip satisfaction, suggest that building well-connected multi-modal networks that incorporate active transportation can improve the travel experience of all commuters and impact their overall life satisfaction.

**Keywords** Trip satisfaction · Life satisfaction · Cycling · Walking · Public transport · Driving

L. Fordham · D. van Lierop · A. El-Geneidy (✉)
McGill University, Montreal, Canada
e-mail: lesley.fordham@mail.mcgill.ca; dea.vanlierop@mail.mcgill.ca; ahmed.elgeneidy@mcgill.ca

© Springer International Publishing AG, part of Springer Nature 2018
M. Friman et al. (eds.), *Quality of Life and Daily Travel*, Applying Quality of Life Research, https://doi.org/10.1007/978-3-319-76623-2_9

## 9.1  Introduction

Individuals' quality of life (QOL) and subjective well-being (SWB) are influenced by many factors. One of these factors is an individual's commuting experience, which is often perceived as both unpleasant and fatiguing, as well as a mandatory part of life (Mokhtarian et al. 2015; Ory and Mokhtarian 2009). However, not all commuters perceive their daily trips to be negative, and many people enjoy their commutes (Manaugh and El-Geneidy 2013). Furthermore, a positive commuting experience can contribute to overall life satisfaction (De Vos and Witlox 2017; Olsson et al. 2013; Ory and Mokhtarian 2005). In other words, commuting can be a favorable experience that positively contributes to an individual's happiness. In contrast to the work commute, travel can be undirected, meaning that instead of being derived by demand, individuals travel for enjoyment (Mokhtarian and Salomon 2001). One reason that satisfaction can result from commuting is due to the ability to engage in multiple activities while traveling, such as working, reading, listening to music or simply gazing out the window (Ettema et al. 2012). Personality and attitude can also influence the enjoyment derived from travel, and individuals who do not enjoy travel will often try to reduce it, in contrast to an individual who enjoys travel (Ory and Mokhtarian 2009). Therefore, not all individuals seek to minimize their travel (Manaugh and El-Geneidy 2013; Mokhtarian and Salomon 2001).

Research on QOL and travel were first integrated in the 1970s by Stokols et al. who examined the relationship between commuting and stress (Stokols et al. 1978). These researchers found that commuters with longer distances and travel times felt more inconvenienced and annoyed, and were less satisfied with their commute. Later, Diener and Suh (1997) defined and measured QOL based on social and economic components, as well as SWB. These authors also found that QOL is shaped by cultural norms and individuals' preferences and experiences. Furthermore, SWB is defined as a reflection of an individual's evaluation of their life in positive terms, which is understood as life satisfaction (Diener 1984; Diener et al. 1985, 1999). Consequently, satisfaction is one of the components of SWB that influences individuals' overall QOL. Therefore, satisfaction with travel is considered a form of stated SWB, and life satisfaction measures inherently rely on an individual's subjective assessment. The impact of SWB on QOL on both individuals and communities (Diener et al. 2003) has led to the argument that SWB should be a key indicator in evaluating planning and policy (Cao and Zhang 2016; Stanley and Stanley 2007). Because commuting is a daily experience for many individuals, it likely contributes to many people's SWB and QOL. The purpose of this study is to analyze the relationship between individuals' satisfaction with their commuting trips and its reported impact on their overall life satisfaction.

## 9.2 Literature Review

Travel can influence the SWB and QOL of individuals (Delbosc 2012). More specifically, commuting can have negative impacts on home life and work, including having a bad mood at home and increased work related stress (Novaco et al. 1991; Wener et al. 2005). Commuters can experience stress during travel, influenced by objective and subjective experiences (Novaco et al. 1990). Increased mobility in urban environments has been associated with higher reported QOL in both young adults (Xiong and Zhang 2016) and the elderly (van den Berg et al. 2016). Establishing the impact that transport can have on SWB has led researchers to further examine satisfaction through trip purpose and mode.

Different aspects of travel influence commuters' perceived satisfaction. For example, trip purpose can have a strong influence on satisfaction, and Bergstad et al. investigated the role of routine activities on life satisfaction. These authors found that positive sentiments were often a result of trips that were for sports, exercise and outdoor activities, and that alternatively, work and school activities were associated with more negative sentiments (Bergstad et al. 2012). The negative affect associated with trips to work has been corroborated by other researchers who have similarly found that trips made for work are the most fatiguing and are viewed as less pleasant compared to taking trips for any other purpose (Mokhtarian et al. 2015). Furthermore, work and school trips are associated with more negative moods and are liked less compared to trips that are for socializing, or sports and leisure (Morris and Hirsch 2016; Ory and Mokhtarian 2005). These results could be due to the fact that commuting is perceived as mandatory and unenjoyable travel in which the commuter has little choice in the decision to travel (Ory and Mokhtarian 2009).

Other factors influencing commuters' enjoyment of travel and commute related stress is the predictability and length of a trip (Olsson et al. 2013; Ory et al. 2004). Commuters that experience a lack of control from delays, congestion and unpredictability during the commute show increased stress (Evans et al. 2002; Gatersleben and Uzzell 2007; Gottholmseder et al. 2009). A less positive mood is associated with driving in larger cities during the peak of peak hours (Morris and Hirsch 2016). Long commuting lengths have been associated with decreased trip satisfaction (Olsson et al. 2013; Ory et al. 2004), lower life satisfaction (Choi et al. 2013; Stutzer and Frey 2008), overall mood (Morris and Guerra 2015), and more stress (Legrain et al. 2015). In contrast, many commuters favor moderate commute times rather than short or long times, or eliminating the commute completely (Ory et al. 2004; Redmond and Mokhtarian 2001). This could be because of the time buffer created between work and home (Jain and Lyons 2008) and the ability to multi-task (Ettema and Verschuren 2007). Additionally, subgroups of commuters have been found to enjoy their school or work related travel (Ory and Mokhtarian 2005) and attitudes about the commute to work can contribute to overall life satisfaction, with positive feelings about the commute leading to positive affect towards life satisfaction (Olsson et al. 2013).

The mode used for travel may also impact travel satisfaction. For example, while Legrain et al. (2015) found that the stress of travelling is strongly associated with the mode of the trip, Morris and Guerra (2015) found that the relationship between mood, including stress, and mode is weak. Perhaps this discrepancy is due to the type of survey data used for analysis. The former used data from a Canadian university survey focused on commuting and the latter used survey data that measured how much time Americans spend on different activities. Studies have also found that those who like the mode they use during a trip are more likely to be satisfied with the trip (Choo et al. 2005), and that people who prefer a certain mode will tend to make choices regarding their home location and self-select to accommodate their travel preferences (Bhat and Guo 2007).

In assessments of mode on travel satisfaction, walking and cycling have been found to elicit more positive emotion than motorized travel (Duarte et al. 2010; Legrain et al. 2015; Mokhtarian et al. 2015; Mokhtarian and Salomon 2001; Olsson et al. 2013). This could be attributed to these active forms of transportation being both relaxing and exciting, as well as a source of physical exercise (Duarte et al. 2010; Gatersleben and Uzzell 2007). The high satisfaction of cyclists has been explored and explained through the convenience of the mode and seasonal variation (Willis et al. 2013). Previous research indicates that bus users are the most unsatisfied mode users (St-Louis et al. 2014). Those who travel by bus may experience low trip satisfaction and a negative impact on mood associated with concerns about safety, crowding, delays, and convenience (Gatersleben and Uzzell 2007; Ory et al. 2004; Stradling et al. 2007). However, taking the bus has the most positive impact on mood when the conditions include short travel times and high access to bus stops (Ettema et al. 2011). Happiness has been found to have a U-shaped or parabolic relationship with access to public transportation. Those with good access and bad access are happy, suggesting that those with poor access are dependent on automobiles (Guo et al. 2016). In terms of automobile use, those that enjoy their automobile trip do so because of a sense of freedom, control, and reliability (Gardner and Abraham 2007; Mann and Abraham 2006), while those who do not enjoy their automobile trip feel that driving is mentally tiring, unpleasant, and stressful (Gatersleben and Uzzell 2007; Legrain et al. 2015; Mokhtarian et al. 2015). It has been suggested, through an analysis of budgeted travel time, that automobile drivers experience more unreliability than pedestrians, cyclists and transit users (Loong and El-Geneidy 2016). Multi-modal trips are more often seen as unpleasant, and mentally and physically tiring, with multi-modal trips involving public transportation being the most fatiguing (Mokhtarian et al. 2015). Though, those who have used multiple modal options feel less stressed (Legrain et al. 2015).

The methods used to measure the relationships between satisfaction and travel include structural equation models (Ory and Mokhtarian 2009), linear regression (Bergstad et al. 2011; Ory and Mokhtarian 2005), satisfaction with life scales (Cao 2016; Diener et al. 1985; Ettema and Schekkerman 2016), as well as through sentiment analysis of social media posts (Guo et al. 2016). Pertinent to the current study, clustering techniques have been used to assess the trip satisfaction of pedestrians (Willis et al. 2013). There are examples of both objective measures (Stanley et al. 2011) and subjective measures (Bergstad et al. 2011) of mobility being used in the study of well-being and transportation. The advantages and disadvantages of using subjective and objective measures of satisfaction in transportation research is discussed by Delbosc, who reminds us that satisfaction can mean different things to different people (Delbosc 2012). Mokhtarian and Salomon also warn of the complexity of measuring affect in transportation studies and state that respondents of self-reported studies often confuse feelings about activities performed at the destination or during travel when reporting their affect for travel (Mokhtarian and Salomon 2001).

Another challenge associated with studying commuting and life satisfaction is the causal direction. Several studies have analyzed how satisfaction with travel influences SWB or QOL. Olsson et al. and Bergstad et al. operate under the assumption that causal direction is from commute satisfaction to overall happiness (Bergstad et al. 2012; Olsson et al. 2013). This assumption is present in other studies that focus on the impact of mobility on perceptions of QOL for the elderly (Banister and Bowling 2004) and study the effect of satisfaction with travel on affective and cognitive SWB (Bergstad et al. 2011). Olsson et al. do acknowledge that the causal direction could go the other way (Olsson et al. 2013) and overall happiness could influence the perception of trip satisfaction. However, Bergstad et al. (2012) assume that the causal direction is from commute satisfaction to overall happiness. They base their assumption on the results of a study by Schimmack (2008) that found a stronger association between the influence of domain satisfaction and life satisfaction compared to the influence of life satisfaction on domain satisfaction. Accordingly, the present study operates under the first assumption that travel impacts SWB and QOL, similarly to the studies by Olsson et al. (2013), Bergstad et al. (2012), and Banister and Bowling (2004). Furthermore, this study adds to the literature that discusses the impact of commuting on overall life satisfaction by exploring the relationship and identifying patterns based on mode used through a factor-cluster analysis. It is not the intention to confirm this causality, but rather to explore the relationship.

## 9.3 Data

McGill University is located in Montreal, Canada, with approximately 40,000 students and 1600 faculty members and staff. The university has two campuses; one is centrally located in downtown Montreal and the other is a much smaller suburban campus. The data for the study are derived from 2015 to 2016 the McGill Commuter Survey, which is an online travel behavior survey that was distributed throughout the 2015/2016 school year to faculty, staff and students. In the fall of 2015 and the winter of 2016, a total of 8383 and 8654 emails were sent to all McGill faculty members and staff, and to one third of the student population. This resulted in a response rate of 35.6%, in which 5094 surveys were fully completed and 974 were partially completed.

The survey captured the commuting habits of faculty, staff and students of McGill, and is therefore focused on utilitarian travel. Respondents were asked questions related to their personal characteristics, including their gender, age, income, home location, and household composition. They were also asked, on a scale of 1–10, to take all things into account and rate their life satisfaction. Other questions were focused on their general commuting habits, including how many years they have been commuting to McGill, how many times a week they commute, how many modes they have access to and which modes they consider reasonable for getting from their home location to McGill. Furthermore, on a five point Likert scale ranging from 'very unsatisfied' to 'very satisfied' respondents were asked, how satisfied they were with their most recent trip overall, and whether their commuting experience has an impact on their life satisfaction. This question operates under the assumption that trip satisfaction influences overall life satisfaction (Banister and Bowling 2004; Bergstad et al. 2011, 2012; Olsson et al. 2013). Several questions about the most recent commute to McGill examined trip characteristics, including length, time of day, and the modes used. Respondents were then asked a series of questions about their main mode. This series of questions targeted both the satisfaction with and the importance of certain components of the trip, including infrastructure, safety, efficiency, service quality, parking facilities and comfort.

In this study, we include only trips to McGill's downtown campus. Responses that did not include the respondents' gender and age were eliminated, as were responses from those under the age of 18 years old. Furthermore, visitors and exchange students were also eliminated because the survey does not indicate the how long these students and visitors were at McGill and their travel behavior may not be indicative of the McGill population as whole. Trips longer than 2 h in length were also eliminated in an attempt to remove commuters living outside of the Greater Montreal Area. Finally, due to small sample sizes, any trips made with the McGill intra-campus shuttle, a motorcycle or scooter, taxi, carpool as a passenger, or "other" were eliminated. This resulted in 3747 trips in which the main modes of transportation were walking, cycling, bus, metro, commuter train or automobile as a driver. The distribution was 841 pedestrians, 293 cyclists, 753 bus users, 1033 metro users, 373 train users and 454 automobile drivers. Although public transit is often looked at as one group, a decision was made to keep bus, metro and commuter train users separate in the hope of creating a more nuanced analysis (St-Louis et al. 2014).

## 9.4   Methodology and Results

### 9.4.1   Factor Analysis

A factor analysis was conducted for each mode to group similar variables together and identify how variables from the survey questions relate to one another. Using the rotated component matrix, several factors were identified for each mode. Variables for each factor were selected based on a factor loading threshold of .5 or above or −.5 or below. These factors, a description of the variables within each factor, and the factor loadings are shown in Tables 9.1, 9.2, and 9.3.

**Table 9.1** Factor analysis for walking and cycling

| Factor | Variable from survey | Walking | Cycling |
|---|---|---|---|
| Satisfaction with safety and quality | Satisfaction with the presence of other pedestrians | 0.53 | |
| | Satisfaction with the quality of sidewalks | 0.60 | |
| | Satisfaction with the safety at intersections | 0.78 | |
| | Satisfaction with the reduced speed of cars | 0.79 | |
| | Satisfaction with the clarity of crosswalks | 0.80 | |
| | Satisfaction with the lighting of sidewalks | 0.83 | |
| Satisfaction with safety and infrastructure | Satisfaction with the quality of bicycle paths | | 0.75 |
| | Satisfaction with the signage for bicycles | | 0.78 |
| | Satisfaction with the reduced speed of cars | | 0.71 |
| | Satisfaction with the lighting of bicycling paths | | 0.67 |
| Importance of safety and quality | Importance of the presence of other pedestrians | 0.60 | |
| | Importance of the quality of sidewalks | 0.65 | |
| | Importance of the safety at intersections | 0.79 | |
| | Importance of the reduced speed of cars | 0.73 | |
| | Importance of the clarity of crosswalks | 0.79 | |
| | Importance of the lighting of sidewalks | 0.65 | |
| Importance of efficiency | Importance of the length of time spent commuting | 0.81 | 0.71 |
| | Importance of the predictability of time spent commuting | 0.77 | 0.78 |
| | Importance of the directness of route | 0.57 | 0.56 |
| Importance of safety and infrastructure | Importance of the quality of bicycle paths | | 0.70 |
| | Importance of the signage for bicycles | | 0.76 |
| | Importance of the reduced speed of cars | | 0.73 |
| | Importance of the lighting of bicycling paths | | 0.74 |
| Satisfaction with parking | Satisfaction with the availability of bicycle parking at destination | | 0.89 |
| | Satisfaction with the quality of bicycle parking at destination | | 0.89 |
| Importance of parking | Importance of the availability of bicycle parking at destination | | 0.87 |
| | Importance of the quality of bicycle parking at destination | | 0.88 |
| Need shower facilities | Importance of the availability of showers and changing facilities at destination | | 0.60 |
| | Willingness to pay for shower facilities (binomial) | | 0.82 |
| | Satisfaction with the availability of showers and changing facilities at destination | | −0.61 |

(continued)

**Table 9.1** (continued)

| Factor | Variable from survey | Walking | Cycling |
|---|---|---|---|
| Seniority at McGill | Status as a member of faculty at McGill (binomial) | 0.76 | 0.65 |
| | Number of years at their current position at McGill (continuous) | 0.82 | 0.80 |
| | Age (continuous) | 0.87 | 0.87 |
| Self-selected not to drive | Importance of the cost of parking when moving to your current residence | −0.72 | −0.56 |
| | Importance of being in a location where I wouldn't have to drive when moving to your home | 0.84 | 0.77 |
| | Importance of being in proximity to public transportation when moving to your home | 0.81 | 0.81 |
| Other modes viable | Driving is a viable option to get to McGill (binomial) | 0.62 | |
| | McGill is within reasonable cycling distance to McGill (binomial) | 0.67 | |
| | Transit is a viable option to get to McGill (binomial) | 0.69 | |
| Short trip and chose to be close to McGill | Importance of being in close proximity to McGill when moving to your home | 0.78 | |
| | Trip length in minutes (continuous) | −0.68 | |
| Short trip where walking is viable and chose to be close to McGill | Trip length in minutes (continuous) | | −0.75 |
| | McGill is within reasonable walking distance to McGill (binomial) | | 0.75 |
| | Importance of being in close proximity to McGill when moving to your home | | 0.57 |
| Multi-modal measure | Number of modes used in the most recent trip (continuous) | 0.72 | 0.85 |
| | Number of modes respondent has access to (continuous) | 0.71 | |
| Frequency of trip | Number of commutes per week (continuous) | 0.69 | 0.79 |
| | Full-time status at McGill (binomial) | 0.75 | 0.78 |
| Variance | | 61% | 67% |

In order to acknowledge heterogeneity in travel behavior between and within modes, a factor analysis was conducted independently for each mode. Therefore, because survey respondents were asked different questions based on their main mode of transportation for the trip, several mode specific factors resulted from the analysis. For some modes, the analysis revealed similar factors. For example, bus users, metro users and train users all revealed an 'Importance with Comfort' and 'Satisfaction with Comfort' factor. Furthermore, a factor called the 'Multi-Modal Measure' was created. With the exception of cyclists, this measure included the number of modes the respondent has access to and the number of modes used to

**Table 9.2** Factor analysis for bus, metro and train

| Factor | Variable from survey | Bus | Metro | Train |
|---|---|---|---|---|
| Satisfaction with service | Satisfaction with the length of time spent on bus/metro | 0.61 | 0.77 | |
| | Satisfaction with the service reliability | 0.86 | 0.79 | |
| | Satisfaction with the consistency (predictability) of time spend on the bus/metro | 0.79 | 0.81 | |
| | Satisfaction with the waiting time for the bus/metro | 0.81 | 0.80 | |
| | Satisfaction with the length of time spent to reach the bus/metro | 0.52 | 0.68 | |
| | Satisfaction with the frequency of service | 0.81 | | |
| Satisfaction with wait time and reliability | Satisfaction with the service reliability | | | 0.80 |
| | Satisfaction with the waiting time for the commuter train | | | 0.78 |
| Importance of service | Importance of the length of time spent on bus/metro/train | 0.69 | 0.81 | 0.80 |
| | Importance of the service reliability | 0.84 | 0.70 | 0.66 |
| | Importance of the consistency (pre-dictability) of time spend on the bus/metro/train | 0.78 | 0.85 | 0.82 |
| | Importance of the length of time spent to reach the bus | 0.63 | 0.73 | 0.69 |
| | Importance of the waiting time for bus | 0.78 | 0.71 | 0.73 |
| | Importance of the frequency of service | 0.79 | | |
| Satisfaction with comfort | Satisfaction with the comfort of seating | 0.76 | 0.79 | 0.86 |
| | Satisfaction with the comfort of standing space | 0.85 | 0.80 | 0.86 |
| | Satisfaction with the comfort of being in proximity to others | 0.84 | 0.75 | 0.89 |
| Importance of comfort | Importance of the comfort of seating on the bus | 0.79 | 0.82 | 0.67 |
| | Importance of the comfort of standing space on the bus | 0.88 | 0.81 | 0.76 |
| | Importance of the comfort of being in proximity to others on the bus | 0.84 | 0.64 | 0.73 |
| Satisfaction and importance of parking at station | Satisfaction with the availability of parking close to commuter train station of origin | | | 0.52 |
| | Satisfaction with the cost of parking close to commuter train station of origin | | | 0.65 |

(continued)

**Table 9.2** (continued)

| Factor | Variable from survey | Bus | Metro | Train |
|---|---|---|---|---|
| | Importance of the availability of parking close to commuter train station of origin | | | 0.79 |
| | Importance of the cost of parking close to commuter train station of origin | | | 0.78 |
| Seniority at McGill | Status as a member of faculty at McGill (binomial) | 0.70 | 0.64 | 0.59 |
| | Number of years at their current position at McGill (continuous) | 0.84 | 0.84 | 0.83 |
| | Age (continuous) | 0.86 | 0.85 | 0.81 |
| Self-selected not to drive | Importance of the cost of parking when moving to your current residence | −0.72 | −0.75 | |
| | Importance of being in a location where I wouldn't have to drive when moving to your home | 0.67 | 0.72 | |
| | Importance of being in proximity to public transportation when moving to your home | 0.86 | 0.85 | |
| Self-selected to be close to McGill and with transit access | Importance of being in proximity to public transportation when moving to your current residence | | | 0.77 |
| | Importance of being in close proximity to McGill when moving to your home | | | 0.77 |
| Short trip where walking and cycling are viable and chose to be close to McGill | Trip length in minutes (continuous) | −0.82 | −0.68 | |
| | McGill is within reasonable walking distance to McGill (binomial) | 0.70 | 0.63 | |
| | McGill is within reasonable cycling distance to McGill (binomial) | 0.76 | 0.67 | |
| | Importance of being in close proximity to McGill when moving to your home | 0.55 | 0.58 | |
| Short trip where walking and cycling are viable | Trip length in minutes (continuous) | | | −0.49 |
| | McGill is within reasonable walking distance to McGill (binomial) | | | 0.72 |
| | McGill is within reasonable cycling distance to McGill (binomial) | | | 0.47 |
| Multi-modal measure | Number of modes used in the most recent trip (continuous) | 0.74 | 0.74 | 0.54 |
| | Number of modes respondent has access to (continuous) | 0.74 | 0.73 | 0.77 |
| Frequency of trip | Number of commutes per week (continuous) | 0.79 | 0.78 | 0.77 |
| | Full-time status at McGill (binomial) | 0.80 | 0.80 | 0.75 |
| Variance | | 66% | 63% | 67% |

**Table 9.3** Factor analysis for driving

| Factor | Variable from survey | Drive |
|---|---|---|
| Satisfaction with parking at destination | Satisfaction with the cost of parking close to destination | 0.67 |
| | Satisfaction with the availability of parking close to destination | 0.89 |
| | Satisfaction with the length of time spent looking for parking | 0.91 |
| | Satisfaction with the consistency (predictability) of time spent looking for parking | 0.91 |
| Importance of parking at destination | Importance of the cost of parking close to destination | 0.79 |
| | Importance of the availability of parking close to destination | 0.89 |
| | Importance of the consistency (predictability) of time spent looking for parking | 0.82 |
| Seniority at McGill | Status as a member of faculty at McGill (binomial) | 0.66 |
| | Number of years at their current position at McGill (continuous) | 0.80 |
| | Age (continuous) | 0.86 |
| Self-celected to be close to McGill and with access to transit and parking | Importance of being in close proximity to McGill when moving to your home | 0.58 |
| | Importance of being in proximity to public transportation when moving to your home | 0.75 |
| | Importance of the cost of parking when moving to your home | 0.79 |
| Short trip and satisfaction with trip length and predictability | Trip length in minutes (continuous) | −0.67 |
| | Satisfaction with the predictability of time spent travelling in the vehicle | 0.88 |
| | Satisfaction with the length of time spent travelling in the vehicle | 0.90 |
| Have access to other modes and walking and cycling are viable | Number of modes respondent has access to (continuous) | 0.65 |
| | McGill is within reasonable walking distance to McGill (binomial) | 0.64 |
| | McGill is within reasonable cycling distance to McGill (binomial) | 0.70 |
| Frequency of trip | Number of commutes per week (continuous) | 0.83 |
| | Full-time status at McGill (binomial) | 0.87 |
| Variance | | 69% |

make their most recent trip. For cyclists, this measure only included the number of modes used in the most recent trip. For drivers, the number of modes the respondent had access to factored with other modes being reasonable options (see Tables 9.1, 9.2, and 9.3 for details).

It is important to note that the respondents were asked mode specific questions based on their main mode. For example, pedestrians were asked about their satisfaction with the quality of sidewalks and cyclists were asked about their satisfaction with the quality of cycle paths. The factors analysis was used because it revealed which components of the trip were important to the different mode users. Therefore, we are not comparing the individual questions. Rather, we are comparing the factors, which contain important trip components for the different mode users.

### 9.4.2   Cluster Analysis

The results of the factor analysis for each mode were used to develop a k-means cluster analysis. The purpose of the cluster analysis is to identify heterogeneity within users of the same mode by clustering similar users together. Clustering was tried using three to five groups for each mode. The best number of groupings for each mode was determined based on the characteristics of the factors in each cluster, previous research on mode user typology, and the authors' judgment. The best segmentation was found through four unique clusters for pedestrians, cyclists, bus users, metro users, and drivers, and three for commuter train users, resulting in 23 clusters total. The results of the cluster analysis are presented in Figs. 9.1 and 9.2. In these figures, each cluster is given a name based on mode. For example, the cyclist clusters are C1, C2, C3 and C4. The number of respondents in each cluster is shown under each name in Figs. 9.1 and 9.2. Summary statistics for the clusters are presented in Table 9.4.

Each cluster corresponds to a similar group of users of the same mode, represented by similar commuting habits, such as travelling frequently, or commuting preferences, such as the satisfaction with service. The following is a description of each cluster that highlights some of the main characteristics.

#### 9.4.2.1   Walking

*W1:* This cluster is satisfied and concerned with safety and quality. Furthermore, they chose to be close to McGill when choosing their home.

*W2:* This group has a long trip length and did not consider being close to McGill as important when choosing their home location.

*W3:* This cluster of pedestrians is unsatisfied and unconcerned with safety and quality, but efficiency is important. Other modes are reasonable options but they do not use or have access to modes.

**PEDESTRIANS**

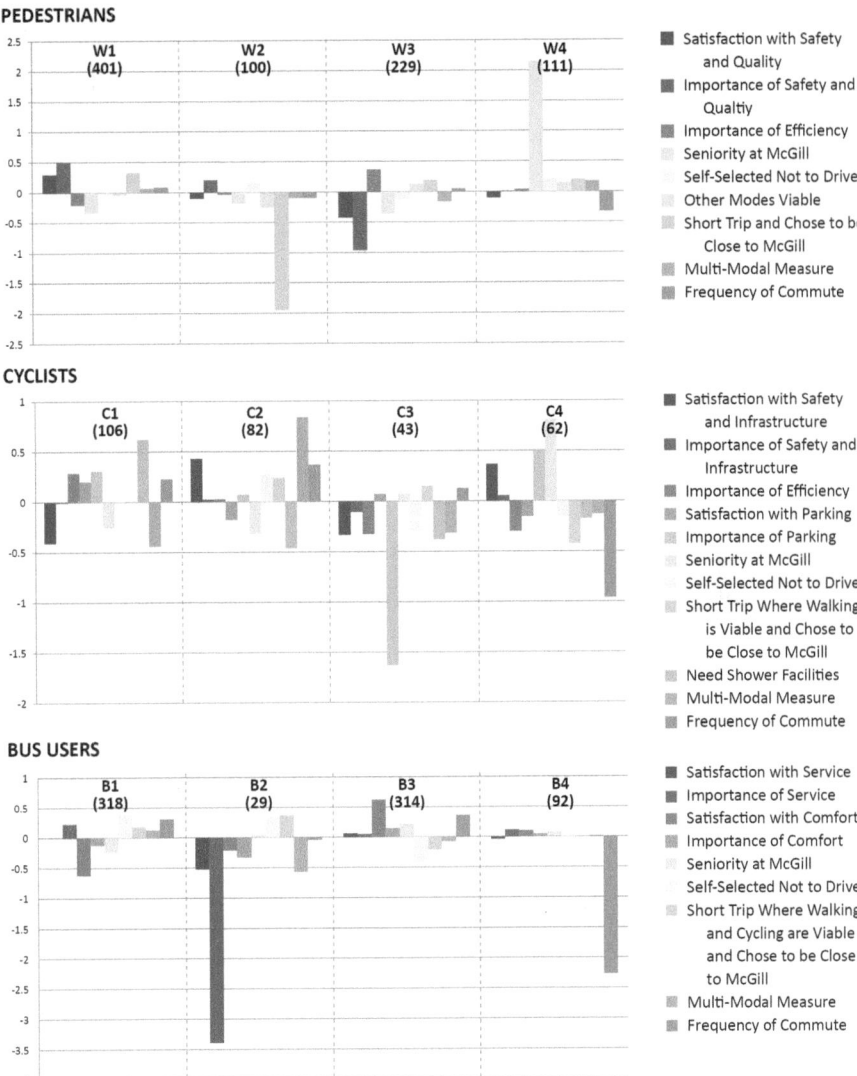

**Fig. 9.1** Clusters for pedestrians, cyclists and bus users

*W4:* These commuters are characterized by seniority at McGill and commute infrequently.

### 9.4.2.2   Cycling

*C1:* These cyclists are concerned about shower facilities and parking and do not use many modes.

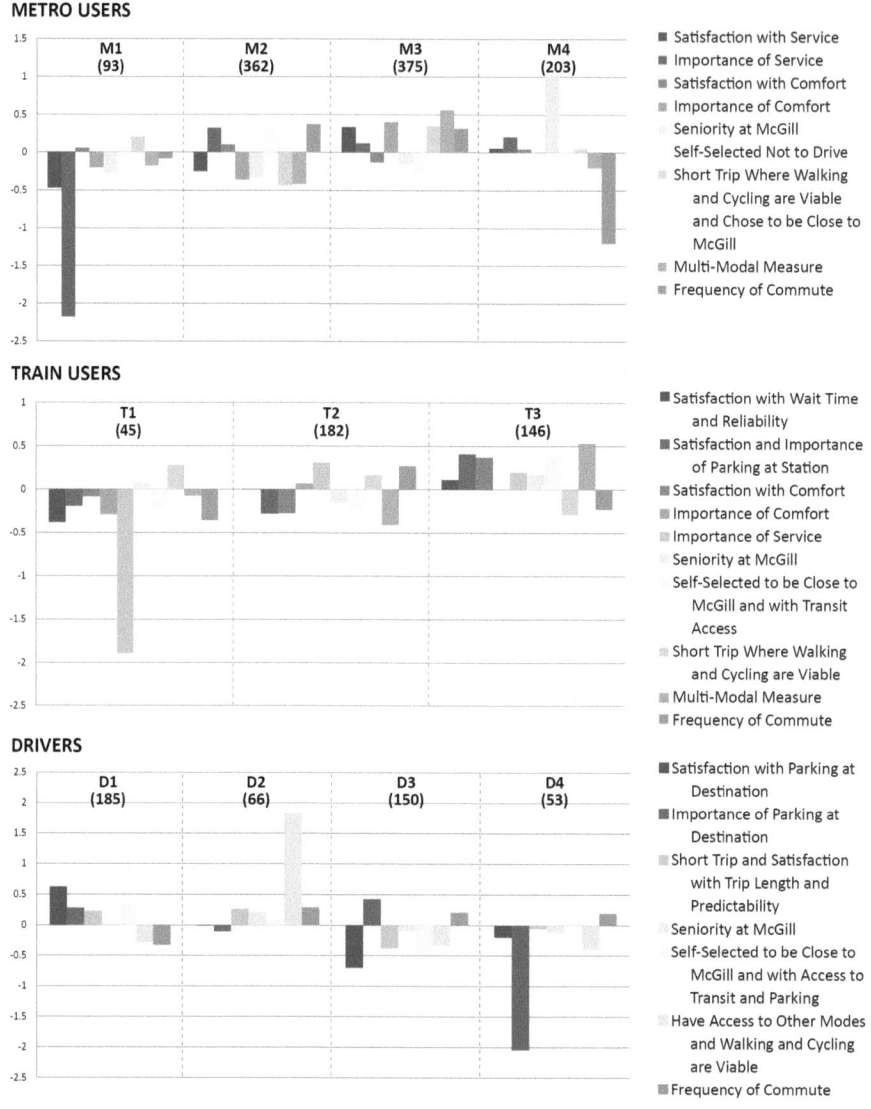

**Fig. 9.2** Clusters for metro users, commuter train users and drivers

*C2:* Cyclists in this cluster are satisfied with safety and infrastructure, use many modes on the trip and report that walking is a reasonable option.

*C3:* This group is concerned with safety, infrastructure and efficiency and have a short trip in which they could walk.

*C4:* The cyclists in this cluster commute infrequently, have seniority at McGill and have a long trip in which they use few modes.

**Table 9.4** Cluster summary statistics

| | Personal characteristics | | | | | | Satisfaction | | | Commute characteristics | | | | Trip characteristics | | |
|---|---|---|---|---|---|---|---|---|---|---|---|---|---|---|---|---|
| Cluster | Age | Gender (% male) | Income (1–10) | Faculty (%) | Staff (%) | Student (%) | Life satisfaction (1–10) | Trip satisfaction (1–5) | Commute impacts my life satisfaction (1–5) | Number of years at McGill | Commutes per week | Full time (%) | Number of modes they have access to | Trip length (minutes) | Left during AM peak (%) | Number of modes used |
| W1 | 25.4 | 41.1 | 1.5 | 0.5 | 9.7 | 89.8 | 7.5 | 4.1 | 4.2 | 2.4 | 5.4 | 95.5 | 1.9 | 16.1 | 40.4 | 1.8 |
| W2 | 32.6 | 40.0 | 2.1 | 3.0 | 29.0 | 68.0 | 7.3 | 3.9 | 4.1 | 4.3 | 4.5 | 93.0 | 1.6 | 37.3 | 47.0 | 1.9 |
| W3 | 24.6 | 41.5 | 1.6 | 0.9 | 10.5 | 88.6 | 7.3 | 3.9 | 4.0 | 2.5 | 5.1 | 98.3 | 1.8 | 17.7 | 37.1 | 1.6 |
| W4 | 50.5 | 52.3 | 5.8 | 80.2 | 19.8 | 0.0 | 8.1 | 4.3 | 4.6 | 14.1 | 4.3 | 83.8 | 2.2 | 29.0 | 71.2 | 1.6 |
| C1 | 34.8 | 53.8 | 2.7 | 17.9 | 23.6 | 58.5 | 7.7 | 4.1 | 4.6 | 3.8 | 5.0 | 98.1 | 2.4 | 24.1 | 0.7 | 1.5 |
| C2 | 31.6 | 56.1 | 2.6 | 11.0 | 28.0 | 61.0 | 7.7 | 4.1 | 4.3 | 3.9 | 5.1 | 98.8 | 2.4 | 23.5 | 0.5 | 2.9 |
| C3 | 33.3 | 65.1 | 2.9 | 25.6 | 16.3 | 58.1 | 8.0 | 4.4 | 4.5 | 6.4 | 4.8 | 100.0 | 2.4 | 22.3 | 0.5 | 1.6 |
| C4 | 44.4 | 66.1 | 4.6 | 53.2 | 30.6 | 16.1 | 8.1 | 4.0 | 4.6 | 9.6 | 3.5 | 67.7 | 2.6 | 32.6 | 0.6 | 1.6 |
| B1 | 32.6 | 30.5 | 2.4 | 8.5 | 33.3 | 58.2 | 7.4 | 3.5 | 4.2 | 5.0 | 4.8 | 100.0 | 1.9 | 45.0 | 62.6 | 2.7 |
| B2 | 38.1 | 58.6 | 2.5 | 13.8 | 34.5 | 51.7 | 7.1 | 2.7 | 3.6 | 7.3 | 4.5 | 89.7 | 1.5 | 44.0 | 55.2 | 2.2 |
| B3 | 40.6 | 36.0 | 3.0 | 16.9 | 44.9 | 38.2 | 7.6 | 3.6 | 4.2 | 9.5 | 4.8 | 99.7 | 1.7 | 52.4 | 59.9 | 2.4 |
| B4 | 40.1 | 31.5 | 2.9 | 22.8 | 21.7 | 55.4 | 7.5 | 3.7 | 4.3 | 6.2 | 1.8 | 38.0 | 2.1 | 45.6 | 39.1 | 2.5 |
| M1 | 31.9 | 45.2 | 2.1 | 3.2 | 24.7 | 72.0 | 7.3 | 3.3 | 3.7 | 3.2 | 4.1 | 87.1 | 1.6 | 44.1 | 59.1 | 2.4 |
| M2 | 31.3 | 33.4 | 2.1 | 0.8 | 35.6 | 63.5 | 7.4 | 3.5 | 4.1 | 3.8 | 4.8 | 99.4 | 1.3 | 50.1 | 60.8 | 2.4 |
| M3 | 34.3 | 36.3 | 2.7 | 5.6 | 47.5 | 46.9 | 7.5 | 3.9 | 4.3 | 4.8 | 4.8 | 98.4 | 2.2 | 37.7 | 70.4 | 3.0 |
| M4 | 46.8 | 38.9 | 3.9 | 40.4 | 31.0 | 28.6 | 7.4 | 3.7 | 4.2 | 11.7 | 2.9 | 55.7 | 1.7 | 43.5 | 59.1 | 2.2 |
| T1 | 47.6 | 55.6 | 3.7 | 13.3 | 71.1 | 15.6 | 7.8 | 3.6 | 3.8 | 12.0 | 4.4 | 80.0 | 1.8 | 69.6 | 57.8 | 2.4 |
| T2 | 43.4 | 37.9 | 3.3 | 4.4 | 72.5 | 23.1 | 7.5 | 3.7 | 4.4 | 8.6 | 4.7 | 97.8 | 1.5 | 68.0 | 59.9 | 2.4 |
| T3 | 42.8 | 41.8 | 3.9 | 26.0 | 50.0 | 24.0 | 7.9 | 3.8 | 4.4 | 10.5 | 4.2 | 85.6 | 2.1 | 70.8 | 66.4 | 3.1 |
| D1 | 46.5 | 36.8 | 4.5 | 36.2 | 43.2 | 20.5 | 7.8 | 3.7 | 4.2 | 11.6 | 3.5 | 63.8 | 1.8 | 40.4 | 52.4 | 1.6 |
| D2 | 44.6 | 63.6 | 5.4 | 65.2 | 16.7 | 18.2 | 7.6 | 3.5 | 4.2 | 12.2 | 4.3 | 90.9 | 2.5 | 30.2 | 71.2 | 1.9 |
| D3 | 43.6 | 39.3 | 4.0 | 18.0 | 48.0 | 34.0 | 7.4 | 3.2 | 4.0 | 9.7 | 3.9 | 81.3 | 1.7 | 50.9 | 52.0 | 1.7 |
| D4 | 47.3 | 39.6 | 4.4 | 24.5 | 58.5 | 17.0 | 7.6 | 3.1 | 3.9 | 10.9 | 4.4 | 81.1 | 1.6 | 45.9 | 62.3 | 1.4 |
| Total | 36.5 | 40.3 | 2.9 | 15.6 | 34.4 | 50.0 | 7.5 | 3.7 | 4.2 | 6.7 | 4.5 | 89.7 | 1.9 | 40.5 | 56.9 | 2.2 |

### 9.4.2.3   Bus Users

*B1:* This group is satisfied with service quality, even though it is unimportant to them. They report that walking and cycling are reasonable options and they have access to modes.

*B2:* These bus users are unsatisfied with service and comfort. Walking and cycling are viable options for them but they do not have access to nor use many modes.

*B3:* These commuters are satisfied with their trip components, which are important to them. They are limited in their modal options.

*B4:* This cluster commutes infrequently at less than two times per week, and services are important to them.

### 9.4.2.4   Metro Users

*M1:* This cluster is unsatisfied and unconcerned with metro service and walking and cycling are reasonable options. They do not use or have access to many modes.

*M2*: They are unsatisfied with service, self-selected to not drive, are limited in their modal options and have low access to other modes.

*M3:* These metro users are satisfied with service and unsatisfied with comfort. Walking and cycling are reasonable options for them and they have access to other modes.

*M4:* They have seniority status at McGill and commute infrequently.

### 9.4.2.5   Train Users

*T1:* These commuters report low satisfaction with several trip components but are unconcerned with service. They have short trips relative to other train users, in which they could walk or cycle and do not have access to many modes.

*T2:* This cluster did not self-select when choosing their home, have a short trip relative to other train users in which walking and cycling are options, and have low access.

*T3:* These train users are satisfied with trip components, self-selected to be close to McGill with transit access and a long trip. Walking and cycling are not reasonable options but they do have access to modes.

### 9.4.2.6   Automobile Drivers

*D1:* This group of drivers is satisfied with their trip components and self-selected to be close to McGill with access to both transit and parking. Walking and cycling are not viable options and they do not have access to modes.

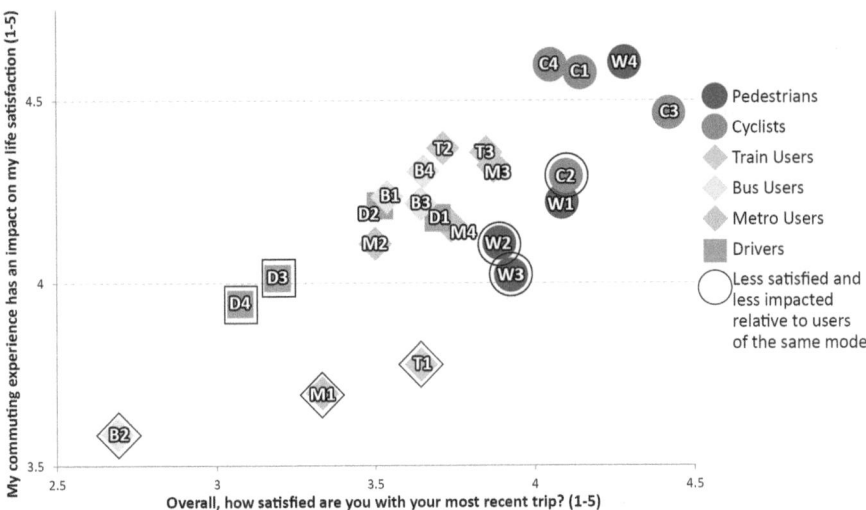

**Fig. 9.3** Trip satisfaction and the impact of commute on life satisfaction

*D2:* Walking and cycling are reasonable options for these drivers and they have access to a high number of modes.

*D3:* This cluster is unsatisfied and concerned with parking and did not self-select when choosing their home. Walking and cycling are reasonable options and they have access to modes.

*D4:* Similar to the above cluster, walking and cycling are reasonable options for these drivers and they have access to a high number of modes.

Trip satisfaction and the impact of commuting on life satisfaction were not included in the factor-cluster analysis. This way, the various clusters could be plotted against trip satisfaction and the impact of commuting on life satisfaction. Accordingly, Fig. 9.3 demonstrates the relationship between life satisfaction and the impact of commuting on life satisfaction for each cluster. However, while the following analysis addresses the relationship between these two aspects of satisfaction, it is not our intention to confirm causality. Rather, this study is an exploratory analysis of the relationship between commuting and its impact on life satisfaction.

### 9.4.3 Trip Satisfaction and the Impact of Commute on Life Satisfaction

Figure 9.3 demonstrates the relationship between the variables measuring overall trip satisfaction and the impact of commuting on overall life satisfaction. Clusters which on average exhibit high trip satisfaction also show that life satisfaction is highly impacted by commuting. Conversely, clusters with lower trip satisfaction show that commuting does not strongly impact life satisfaction. Furthermore, clusters located in the lower left-hand corner of Fig. 9.3 also exhibit below-average overall life satisfaction on a scale of 1–10 (See Table 9.4). For example, cluster B2 has the lowest reported life satisfaction at 7.1/10, the lowest reported trip satisfaction of 2.7/5, and report their life satisfaction is the least impacted by commuting. On the other end of the spectrum, cluster W4 has the highest life satisfaction, as well as high trip satisfaction, and has a life satisfaction that is one of the most influenced by their commuting experience. This is consistent with previous research that found that happiness with commuting can contribute to overall happiness (Olsson et al. 2013) and suggests that as users' trip satisfaction increases, they may be more likely to report that their life satisfaction is influenced by their commute.

These findings might suggest that commuters who are unsatisfied with their trip could be unaware of the negative impact that commuting has on their overall life satisfaction. Alternatively, the results may be suggesting that those who reported a low trip satisfaction may not want to admit that their commute is impacting their overall life satisfaction. In either case, it appears as though the perceived association between commuting and overall life satisfaction decreases with trip satisfaction. In other words, as trip satisfaction decreases, respondents assign a lower level of association between commuting and life satisfaction. Since personality and attitude can play a role in the enjoyment of travel (Mokhtarian and Salomon 2001; Ory and Mokhtarian 2005), it is possible that personality traits influence the decision to report both low trip satisfaction and low life satisfaction. However, personality traits were not captured in the survey. Therefore, the impact of personality and attitude cannot be examined in this study.

The top right-hand corner of Fig. 9.3 represents high trip satisfaction and high impact of commuting on life satisfaction. This corner is dominated by active transportation clusters, which is consistent with previous findings that report high satisfaction and happiness among cyclists and pedestrians (Duarte et al. 2010; Legrain et al. 2015; Mokhtarian et al. 2015; Mokhtarian and Salomon 2001; Olsson et al. 2013). These clusters have been able to derive the enjoyment from their utilitarian work commute that has previously been identified in undirected travel (Mokhtarian and Salomon 2001). Also similar to previous findings about the dissatisfaction of bus users (St-Louis et al. 2014), the least satisfied cluster is B2.

### 9.4.4  Relatively Less Satisfied Clusters

Overall, Fig. 9.3 demonstrates that active transport users tend to be both more satisfied with their trips and believe that their overall life satisfaction is strongly influenced by their commute. On the other hand, public transit and automobile users tend to be less satisfied overall and their life satisfaction is less influenced by their trip. However, Fig. 9.3 reveals that although there is a general pattern, there are modal clusters that are less satisfied and less impacted by commuting, compared to users of the same mode. These clusters are W2, W3, C2, B2, M1, T1, D3 and D4.

Commuters in these clusters were identified as being less satisfied with their trip and their life satisfaction is less impacted by commuting relative to other clusters of the same mode. The clusters that are less satisfied and less impacted by commuting are identified by a black outline in Fig. 9.3. This finding suggests that, while mode choice does influence satisfaction (St-Louis et al. 2014), not all users of the same mode are similar. With the exception of C2, a commonality among the less satisfied and less impacted by commuting modal clusters is that the factor measuring access to and use of multiple modes is negative. Therefore, clusters that are less satisfied and less impacted by commuting tend to report having access to and/or using fewer modes than the other clusters using the same mode (Figs. 9.1 and 9.2). Therefore, clusters with both lower trip satisfaction and a lower impact of commuting on life satisfaction are limited in their travel options, relative to clusters of the same mode. Taking into consideration previous findings that commutes are often viewed as mandatory and unenjoyable (Ory and Mokhtarian 2009), these clusters may have low satisfaction because of the lack of control and flexibility in a trip that is viewed as obligatory. This is a significant finding because it emphasizes the importance of giving commuters different modal options that are flexible, reliable and accessible. This finding is similar to previous research concentrating on trip satisfaction and flexibility in choice in Beijing context (Mao et al. 2016).

Commuters in clusters that are less satisfied and less impacted by commuting are not the only respondents with access to fewer modes. There are several clusters with low access even though they are not identified as less satisfied in Fig. 9.3. It is possible that their relatively high satisfaction is explained through self-selection measures, as users in these clusters considered their proximity to McGill or access to transit, when choosing their home location. Through these self-selection strategies, respondents have been able to choose a home that makes their chosen mode a reasonable option. This is likely influencing their trip satisfaction to be relatively high, despite clustering negatively for the factor measuring access to and use of multiple modes. Taking into account previous findings that those who like the mode they are using have higher satisfaction and that people tend to choose home locations where their preferred modes are reasonable options (Bhat and Guo 2007; Choo et al. 2005), the effect of low access appears to be mitigated through self-selection strategies.

## 9.5  Policy Recommendations

The results of this study reveal that those whose life satisfaction is impacted by their commute are relatively more satisfied with their trip, while those whose life satisfaction is less impacted by their commute are less satisfied with their trip. Accordingly, since the life satisfaction of those who are less impacted is lower than those who are impacted, it can be assumed that increasing trip satisfaction could increase the impact of commuting and result in a higher life satisfaction. This is based on respondents with high trip satisfaction also reporting high overall life satisfaction.

Based on this analysis, increasing an individual's SWB could be done through improving their commute.

The above analysis revealed that there is variation among clusters in terms of trip satisfaction, the impact of commuting on life satisfaction and having access to and using different modes. To increase satisfaction among those who are relatively less satisfied, planners and policy makers should develop strategies that provide increase the number of options from a single mode and/or increase access to multi-modal trips that are more reasonable, flexible, and reliable. Additionally, these strategies should encourage multi-modal trips that include more walking and cycling. Strategies for improving multi-modality include developing integrated payment systems for public services such as transit and bicycle-share systems, as well as by integrating bicycle and car parking at transit hubs, and by better integrating pedestrian areas. Other strategies include investing in cycling, pedestrian and transit infrastructure, prioritizing transit connectivity, and creating route findings systems that incorporate multiple modes (Henao et al. 2015; Mishra et al. 2012; Terveen 2013). These approaches have been shown to increase mode share for walking and cycling and allow users to express their modal preference. Since those who walk and cycle to work tend to be the most satisfied, with both their trip and their life, increasing the mode share of walking and cycling could have a positive impact on life satisfaction. Additionally, since those who like the mode they use during a trip are more likely to be satisfied with the trip (Choo et al. 2005), a well-connected multi-modal network would allow commuters to use their preferred mode. Multi-modal trips are sometimes viewed as unpleasant (Mokhtarian et al. 2015), however, strategies to improve the multi-modal experience could encourage the modes that result in high trip satisfaction.

## 9.6   Limitations

Similarly to previous research, this study has shown that commuting can influence life satisfaction (Banister and Bowling 2004; Bergstad et al. 2011, 2012; Olsson et al. 2013) and adds to the literature by exploring this relationship through a factor-cluster analysis based on mode. However, commuting is only one of many components that impact a person's SWB. Many other social and economic factors impact life satisfaction and SWB, including income, unemployment, education and quality personal relationships (Clark and Oswald 1996; Delbosc and Currie 2011; Diener et al. 1999; Ferrer-i-Carbonell 2005; Helliwell 2003; Myers 2000). However, due to data limitations, these factors could not be included in this study. Additionally, personal factors, including personality and attitude can influence SWB (Ory and Mokhtarian 2009). Based on the results of the literature review, as well the findings from the present study, conclusions cannot be drawn that all types of people would benefit from a mode change.

Question and sample bias are potential limitations of this study. Diener et al. (2013). present a review of the reliability of satisfaction with life scales and find that the results of the scales can be representative of an individual's actual QOL. However, results can be effected by factors such as current mood, question order and method of presentation. Therefore, it is important to note the potential sample bias in the self-reported trip satisfaction and life satisfaction, as self-reported satisfaction and subjective measures rely on the respondents' subjective meaning of satisfaction and trip satisfaction may be biased by the destination itself (Delbosc 2012; Mokhtarian and Salomon 2001). Additionally, the sample is comprised of faculty, staff and students of a university, meaning the sample is both educated and employed. As noted above, education and employment have a positive impact on satisfaction (Clark and Oswald 1996; Delbosc and Currie 2011; Helliwell 2003), and it should therefore be expected that the sample would report a higher life satisfaction compared to the general population. Finally, the survey question that asked the respondents to agree or disagree, on a scale of one to five, with the statement about commuting impacting life satisfaction was asked immediately after the respondent was asked to rate their trip satisfaction. The close proximity of these two questions in the survey could have induced further response bias.

## 9.7  Conclusion

To conclude, previous research has shown that transportation and commuting can have an impact on overall life satisfaction (Banister and Bowling 2004; Bergstad et al. 2011, 2012; Olsson et al. 2013). Furthermore, results of this study have revealed that commuters with high trip satisfaction also tend to report that commuting has an impact on their life satisfaction. While the results of this study have revealed relationships between variables, based on the current findings, causality cannot be confirmed. Therefore, in the future, researchers should focus on developing methods to more comprehensively study the impact that commutes have on life satisfaction and focus on assessing causality. While the present study assessed the impact of commuting on life satisfaction, further research could focus on analyzing whether overall QOL and SWB impact the satisfaction with commuting. In addition, researchers studying life satisfaction in different fields should be collaborating with the goal of painting a better overall picture of the factors influencing overall satisfaction and QOL.

The findings of the study reveal that there is a relationship between individuals' overall life satisfaction, their reported trip satisfaction, and the perception that trip satisfaction impacts their life satisfaction. Findings suggest that commuters who are satisfied with their trip also report that their commute impacts their life satisfaction. In contrast, less satisfied commuters report a lower association between trip satisfaction and life satisfaction. This suggests that as users' trip satisfaction increases, they may be more likely to report that their life satisfaction is influenced by their commute.

This study has added to the literature by exploring the relationship between commuting and overall life satisfaction through modal clusters. Exploring the relationship between trip satisfaction and the impact of commuting on life satisfaction has resulted in policy recommendations that advocate for the building of a well-connected multi-modal transportation network that incorporates active transportation. This would allow commuters to use their preferred mode and diminish the negative impact of being constrained in their modal options.

**Acknowledgements** The authors would like to thank the Social Sciences and Humanities Research Council (SSHRC) and the Natural Sciences and Engineering Research Council of Canada (NSERC) for their financial support. We would also like to acknowledge Kathleen Ng and Brian Karasick from the McGill Office of Sustainability for their assistance with the various phases of this project, Prof. Kevin Manaugh and Charis Loong from McGill University for their help in designing the survey and Daniel Schwartz from IT Customer Services for his support in developing the online survey and managing the distribution of the survey to the McGill community.

# References

Banister, D., & Bowling, A. (2004). Quality of life for the elderly: The transport dimension. *Transport Policy, 11*(2), 105–115.

Bergstad, C., Gamble, A., Gärling, T., Hagman, O., Polk, M., Ettema, D., et al. (2011). Subjective well-being related to satisfaction with daily travel. *Transportation, 38*(1), 1–15.

Bergstad, C., Gamble, A., Hagman, O., Polk, M., Gärling, T., Ettema, D., et al. (2012). Influences of affect associated with routine out-of-home activities on subjective well-being. *Applied Research in Quality of Life, 7*(1), 49–62.

Bhat, C., & Guo, J. (2007). A comprehensive analysis of built environment characteristics on household residential choice and auto ownership levels. *Transportation Research Part B: Methodological, 41*(5), 506–526.

Cao, X. (2016). How does neighborhood design affect life satisfaction? Evidence from Twin Cities. *Travel Behaviour and Society, 5*, 68–76.

Cao, J., & Zhang, J. (2016). Built environment, mobility, and quality of life. *Travel Behaviour and Society, 5*, 1–4.

Choi, J., Coughlin, J., & D'Ambrosio, L. (2013). Travel time and subjective well-being. *Transportation Research Record: Journal of the Transportation Research Board, 2357*, 100–108.

Choo, S., Collantes, G., & Mokhtarian, P. (2005). Wanting to travel, more or less: Exploring the determinants of the deficit and surfeit of personal travel. *Transportation, 32*(2), 135–164.

Clark, A., & Oswald, A. (1996). Satisfaction and comparison income. *Journal of Public Economics, 61*(3), 359–381.

De Vos, J., & Witlox, F. (2017). Travel satisfaction revisited: On the pivotal role of travel satisfaction in conceptualising a travel behaviour process. *Transportation Research Part A: Policy and Practice, 106*, 364–373.

Delbosc, A. (2012). The role of well-being in transport policy. *Transport Policy, 23*, 25–33.

Delbosc, A., & Currie, G. (2011). Exploring the relative influences of transport disadvantage and social exclusion on well-being. *Transport Policy, 18*(4), 555–562.

Diener, E. (1984). Subjective well-being. *Psychological Bulletin, 95*, 276–302.

Diener, E., & Suh, E. (1997). Measuring quality of life: Economic, social and subjective indicators. *Social Indicators Research, 40*, 189–216.

Diener, E., Emmons, R., Larsen, R., & Griffin, S. (1985). The satisfaction with life scale. *Journal of Personality Assessment, 49*, 71–75.

Diener, E., Suh, R., & Smith, H. (1999). Subjective well-being: Three decades of progress. *Psychological Bulletin, 125*, 276–302.

Diener, E., Oishi, S., & Lucas, R. (2003). Personality, culture, and subjective well-being: Emotional and cognitive evaluations of life. *Annual Review of Psychology, 54*(1), 403–425.

Diener, E., Inglehart, R., & Tay, L. (2013). Theory and validity of life satisfaction scales. *Social Indicators Research, 112*(3), 497–527.

Duarte, A., Garcia, C., Giannarakis, G., Limão, S., Polydoropoulou, A., & Litinas, N. (2010). New approaches in transportation planning: Happiness and transport economics. *NETNOMICS: Economic Research and Electronic Networking, 11*(1), 5–32.

Ettema, D., & Schekkerman, M. (2016). How do spatial characteristics influence well-being and mental health? Comparing the effect of objective and subjective characteristics at different spatial scales. *Travel Behaviour and Society, 5*, 56–67.

Ettema, D., & Verschuren, L. (2007). Multitasking and value of travel time savings. *Transportation Research Record: Journal of the Transportation Research Board, 2010*, 19–25.

Ettema, D., Gärling, T., Eriksson, L., Friman, M., Olsson, L., & Fujii, S. (2011). Satisfaction with travel and subjective well-being: Development and test of a measurement tool. *Transportation Research Part F: Traffic Psychology and Behaviour, 14*(3), 167–175.

Ettema, D., Friman, M., Gärling, T., Olsson, L., & Fujii, S. (2012). How in-vehicle activities affect work commuters' satisfaction with public transport. *Journal of Transport Geography, 24*, 215–222.

Evans, G., Wener, R., & Phillips, D. (2002). The morning rush hour predictability and commuter stress. *Environment and Behavior, 34*(4), 521–530.

Ferrer-i-Carbonell, A. (2005). Income and well-being: An empirical analysis of the comparison income effect. *Journal of Public Economics, 89*(5), 997–1019.

Gardner, B., & Abraham, C. (2007). What drives car use? A grounded theory analysis of commuters' reasons for driving. *Transportation Research Part F: Traffic Psychology and Behaviour, 10*(3), 187–200.

Gatersleben, B., & Uzzell, D. (2007). Affective appraisals of the daily commute comparing perceptions of drivers, cyclists, walkers, and users of public transport. *Environment and Behavior, 39*(3), 416–431.

Gottholmseder, G., Nowotny, K., Pruckner, G., & Theurl, E. (2009). Stress perception and commuting. *Health Economics, 18*(5), 559–576.

Guo, W., Gupta, N., Pogrebna, G., & Jarvis, S. (2016). Understanding happiness in cities using Twitter: Jobs, children and transport. *IEEE International Smart Cities Conference*, Trento, Italy, 12–15 Sep 2016.

Helliwell, J. (2003). How's life? Combining individual and national variables to explain subjective well-being. *Economic Modelling, 20*(2), 331–360.

Henao, A., Piatkowski, D., Luckey, K., Nordback, K., Marshall, W., & Krizek, K. (2015). Sustainable transportation infrastructure investments and mode share changes: A 20-year background of Boulder, Colorado. *Transport Policy, 37*, 64–71.

Jain, J., & Lyons, G. (2008). The gift of travel time. *Journal of Transport Geography, 16*(2), 81–89.

Legrain, A., Eluru, N., & El-Geneidy, A. (2015). Am stressed, must travel: The relationship between mode choice and commuting stress. *Transportation Research Part F: Traffic Psychology and Behaviour, 34*, 141–151.

Loong, C., & El-Geneidy, A. (2016). *It's a matter of time: An assessment of additional time budgeted for commuting across modes.* Paper presented at the Transportation Research Board 95th Annual Meeting.

Manaugh, K., & El-Geneidy, A. (2013). Does distance matter? Exploring the links among values, motivations, home location, and satisfaction in walking trips. *Transportation Research Part A: Policy and Practice, 50*, 198–208. https://doi.org/10.1016/j.tra.2013.01.044.

Mann, E., & Abraham, C. (2006). The role of affect in UK commuters' travel mode choices: An interpretative phenomenological analysis. *British Journal of Psychology, 97*(2), 155–176.

Mao, Z., Ettema, D., & Dijst, M. (2016). Commuting trip satisfaction in Beijing: Exploring the influence of multimodal behavior and modal flexibility. *Transportation Research Part A: Policy and Practice, 94*, 592–603.

Mishra, S., Welch, T., & Jha, M. (2012). Performance indicators for public transit connectivity in multi-modal transportation networks. *Transportation Research Part A: Policy and Practice, 46* (7), 1066–1085.

Mokhtarian, P., & Salomon, I. (2001). How derived is the demand for travel? Some conceptual and measurement considerations. *Transportation Research Part A: Policy and Practice, 35*(8), 695–719.

Mokhtarian, P., Papon, F., Goulard, M., & Diana, M. (2015). What makes travel pleasant and/or tiring? An investigation based on the French National Travel Survey. *Transportation, 42*(6), 1103–1128.

Morris, E., & Guerra, E. (2015). Mood and mode: Does how we travel affect how we feel? *Transportation, 42*(1), 25–43.

Morris, E., & Hirsch, J. (2016). Does rush hour see a rush of emotions? Driver mood in conditions likely to exhibit congestion. *Travel Behaviour and Society, 5*, 5–13.

Myers, D. (2000). The funds, friends, and faith of happy people. *American Psychologist, 55*(1), 56.

Novaco, R., Stokols, D., & Milanesi, L. (1990). Objective and subjective dimensions of travel impedance as determinants of commuting stress. *American Journal of Community Psychology, 18*(2), 231–257.

Novaco, R., Kliewer, W., & Broquet, A. (1991). Home environmental consequences of commute travel impedance. *American Journal of Community Psychology, 19*(6), 881–909.

Olsson, L., Gärling, T., Ettema, D., Friman, M., & Fujii, S. (2013). Happiness and satisfaction with work commute. *Social Indicators Research, 111*(1), 255–263.

Ory, D., & Mokhtarian, P. (2005). When is getting there half the fun? Modeling the liking for travel. *Transportation Research Part A: Policy and Practice, 39*(2), 97–123.

Ory, D., & Mokhtarian, P. (2009). Modeling the structural relationships among short-distance travel amounts, perceptions, affections, and desires. *Transportation Research Part A: Policy and Practice, 43*(1), 26–43.

Ory, D. T., Mokhtarian, P. L., Redmond, L. S., Salomon, I., Collantes, G. O., & Choo, S. (2004). When is commuting desirable to the individual? *Growth and Change, 35*(3), 334–359.

Redmond, L., & Mokhtarian, P. (2001). The positive utility of the commute: Modeling ideal commute time and relative desired commute amount. *Transportation, 28*(2), 179–205.

Schimmack, U. (2008). The structure of subjective well-being. In *The science of subjective well-being* (pp. 97–123). New York: Guilford Press.

Stanley, J., & Stanley, J. (2007). Public transport and social policy goals. *Road & Transport Research: A Journal of Australian and New Zealand Research and Practice, 16*(1), 20.

Stanley, J., Hensher, D., Stanley, J., & Vella-Brodrick, D. (2011). Mobility, social exclusion and well-being: Exploring the links. *Transportation Research Part A: Policy and Practice, 45*(8), 789–801.

St-Louis, E., Manaugh, K., van Lierop, D., & El-Geneidy, A. (2014). The happy commuter: A comparison of commuter satisfaction across modes. *Transportation Research Part F: Traffic Psychology and Behaviour, 26*, 160–170.

Stokols, D., Novaco, R., Stokols, J., & Campbell, J. (1978). Traffic congestion, type A behavior, and stress. *Journal of Applied Psychology, 63*(4), 467.

Stradling, S., Anable, J., & Carreno, M. (2007). Performance, importance and user disgruntlement: A six-step method for measuring satisfaction with travel modes. *Transportation Research Part A: Policy and Practice, 41*(1), 98–106.

Stutzer, A., & Frey, B. (2008). Stress that doesn't pay: The commuting paradox. *The Scandinavian Journal of Economics, 110*(2), 339–366.

Terveen, L. (2013). *Bike, bus, and beyond: Extending cyclopath to enable multi-modal routing.* Minnesota Department of Transprtation: Twin Cities, Minnesota.

van den Berg, P., Kemperman, A., de Kleijn, B., & Borgers, A. (2016). Ageing and loneliness: The role of mobility and the built environment. *Travel Behaviour and Society, 5*, 48–55.

Wener, R., Evans, G., & Boately, P. (2005). Commuting stress: Psychophysiological effects of a trip and spillover into the workplace. *Transportation Research Record: Journal of the Transportation Research Board, 1924*, 112–117.

Willis, D., Manaugh, K., & El-Geneidy, A. (2013). Uniquely satisfied: Exploring cyclist satisfaction. *Transportation Research Part F: Traffic Psychology and Behaviour, 18*, 136–147.

Xiong, Y., & Zhang, J. (2016). Effects of land use and transport on young adults' quality of life. *Travel Behaviour and Society, 5*, 37–47.

# Chapter 10
# A Case Study Exploring Associations of Quality of Life Measures with Car and Active Transport Commute Modes in Sydney

Nicholas Petrunoff, Melanie Crane, and Chris Rissel

**Abstract** Several dimensions of commuting influence perceived stress, such as impedance (a measure of distance and time which is impacted by the number of transport nodes), and control over and predictability of commuting. Research into commuting mode and stress has generated mixed results. The case study in this chapter used baseline survey data from a 3-year workplace travel plan intervention. Workplace travel plans aim to promote active and sustainable forms of transport and reduce driving to work. An on-line cross-sectional survey of staff travel behaviour was conducted in September 2011 at Liverpool Hospital in Sydney, Australia. A total of 675 respondents provided data on the items of interest for this analysis (travel behaviour, self-reported stress, occupation type, demographics). Approximately one in six respondents (15%) actively commuted to work (walking 4%, cycling 2% or using public transport 9%). There was a large (15%) difference between active commuters' (10.1%) and drivers' (25%) perceptions that the commute to work was more stressful than the rest of their day that remained statistically significant (adjusted odds ratio 0.35, 95% confidence interval 0.17–0.73) after adjusting for factors including gender, age, physical activity levels and occupational type (clinical vs non-clinical). These findings support international research which has shown that active travel to work may be less stressful than car commuting.

**Keywords** Active travel · Bicycling · Walking · Travel planning · Physical activity · Stress · Quality of life · Health promotion

N. Petrunoff · M. Crane · C. Rissel (✉)
The University of Sydney, Sydney, Australia
e-mail: melanie.crane@sydney.edu.au; chris.rissel@sydney.edu.au

© Springer International Publishing AG, part of Springer Nature 2018
M. Friman et al. (eds.), *Quality of Life and Daily Travel*, Applying Quality of Life
Research, https://doi.org/10.1007/978-3-319-76623-2_10

## 10.1 Elements of the Quality of Life Concept Explored in This Case Study

This chapter presents a case study of an investigation into the relationship between stress, and the daily commute to work by car and by active modes of transport (Rissel et al. 2014b). Stress is an aspect of quality of life, often investigated singularly, and at other times embedded alongside other indicators of quality of life to measure affect or aspects of mental wellbeing. This chapter specifically explores stress as it relates directly to the psychological health component of quality of life (Novaco and Gonzalez 2009).

Several dimensions of the commuting situation influence perceived stress, such as impedance (a measure of distance and time which is impacted by the number of transport nodes), and control over and predictability of commuting. In this case study, perceptions of stress is compared between commuters who travel to work by car and by active modes.

## 10.2 Definition of the Problem

In developing and developed countries the majority of the world's citizens now live in urban areas (WHO/UN-HABITAT 2010). Although evidence suggests the steep rise in private motor vehicle ownership that occurred over the last 60 years in most developed countries has plateaued, (Newman and Kenworthy 2015) the global trend is still toward private car ownership growing faster than any other form of transport (Dargay et al. 2007). In many countries cars are currently the dominant form of transport for trips to work (Newman and Kenworthy 2015). Commuting to work by car contributes negligible physical activity (Ding et al. 2014; Petrunoff et al. 2013b). Public health advocates are concerned about this because physical inactivity has reached a state of what has been described as global pandemic. Physical inactivity, it is a major risk factor for chronic diseases including ischemic heart disease, stroke, diabetes and some cancers, and is the fourth leading risk factor for death worldwide (Kohl et al. 2012).

As well as reducing opportunities for physical activity, this global increase in car ownership and urbanisation inevitably creates greater traffic congestion, if more cars traveling on existing road infrastructure within the built environment. Traffic impedance, personal control over the journey, and predictability of the work commute are all factors contributing to stress of the commuting trip (Gottholmseder et al. 2009). Commuting to work by car may be more stressful than other modes of travel because of the impedance associated with traffic congestion that is largely avoided by active travel modes (Novaco and Gonzalez 2009). In previous research, car commuters have report higher stress levels than other transport mode users, (Gatersleben and Uzzell 2007; Legrain et al. 2015).

Other research has found that public transport users also report stress, but are more likely to reported greater boredom (Gatersleben and Uzzell 2007). Part of the reason for this may be due to distance travelled, with longer distances, greater than 30 min, associated with higher amounts of perceived stress and poorer life satisfaction (Gottholmseder et al. 2009; St-Louis et al. 2014; Wheatley 2014). The findings are however mixed and other studies have shown commuting times over 60 min to be less stressful and indeed variable, according to residential location and time (Hansson et al. 2011; Mattisson et al. 2016). In the case of public transport, social and entertainment technologies may be helping to counteract potential stress and boredom (Ettema et al. 2012). Much more needs to be understood about the relationship between stress and commuting, particularly in regards to the variability across different transport environments, travel modes and work employment situations.

## 10.3 Explanation of Why the Problem Is Important

There is an urgent need to consider how to incorporate physical activity into our daily lives and one promising way to do this is to promote active commuting to work (Petrunoff et al. 2016a). Active commuting, allows people to participate in amounts of physical activity that are important for maintaining health (Petrunoff et al. 2013b; Sahlqvist et al. 2012; Yang et al. 2012). Walking and cycling are inherently active forms of commuting. Using public transport to travel to work can also be considered active commuting when the journey between the worksite or home and the public transport interchange includes for example a 10-min brisk walk each way (WHO 2010). If active travel options are not available and workers have little choice but to commute by car, then stress-related health issues and associated healthcare costs can only increase.

Strong evidence supports that adults who change from inactive transport to more active forms of transport significantly reduce their cardiovascular disease risk (Celis-Morales et al. 2017; Gordon-Larsen et al. 2009; Møller et al. 2011; Wennberg et al. 2006; Xu et al. 2013). Good evidence also suggests active travel can lead to significant reductions in body mass index (weight in kilograms divided by height in meters squared – a population measure used to classify people's weight).(Flint and Cummins 2015; Martin et al. 2015; Mytton et al. 2016; Sato et al. 2007; Sugiyama et al. 2012, 2013; Wanner et al. 2012; Wen et al. 2006; Xu et al. 2013) While important as a way of achieving physical activity, interventions to encourage active commuting, as an alternative to car-based travel might also reduce stress and have positive effects on overall mental health (Ohta et al. 2007; Rissel et al. 2014a, b) as well as improve wellbeing more broadly (Crane et al. 2014).

The workplace setting is a valid place to promote active travel since in many developed countries the majority of adults travel to a workplace, (OECD 2013) and the trip is generally repetitive. A large proportion of journeys to work which are made by private motor vehicles are relatively short distances of less than 5 km and could be made by walking and cycling modes, or supported by public travel for longer distances (BTS 2013; Goodman 2013). A shift from driving private motor vehicles towards active travel to workplace settings could achieve population level increases in physical activity, lead to associated reductions in chronic disease risk, and a large decrease in traffic volume.

The workplace setting is also a valid target for active travel interventions as a way to improve workplace health. Workforce well-being is affected by many factors, such as job demand and control, support, organisational justice and the effort–reward balance; as well as personal factors such as health, socioeconomic and other demographics (Nieuwenhuijsen et al. 2010). The association between perceived stress and work productivity, absenteeism and presenteeism is well recognised, and attention has focused on workplace interventions to manage stress and improve employee health (Bhui et al. 2012; Jacobson et al. 1996; Noblet and LaMontagne 2006). This is important given mental illness is a significant global disease burden. Stress-related workers compensation claims are estimated to cost Australia between $10 and 20 billion in loss of work productivity and participation (Safe, Work, & Australia 2013).

Research into the association between work productivity and stress has tended to focus only on the stress accumulated within the work environment. The contribution of the commute to work to workplace stress is often under-recognised or ignored in studies investigating workplace stress, productivity and absenteeism. To some extent this is attributable to the perception that how individuals get to work is a personal choice, and that individual attitudes and perceptions towards transportation affect transport choices (Friman et al. 2017; Popuri et al. 2011). Yet it must be recognised that the commuting stress transfer beyond the individual to impact work and home life (Novaco and Gonzalez 2009). The relationship between stress reported by workers therefore needs to be considered holistically, and that includes an assessment of how the journey to work might contribute to that stress. This case study aims to address this gap in the literature and explore the association between perceptions of work-related stress and the work commute.

## 10.4   Steps Taken to Address the Problem

The case study in this chapter used baseline survey data from a 3-year workplace travel plan intervention. Workplace travel plans aim to promote active and sustainable forms of transport and reduce driving to work. Workplace travel plans can achieve between 10% and 20% reductions in driving to work, (Bamberg and Möser 2007; Cairns et al. 2010; De Gruyter et al. 2018; Hosking et al. 2010; Macmillan et al. 2013; Marsden et al. 2011). Some studies have also demonstrated significant increases in active travel to work, (Brockman and Fox 2011; Petrunoff et al. under review) but only one robust experimental study of these effects (Higgins 1996). Workplace travel plans are a delivery mechanism for actions which often include policy (e.g. parking management policy, public transport ticket subsidies), infrastructure (e.g. provision of end of trip facilities, creation of maps) and behaviour change programs (e.g. cycling and walking programs) (Enoch 2012).

There is no internationally accepted term for workplace travel plans. The term is used in Australia, New Zealand, the United Kingdom, Singapore and some other countries. In North America they are sometimes referred to as travel demand management plans and in some parts of Europe and Scandinavia site-based mobility management plans. In some regions they can be required as a condition of planning consent for new or expanded developments typically occupied by medium-large organisations (Rye et al. 2011a, b; Wynne 2015). However, even where systematic government support for their adoption exists, take-up of these promising interventions has been modest, which has led experts to recommend they be marketed to organisations in terms of their benefit to the organisation (Enoch 2012; Petrunoff et al. 2017).

The baseline study included the quality of life construct of stress to assess the relationship between stress and commuting to work by different transport modes (Rissel et al. 2014a, b). Data on reductions in stress and links to associated gains in productivity may assist with engaging these organisations to adopt and support the implementation of travel plans.

### 10.4.1   Research Design

An on-line cross-sectional survey of staff travel behaviour was conducted in September 2011 at Liverpool Hospital in Sydney, Australia (Petrunoff et al. 2013a). The survey was part of a larger study that was repeated in three annual follow-up surveys (Petrunoff et al. 2016b).

### 10.4.2   Setting and Context

Liverpool Hospital is in an outer metropolitan area of Liverpool, south-west Sydney, Australia and is a principal referral teaching hospital. Liverpool Hospital was in the second stage of a major re-development when the travel plan was being developed. The re-development plans forecast the number of staff and hospital beds increasing by approximately one-third between 2006 and 2016, to cope with the increasing health demands of the growing population of the area, identified as one of two 'growth centres' by state government planning departments. At the time the study commenced, the Hospital was well serviced by heavy rail, with two stations within 10-min easy walking distance. Hospital staff also had access to an extensive bus network. There were significant gaps in the cycling network in the immediate surrounds of the hospital (see Fig. 10.1). A more detailed of the regional level cycling network map which clearly shows these gaps is available at a web link in references (Rissel 2010).

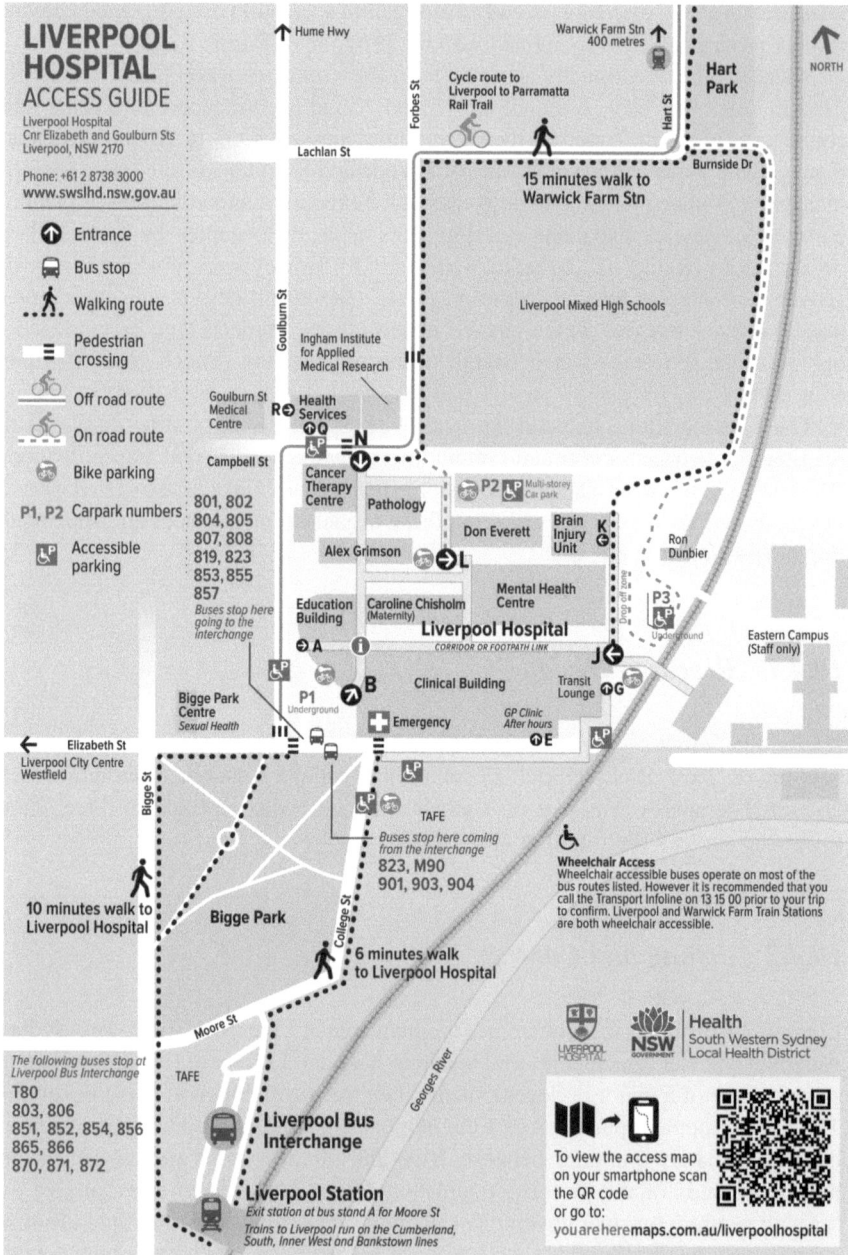

**Fig. 10.1** Liverpool hospital access guide showing local transport context

### 10.4.3   Survey Methods

An email was sent to all staff (approximately n = 3200) via existing staff communication channels. The survey was a self-administered online questionnaire (Qualtrics 2017). All staff were invited via email to participate in the survey, which was supported by the hospital General Manager. A flyer promoting the survey was distributed to all staff via the mail room, posters were placed around the hospital and a prize incentive offered to encourage participation. The survey ran for 2 weeks, with a reminder sent 7 days after the survey started. Paper copies of the survey were made available to General Services staff who did not have regular access to work emails.

Participants were asked: "How did you travel to work this week? (If you used more than one form of transport, show the method used for the longest (distance) part of the journey)". Response options for each day of the week were walked, cycled, drove a car, car passenger, bus, ferry, train, taxi, truck, motorbike or scooter, worked at home, other, and I did not go to work. This question was tested with a sub-sample of staff and was shown to be valid and reliable (Petrunoff et al. 2013b).

Walking, cycling and public transport categories were considered "active travel." Public transport users were included here because this typically included an approximate 10-min walk to major bus and train interchanges. Car categories including car as a driver or passenger, motorbike and scooter were considered "non-active travellers" since for the majority of car drivers their commute was likely to be inactive, and this was demonstrated using objective accelerometer data with a sub-sample of staff in the survey validation study (Petrunoff et al. 2013b). Participants were categorised as "active travellers" overall if they travelled using an active travel mode on half or more of the working days recorded in their travel diary.

Participants were also asked about the relative stress of their commute: "Compared to other parts of your day, how stressful do you find the journey to and from work?" with response options being "More stressful", "Less stressful" or "About the same". Demographic information (age, sex, and whether they had mainly a clinical or administrative role) was also collected, as was the amount of physical activity over the previous week (using the International Physical Activity Questionnaire-short version) (Booth et al. 2003). Transport-related physical activity was included in the measurement of physical activity. Total moderate to vigorous physical activity time has been used to assess adequate physical activity, which is defined as 150 min/week for consistency with international physical activity guidelines.

Statistical methods were used to test the strength of associations between the different commute modes to work and participants' self-reported levels of stress after adjusting for differences in some of the factors which could impact the results. Specifically, Chi square statistics were also used to examine the association between demographic characteristics of the sample and travel mode to work. Then, logistic regression was used to investigate the association of travel mode to work with self-reported stress ("more stressful" vs "about the same"/"less stressful"), adjusting for age, sex, clinical or non-clinical role, and adequate weekly physical activity (150 min/week). Odds ratios (ORs) and adjusted odds ratios (AORs) with 95% confidence intervals (CIs) were estimated as a measure of strength of association.

## 10.5   Findings

### 10.5.1   Participant Characteristics and Travel Behaviour

Table 10.1 below shows the characteristics of hospital staff who participated in the survey by active travel status. Overall 804 hospital employees participated in the initial survey (25% response rate), while 675 respondents provided data on the items of interest for this analysis. Approximately one in six respondents (15%) actively commuted to work (walking 4%, cycling 2% or using public transport 9%). Active travelers were almost twice as likely to be older than middle aged (i.e. greater than 55 years), and 60% more likely to work in an administrative rather than a clinical role.

Comparing respondents in the survey to the Sydney region, overall Sydney has a low level of active travel to work, but it varies by proximity to the central business district. Inner city areas have the highest levels of walking (10.1%) and cycling (2.2%) journeys to work (Zander et al. 2013a, b). In the outer areas of Sydney, where this study was conducted, active commuting is much lower at 2.6% of journey being by walking and 0.59% of journeys by bicycle (Zander et al. 2013a, b).

**Table 10.1** Characteristics of hospital staff in south west Sydney 2011 by active travel status

|                                | N   | Non-active (%) | Active travel (%) | P     |
| ------------------------------ | --- | -------------- | ----------------- | ----- |
| Sex                            |     |                |                   |       |
| Males                          | 156 | 81.0           | 16.9              | 0.104 |
| Females                        | 489 | 86.3           | 11.6              |       |
| Age                            |     |                |                   |       |
| 18–34 years                    | 177 | 83.1           | 16.9              | 0.024 |
| 35–54 years                    | 351 | 88.4           | 11.6              |       |
| 55+ years                      | 116 | 78.6           | 21.4              |       |
| Physical activity              |     |                |                   |       |
| Insufficient physical activity | 290 | 84.2           | 15.8              | 0.728 |
| Sufficient physical activity   | 337 | 85.1           | 14.9              |       |
| Occupation                     |     |                |                   |       |
| Administrative                 | 268 | 81.1           | 18.9              | 0.012 |
| Clinical                       | 380 | 88.2           | 11.8              |       |

## 10.5.2   Stress and the Work Commute

One in five respondents (20.5%) said that compared to the rest of their working day, their commute was more stressful. When compared between car commuters and active travel commuters, car commuters reported a higher level of stress, with 26.1% saying the commute trip was more stressful than the rest of their day, while active commuters reported a lower rate of stress (10.1% saying the trip was more stressful than the rest of their day).

Table 10.2 shows that after adjusting for the individual's gender, age physical activity levels and occupational role; active commuters were significantly less likely to report that their commute to work was more stressful than the rest of their day than car commuters. This result was highly statistically significant (AOR 0.35, 95% CI 0.17–0.73). Interestingly, age, sex, physical activity and occupational role were not associated with reporting a greater amount of stress on the journey to work.

**Table 10.2** Odds ratios and adjusted odds ratios of reporting more stressful commuting using multiple logistic regression among hospital staff in South West Sydney 2011

| | N[a] (Total n = 675) | % reporting commuting was the more stressful part of the day | Odds ratio | 95% CI | Adjusted odds ratio[b] | 95% CI |
|---|---|---|---|---|---|---|
| Motor vehicle travel | 576 | 25.0 | 1.0 | | 1.0 | |
| Active travel | 99 | 10.1 | 0.34 | 0.17–0.67 | 0.35* | 0.17–0.73 |
| Males | 156 | 22.4 | 1.0 | | 1.0 | |
| Females | 489 | 22.5 | 0.99 | 0.65–1.54 | 0.95 | 0.60–1.52 |
| 18–34 years | 177 | 20.3 | 1.0 | | 1.0 | |
| 35–54 years | 351 | 24.8 | 1.29 | 0.83–2.00 | 1.20 | 0.76–1.89 |
| 55+ years | 116 | 19.0 | 0.92 | 0.51–1.66 | 0.72 | 0.37–1.40 |
| Insufficient physical activity | 290 | 23.5 | 1.0 | | 1.0 | |
| Sufficient physical activity | 337 | 22.6 | 0.95 | 0.65–1.38 | 0.93 | 0.63–1.37 |
| Administrative | 268 | 20.9 | 1.0 | | 1.0 | |
| Clinical position | 380 | 23.7 | 1.17 | 0.81–1.71 | 1.15 | 0.77–1.73 |

*P < 0.05
[a]May not add up to 675 due to missing data
[b]Adjusted for other variables in the table

## 10.6   Lessons Learned

The large (15%) difference between active commuters' and car commuters' perceptions that the commute to work was more stressful than the rest of their day remained statistically significant after adjusting for factors including gender, age, physical activity levels and occupational type (clinical vs non-clinical). These findings support international research which has shown that active travel to work may be less stressful than car commuting. Car commuting stress has been found to be associated with increased negative moods on arrival at work and the home, lower tolerance threshold, cognitive impairment, greater illness and work absenteeism, job instability and a negative effect on overall life satisfaction (Novaco and Gonzalez 2009). Many of the impedances that have been associated with car commuting stress, such as traffic congestion, have lower impact on active travel modes of transport. For example, in a UK study, where commuting by private car was found to be stressful, walking and cycling by comparison, were found to be relaxing and exciting experiences (Gatersleben and Uzzell 2007).

This case study sought to adjust for the different influences of age, gender, physical activity and the nature of respondents' jobs which might have influence both on their commuting choices and the level of stress they might experience within the work environment. The sample of participants included in this survey were slightly disparate so that active travelers were more likely to be older and have an administrative role. Our data do not answer questions about whether administrative or clinical staff have more stressful jobs, and this may prove to be important in determining the relative stress of mode of travel. Whilst the regression model did adjust for clinical versus non-clinical roles, and a simplistic view may be that some clinical roles might be quite stressful due to high job demands, these roles may also have high levels of job control so on balance the levels of stress may in fact be as high as some administrative roles which have both a high job demand and low levels of perceived job control. We do not have an occupational delineation that allows us to describe in more detail the nature of the work respondents did. Such a study may consider the job demand and job control aspects of different work roles to attain a holistic understanding of stress within the workplace and enroute to work and to better determine the impact of stress and the role of active travel (Jones and Bright 2001).

One of the strengths of this case study is that it was the first time that the association of different travel modes with self-reported stress was confirmed in the Australian transport context. However, the findings of the case study presented was limited by being just one snapshot in time, and this prohibits the assertion of causal relationship. The generalisability of the study findings are also limited due to the study being conducted among hospital staff in southwest Sydney, where the results may be specific to the south-western Sydney transport context. Although, transport studies are always strongly influenced by the local transport and geographical contexts, and these contexts have been described in this chapter and in journal articles associated with the study so that readers can decide if the results are applicable to their local settings (Petrunoff et al. 2013a, 2016a, 2017) The results are also consistent with studies in the USA and other car-centric countries, and add to this relatively sparse area of research (Gatersleben and Uzzell 2007; Gottholmseder et al. 2009). Another limitation was that the sample consisted mostly of women, which is typical of healthcare services in Australia. Women in Australia are less likely to be active commuters than men, (Rissel et al. 2014a) so active travel rates may be lower than in other workplaces.

Assessing the association between active travel mode with self-reported stress with the work commute has important public health implications. A positive relationship between active commuting and lower levels of stress during the commute to work is likely to necessitate support for allocation of funding of infrastructure, policies and programs which support active commuting. This will also have implications for health and wellbeing within the workplace and may lead to greater work productivity and reduced absenteeism however these findings need to be assessed over time.

The findings of this case study form part of a larger piece of research to evaluate the effects of the 3-year workplace travel plan to encourage hospital workers to commute to work by active travel means. The study concluded that a workplace travel plan which included strategies to encourage active travel to work achieved significant increases in active travel (Petrunoff et al. 2016). How interventions like workplace travel plans might impact quality of life beyond the construct of stress is a question which may be investigated as part of future research.

While these findings support the evidence that commuting to work by car is more stressful than other modes of travel the next step is to be able to test the causal association by following participants over time to track these effects and, to determine how important transport for the work commute is to health outcomes such as mental health and cardiovascular disease. This will allow for other factors that cannot be attributed to the role of physical activity to be investigated, such as enjoying the scenery, lack of frustration, or letting the mind drift while travelling, all of which are important factors in why people travel (Mokhtarian et al. 2015; Ory and Mokhtarian 2005).

Stress is an important measure for further consideration in how we value travel and appraise transport options. Increasingly, transport appraisals value transport based on satisfaction with the transport journey as a measure of transport-related wellbeing (Cantwell et al. 2009). This is good, yet investigations of the relationship between the journey to work and quality of life from a health perspective are rare, (Crane et al. 2016) and quality of life measures which capture the health effects of the various transport modes tend to be unsuitable for transport studies, as they are focused primarily on clinical-based measures of physical functioning. Likewise a narrow focus on transport satisfaction to inform policy is a limitation and disregards the larger benefits of active travel to quality of life. To progress in an understanding of the journey to work, transport options and our quality of life, we need to better understand the impact at a broader level, considering not only transport and life satisfaction but measures of life experience such as stress and enjoyment (Rissel et al. 2016).

**Acknowledgments** We wish to convey our appreciation to members of the South Western Sydney and Sydney Health Promotion Services, who supported implementation of the main intervention study. Thanks also to the executives and staff from Liverpool Hospital in Sydney, who supported the study.

# References

Bamberg, S., & Möser, G. (2007). Why are work travel plans effective? Comparing conclusions from narrative and meta-analytical research synthesis. *Transportation, 34*(6), 647–666. https://doi.org/10.1007/s11116-007-9121-0.

Bhui, K. S., Dinos, S., Stansfeld, S. A., & White, P. D. (2012). A synthesis of the evidence for managing stress at work: A review of the reviews reporting on anxiety, depression, and absenteeism. *Journal of Environmental and Public Health, 2012*, 515874.

Booth, M. L., Ainsworth, B. E., Pratt, M., Ekelund, U., Yngve, A., Sallis, J. F., & Oja, P. (2003). International physical activity questionnaire: 12-country reliability and validity. *Medicine and Science in Sports and Exercise, 195*(9131/03), 3508–1381.

Brockman, R., & Fox, K. R. (2011). Physical activity by stealth? The potential health benefits of a workplace transport plan. *Public Health, 125*(4), 210–216. https://doi.org/10.1016/j.puhe.2011.01.005.

BTS. (2013). *2012/13 household travel survey summary report 2013 release*. NSW: Bureau of Transport Statistics. Retrieved from https://www.transport.nsw.gov.au/sites/default/files/media/documents/2017/HTS%20Report%20Sydney%202012-13.pdf

Cairns, S., Newson, C., & Davis, A. (2010). Understanding successful workplace travel initiatives in the UK. *Transportation Research Part A: Policy and Practice, 44*(7), 473–494. https://doi.org/10.1016/j.tra.2010.03.010.

Cantwell, M., Caulfield, B., & O'Mahony, M. (2009). Examining the factors that impact public transport commuting satisfaction. *Journal of Public Transportation, 12*(2), 1.

Celis-Morales, C. A., Lyall, D. M., Welsh, P., Anderson, J., Steell, L., Guo, Y., … Gill, J. M. R. (2017). Association between active commuting and incident cardiovascular disease, cancer, and mortality: Prospective cohort study. *BMJ, 357*. https://doi.org/10.1136/bmj.j1456

Crane, M., Rissel, C., Standen, C., & Greaves, S. (2014). Associations between the frequency of cycling and domains of quality of life. *Health Promotion Journal of Australia, 25*(3), 182–185. https://doi.org/10.1071/HE14053.

Crane, M., Rissel, C., Greaves, S., & Gebel, K. (2016). Correcting bias in self-rated quality of life: An application of anchoring vignettes and ordinal regression models to better understand QoL differences across commuting modes. *Quality of Life Research, 25*(2), 257–266. https://doi.org/10.1007/s11136-015-1090-8.

Dargay, J., Gately, D., & Sommer, M. (2007). Vehicle ownership and income growth, worldwide: 1960–2030. *The Energy Journal, 28*(4), 143–170. https://doi.org/10.2307/41323125.

De Gruyter, C., Rose, G., Currie, G., Rye, T., & van de Graaff, E. (2018). Travel plans for new developments: A global review. *Transport Reviews, 38*(2), 142–161.

Ding, D., Gebel, K., Phongsavan, P., Bauman, A. E., & Merom, D. (2014). Driving: A road to unhealthy lifestyles and poor health outcomes. *PLoS One, 9*(6), e94602. https://doi.org/10.1371/journal.pone.0094602.

Enoch, M. (2012). The development of the travel plan. In M. Enoch (Ed.), *Sustainable transport, mobility management and travel plans*. Surrey: Ashgate Publishing Limited.

Ettema, D., Friman, M., Gärling, T., Olsson, L. E., & Fujii, S. (2012). How in-vehicle activities affect work commuters' satisfaction with public transport. *Journal of Transport Geography, 24*, 215–222.

Flint, E., & Cummins, S. (2015). Does active commuting protect against obesity in mid-life? Cross-sectional, observational evidence from UK Biobank. *The Lancet, 386*(Supplement 2), S8. https://doi.org/10.1016/S0140-6736(15)00846-6.

Friman, M., Olsson, L. E., Ståhl, M., Ettema, D., & Gärling, T. (2017). Travel and residual emotional well-being. *Transportation Research Part F: Traffic Psychology and Behaviour, 49*, 159–176.

Gatersleben, B., & Uzzell, D. (2007). Affective appraisals of the daily commute comparing perceptions of drivers, cyclists, walkers, and users of public transport. *Environment and Behavior, 39*(3), 416–431.

Goodman, A. (2013). Walking, cycling and driving to work in the English and Welsh 2011 census: Trends, socio-economic patterning and relevance to travel behaviour in general. *PLoS One, 8* (8), e71790. https://doi.org/10.1371/journal.pone.0071790.

Gordon-Larsen, P., Boone-Heinonen, J., Sidney, S., Sternfeld, B., Jacobs, D. R., Jr., & Lewis, C. E. (2009). Active commuting and cardiovascular disease risk: The CARDIA study. *Archives of Internal Medicine, 169*(13), 1216–1223.

Gottholmseder, G., Nowotny, K., Pruckner, G. J., & Theurl, E. (2009). Stress perception and commuting. *Health Economics, 18*(5), 559–576.

Hansson, E., Mattisson, K., Björk, J., Östergren, P.-O., & Jakobsson, K. (2011). Relationship between commuting and health outcomes in a cross-sectional population survey in southern Sweden. *BMC Public Health, 11*(1), 834.

Higgins, T. (1996). How do we know employer-based transportation demand management works? The need for experimental design. *Transportation Research Record: Journal of the Transportation Research Board, 1564*, 54–59.

Hosking, J., Macmillan, A., Connor, J., Bullen, C., & Ameratunga, S. (2010). Organisational travel plans for improving health. *Cochrane Database of Systematic Reviews (Online), 3*, CD005575.

Jacobson, B. H., Aldana, S. G., Goetzel, R. Z., Vardell, K., Adams, T. B., & Pietras, R. J. (1996). The relationship between perceived stress and self-reported illness-related absenteeism. *American Journal of Health Promotion, 11*(1), 54–61.

Jones, F., & Bright, J. (2001). *Stress: Myth, theory and research*. London: Prentice Hall.

Kohl, H. W., 3rd, Craig, C. L., Lambert, E. V., Inoue, S., Alkandari, J. R., Leetongin, G., & Kahlmeier, S. (2012). The pandemic of physical inactivity: Global action for public health. *The Lancet, 380*(9838), 294–305. https://doi.org/10.1016/S0140-6736(12)60898-8.

Legrain, A., Eluru, N., & El-Geneidy, A. M. (2015). Am stressed, must travel: The relationship between mode choice and commuting stress. *Transportation Research Part F: Traffic Psychology and Behaviour, 34*, 141–151.

Macmillan, A. K., Hosking, J., Connor, J. L., Bullen, C., & Ameratunga, S. (2013). A Cochrane systematic review of the effectiveness of organisational travel plans: Improving the evidence base for transport decisions. *Transport Policy, 29*(0), 249–256. https://doi.org/10.1016/j.tranpol.2012.06.019.

Marsden, A., Tunny, G., & Fitzgibbons, A. (2011). *Evaluation of the travel smart local government and workplace programs*. Retrieved from Perth, Western Australia: http://www.transport.wa.gov.au/mediaFiles/active-transport/AT_TS_P_Evaluation_LocalGov_Workplace.pdf

Martin, A., Panter, J., Suhrcke, M., & Ogilvie, D. (2015). Impact of changes in mode of travel to work on changes in body mass index: Evidence from the British Household Panel Survey. *Journal of Epidemiology and Community Health, 69*(8), 753–761. https://doi.org/10.1136/jech-2014-205211.

Mattisson, K., Jakobsson, K., Håkansson, C., & Cromley, E. (2016). Spatial heterogeneity in repeated measures of perceived stress among car commuters in Scania, Sweden. *International Journal of Health Geographics, 15*(1), 22.

Mokhtarian, P. L., Salomon, I., & Singer, M. E. (2015). What moves us? An interdisciplinary exploration of reasons for traveling. *Transport Reviews, 35*(3), 250–274.

Møller, N. C., Østergaard, L., Gade, J. R., Nielsen, J. L., & Andersen, L. B. (2011). The effect on cardiorespiratory fitness after an 8-week period of commuter cycling—A randomized controlled study in adults. *Preventive Medicine, 53*(3), 172–177.

Mytton, O. T., Panter, J., & Ogilvie, D. (2016). Longitudinal associations of active commuting with body mass index. *Preventive Medicine, 90*, 1–7. https://doi.org/10.1016/j.ypmed.2016.06.014.

Newman, P., & Kenworthy, J. (2015). Urban transportation patterns and trends in global cities. In *The end of automobile dependence: How cities are moving beyond car-based planning* (pp. 33–76). Washington, DC: Island Press/Center for Resource Economics.

Nieuwenhuijsen, K., Bruinvels, D., & Frings-Dresen, M. (2010). Psychosocial work environment and stress-related disorders, a systematic review. *Occupational Medicine, 60*(4), 277–286.

Noblet, A., & LaMontagne, A. D. (2006). The role of workplace health promotion in addressing job stress. *Health Promotion International, 21*(4), 346–353.

Novaco, R. W., & Gonzalez, O. I. (2009). Commuting and well-being. In Y. Amichai-Hamburger (Ed.), *Technology and well-being* (Vol. 3, pp. 174–205). New York: Cambridge University Press.

OECD. (2013). *OECD skills outlook 2013*. OECD Publishing.

Ohta, M., Mizoue, T., Mishima, N., & Ikeda, M. (2007). Effect of the physical activities in leisure time and commuting to work on mental health. *Journal of Occupational Health, 49*(1), 46–52.

Ory, D. T., & Mokhtarian, P. L. (2005). When is getting there half the fun? Modeling the liking for travel. *Transportation Research Part A: Policy and Practice, 39*(2), 97–123.

Petrunoff, N., Rissel, C., Wen, L. M., Xu, H., Meikeljohn, D., & Schembri, A. (2013a). Developing a hospital travel plan: Process and baseline findings from a western Sydney hospital. *Australian Health Review, 37*(5), 579–584. 10.1071/AH13006.

Petrunoff, N., Xu, H., Rissel, C., Wen, L. M., & van der Ploeg, H. (2013b). Measuring workplace travel behaviour: Validity and reliability of survey questions. *Journal of Environmental and Public Health, 2013*, 6. https://doi.org/10.1155/2013/423035.

Petrunoff, N., Rissel, C., & Wen, L. M. (2016a). The effect of active travel interventions conducted in work settings on driving to work: A systematic review. *Journal of Transport & Health, 3*(1), 61–76. https://doi.org/10.1016/j.jth.2015.12.001.

Petrunoff, N., Wen, L. M., & Rissel, C. (2016b). Effects of a workplace travel plan intervention encouraging active travel to work: outcomes from a three year time-series study. *Public Health, 135*, 38–47.

N. Petrunoff, L.M. Wen, C. Rissel, (2016) Effects of a workplace travel plan intervention encouraging active travel to work: outcomes from a three-year time-series study. Public Health 135:38-47

Petrunoff, N., Rissel, C., & Wen, L. M. (2017). "If You Don't Do Parking Management.. Forget Your Behaviour Change, It's Not Going to Work.": Health and transport practitioner perspectives on workplace active travel promotion. *PLoS One, 12*(1), e0170064.

Popuri, Y., Proussaloglou, K., Ayvalik, C., Koppelman, F., & Lee, A. (2011). Importance of traveler attitudes in the choice of public transportation to work: Findings from the Regional Transportation Authority Attitudinal Survey. *Transportation, 38*(4), 643–661.

Qualtrics. (2017). Qualtrics survey software. Retrieved from www.qualtrics.com

Rissel, C. (2010). Cycling connecting communities: Bicycle route map for fairfield and liverpool. Retrieved from https://cyclingconnectingcommunities.files.wordpress.com/2010/08/bicycle-route-map-fairfield-liverpool-2010.pdf

Rissel, C., Greenaway, M., Bauman, A., & Wen, L. M. (2014a). Active travel to work in New South Wales 2005–2010, individual characteristics and association with body mass index. *Australian and New Zealand Journal of Public Health, 38*(1), 25–29.

Rissel, C., Petrunoff, N., Wen, L., & Crane, M. (2014b). Travel to work and self-reported stress: Findings from a workplace survey in south west Sydney, Australia. *Journal of Transport & Health, 1*(1), 50–53.

Rissel, C., Crane, M., Wen, L. M., Greaves, S., & Standen, C. (2016). Satisfaction with transport and enjoyment of the commute by commuting mode in inner Sydney. *Health Promotion Journal of Australia, 27*(1), 80–83.

Rye, T., Green, C., Young, E., & Ison, S. (2011a). Using the land-use planning process to secure travel plans: An assessment of progress in England to date. *Journal of Transport Geography, 19* (2), 235–243. https://doi.org/10.1016/j.jtrangeo.2010.05.002.

Rye, T., Welsch, J., Plevnik, A., & de Tommasi, R. (2011b). First steps towards cross-national transfer in integrating mobility management and land use planning in the EU and Switzerland. *Transport Policy, 18*(3), 533–543. https://doi.org/10.1016/j.tranpol.2010.10.008.

Safe, Work, & Australia. (2013). *The incidence of accepted workers' compensation claims for mental stress in Australia.* Canberra: Safe Work Australia. Retrieved from https://www.safeworkaustralia.gov.au/system/files/documents/1702/the-incidence-accepted-wc-claims-mental-stress-australia.pdf

Sahlqvist, S., Song, Y., & Ogilvie, D. (2012). Is active travel associated with greater physical activity? The contribution of commuting and non-commuting active travel to total physical activity in adults. *Preventive Medicine, 55*(3), 206–211.

Sato, K. K., Hayashi, T., Kambe, H., Nakamura, Y., Harita, N., Endo, G., & Yoneda, T. (2007). Walking to work is an independent predictor of incidence of type 2 diabetes in Japanese men: The Kansai Healthcare Study. *Diabetes Care, 30*(9), 2296–2298.

St-Louis, E., Manaugh, K., van Lierop, D., & El-Geneidy, A. (2014). The happy commuter: A comparison of commuter satisfaction across modes. *Transportation Research Part F: Traffic Psychology and Behaviour, 26*, 160–170.

Sugiyama, T., Ding, D., & Owen, N. (2012). Sitting in cars for commuting and adults' weight gain over four years. *Journal of Science and Medicine in Sport, 15*, S72. https://doi.org/10.1016/j.jsams.2012.11.173.

Sugiyama, T., Ding, D., & Owen, N. (2013). Commuting by car: Weight gain among physically active adults. *American Journal of Preventive Medicine, 44*(2), 169–173.

Wanner, M., Gotschi, T., Martin-Diener, E., Kahlmeier, S., & Martin, B. W. (2012). Active transport, physical activity, and body weight in adults: A systematic review. *American Journal of Preventive Medicine, 42*(5), 493–502. https://doi.org/10.1016/j.amepre.2012.01.030.

Wen, L. M., Orr, N., Millett, C., & Rissel, C. (2006). Driving to work and overweight and obesity: Findings from the 2003 New South Wales Health Survey, Australia. *International Journal of Obesity, 30*(5), 782–786. https://doi.org/10.1038/sj.ijo.0803199.

Wennberg, P., Lindahl, B., Hallmans, G., Messner, T., Weinehall, L., Johansson, L., ... Jansson, J. H. (2006). The effects of commuting activity and occupational and leisure time physical activity on risk of myocardial infarction. *European Journal of Cardiovascular Prevention & Rehabilitation, 13*(6), 924–930.

Wheatley, D. (2014). Travel-to-work and subjective well-being: A study of UK dual career households. *Journal of Transport Geography, 39*, 187–196.

WHO. (2010). *Global recommendations on physical activity for health.* Geneva: World Health Organisation.

WHO/UN-HABITAT. (2010). *Hidden cities: Unmasking and uncovering health inequities in urban cities.* Geneva: World Health Organisation. Retreived from http://www.who.int/kobe_centre/publications/hiddencities_media/who_un_habitat_hidden_cities_web.pdf

Wynne, L. (2015). *Can we integrate land-use and transport planning? An investigation into the use of travel planning regulation.* Paper presented at the 21st International Conference on Urban Transport and the Environment, Spain. http://www.witpress.com/elibrary/wit-transactions-on-the-built-environment/146/34078

Xu, H., Wen, L. M., & Rissel, C. (2013). The relationships between active transport to work or school and cardiovascular health or body weight: A systematic review. *Asia-Pacific Journal of Public Health, 25*(4), 298–315. https://doi.org/10.1177/1010539513482965.

Yang, L., Panter, J., Griffin, S. J., & Ogilvie, D. (2012). Associations between active commuting and physical activity in working adults: Cross-sectional results from the Commuting and Health in Cambridge study. *Preventive Medicine, 55*(5), 453–457.

Zander, A., Rissel, C., & Bauman, A. (2013a). *Cycling to work in sydney: Analysis of journey-to-work census data from 2001 and 2011.* Camperdown: University of Sydney. Retrieved from http://sydney.edu.au/medicine/public-health/prevention-research/news/Cycling%20to%20work%20in%20Sydney%202001%202011_b.pdf

Zander, A., Rissel, C., Rogers, K., & Bauman, A. (2013b). *Walking to work in Sydney: Analysis of journey-to-work Census data from 2001 and 2011.* Camperdown: University of Sydney. Retrieved from http://sydney.edu.au/medicine/public-health/prevention-research/news/reports/Walking%20to%20work%202001-2011.pdf

# Chapter 11
# Transport and Child Well-Being: Case Study of Quebec City

E. Owen D. Waygood

**Abstract** Transport affects children's well-being differently than adults. This is due to, amongst other things, their restricted use of motorized vehicles. The concept of well-being itself may also be different for children with the addition of cognitive and economic added to the usual physical, psychological, and social domains. Lastly, transport can interact with well-being through access to destinations (traditional concept of transport), during transport (recent considerations), and as an external impact (e.g. danger, air quality, etc.). Different modes will have different impacts on children's well-being, and the use of these modes is known to be different by contexts such as the built environment. In this chapter, a summary is given of how past research has shown links between those five domains of well-being through the three means-of-influence. Then, a case study of children's (aged 9–12 in grade 5 classes) travel in Quebec City, Canada will be examined with respect to those five domains of well-being by mode and built environment. The schools were located in three different types of built environments and children completed travel diaries for all trips during a day. Measures related to all five domains of well-being are examined by mode and built environment. Findings suggest a number of advantages with respect to active and independent travel, with some variation found by built environment type.

**Keywords** Children's travel · Well-being · Physical · Social · Psychological · Cognitive · Economic · Independent mobility · Built environment

## 11.1 Introduction

Transport's impacts on children are not the same as for adults. Children do not legally have access to personal motor vehicles, which are often the primary concern of transport planners (e.g. Gilbert and O'Brien 2005). Their trips are not valued

E. O. D. Waygood (✉)
Laval University, Quebec City, Canada
e-mail: Owen.Waygood@esad.ulaval.ca

© Springer International Publishing AG, part of Springer Nature 2018
M. Friman et al. (eds.), *Quality of Life and Daily Travel*, Applying Quality of Life
Research, https://doi.org/10.1007/978-3-319-76623-2_11

(or not equivalently valued) by transport planning that focuses on value of time. They are not physically as tall as adults (generally), and so cars parked by intersections can limit their line of sight, but also hide them from oncoming traffic. The fear of traffic danger can limit their personal independent mobility. They seem to be more susceptible to lung problems from traffic-based air pollution (e.g. Boothe and Shendell 2008). The experience of travel is also different as exploring one's neighborhood and finding friends to pass time with are perhaps more important or desired by children. These examples are just a few that highlight why transport planning that only (or predominantly) considers adults may fall short of providing systems that function well for marginalized groups such as children.

Transport is traditionally seen as a derived demand, facilitating the access to destinations that contribute to a child's quality of life such as sports, leisure, and education. Relationships such as active travel (travel that involves human effort such as walking, cycling, skateboarding, etc.) as a contribution to physical health have received much attention in the past few years as concerns about childhood obesity have increased (e.g. Schoeppe et al. 2013; Sirard and Slater 2008). Transport can directly take the life of a child through vehicle crashes and collisions and is the number one cause of death of youth around the world (Toroyan and Peden 2007) and Canada is no exception (Gilbert and O'Brien 2005; Waygood et al. 2015). Those three examples demonstrate how transport affects child well-being as a means of access, intrinsic impacts through the mode itself, and how transport has external (the transport decisions of others) impacts.

**Key Point** *Transport affects child well-being through access to activities, through the mode used, and through the external impacts due to others' transport choices.*

The previous examples are frequently studied in children's transport research. This is likely because death is the most severe impact possible and thus data is collected in most every country, transport as a means of access is studied to improve access to activities (though the emphasis is typically put on adults' travel Gilbert and O'Brien 2005), and the minutes of active travel are either directly captured through travel surveys or can be imputed through distances. However, child well-being is not limited to these impacts.

Transport affects children's health and well-being in a multitude of ways (Waygood et al. 2017). The definition of health and well-being is somewhat elusive, but the World Health Organisation gave this definition "a state of complete physical, mental, and social well-being and not merely the absence of disease or infirmity" in 1948.[1] This reflects modern definitions of well-being where the physical, psychological, and social domains are included (e.g. Dodge et al. 2012). Pollard and Lee (2003) in a review of work on child well-being expanded that to include cognitive (a sub-domain of psychology) and economic domains. Pollard and Lee (p.64) define the differences as: "The psychological domain includes indicators that pertain to

---

[1]http://www.who.int/about/mission/en/

emotions, mental health, or mental illness, while the cognitive domain includes those indicators that are considered intellectual or school-related in nature."

**Definition** *Child well-being includes impacts on their physical, psychological, cognitive, social, and economic condition.*

This chapter will give a brief overview of some of the different impacts on children's well-being for each of those domains and by each of the means-of-influence (access, intrinsic, external). It will then use data from a survey conducted with children in Quebec City, Canada that included questions related to each domain.


## 11.2  Background Literature

This is not the first work to examine links between transport (Hillman 1993) or the built environment (Lennard and Lennard 2000) with child well-being or quality of life. As well, research exists that has considered children in urban environments (Davis and Jones 1996), or children and planning (Gilbert and O'Brien 2005; Matthews and Limb 1999). Hillman edited a book (Hillman 1993) containing a collection of articles that deal with many of the topics to be discussed and analysed in this chapter. That work includes both empirical work and think pieces related to safety, children's rights, mental development, independent and escorted travel, and a consideration to costs to society (here, congestion).

Lennard and Lennard (2000) took an architectural approach relating many of their arguments to social and community interaction, amongst others. It discusses issues such as legibility (similar to wayfinding), a variety of uses in one place, the urban environment as a place of social learning, attitudes towards providing public space for children, the role of social capital, and events and improvements that can create a better urban environment for children and adults. The book itself is mostly a think piece making links between sociology and urban form with little empirical evidence of differences by urban form. As a think piece though, it raises many good points that could be incorporated into the built form that would likely improve the quality of life of children.

Davis and Jones (1996) wrote one of the more interesting and compelling arguments on this topic over 20 years ago. They examined children in the urban environment from a public health perspective. They focus on the differences between needs, perceptions, and affordances between children and adults in urban settings. They make important arguments that rather than blaming the victims, children, it would be better to manipulate the built environment rather than children. As well, they put forward compelling points on how children needs are less quantified and are thus largely ignored in policy and development that focuses on adult needs. One example given is that children are taught to be fearful of traffic, but the cause of the problem, traffic is encouraged through promotion of mobility (speed).

Finally, Matthews and Limb (1999) convincingly argue that much of Western planning focuses on the needs of one group, "white, ableist, adult, male, middle-class." The write that much "strong groups exert maximum preferences, and weaker groups are pushed to less desirable environs in place". This is likely evident in how streets are no longer seen as a place for children to play, but rather a place for those with access to vehicles to use to their advantage at the expense of other uses. As such, they argue that children are a sociospatial marginalized group. As well they emphasize key differences between children and adults: rhythms of time and space; use of land and facilities; independent mobility is restricted due to money, physical capabilities, caretaking conventions, etc.; threats are different (e.g. with air quality); even in the same environment, interpretation and perceptions are different; and finally, they are unable to influence decision-makers.

Gilbert and O'Brien (2005) make a similar argument to Matthews and Limb (1999) in their work from 2005. They highlight that planning focuses on the needs of adults, which likely leads to a system where children are more and more dependent on adults for their transport. They argue that children's travel is typically by active transport, which is often not favoured in transportation planning as the emphasis is on speed and moving vehicular traffic. The result though is that children's trips move from active transport to motorised transport, creating more traffic. In their work, they discuss numerous links between transport and child well-being including crashes, financial implications, social interactions, amongst others though the points are not always supported by empirical evidence. The report however offers many constructive guidelines that should be incorporated by transportation planners.

A recent integrative review was conducted with the aim of examining how transport affects child well-being in a holistic way (i.e. include all the domains of well-being) (Waygood et al. 2017). It found research that demonstrates a relationship between transport and each of the domains of well-being. Further to that, for nearly all domains of well-being, an association was found for each of the three transport means-of-influence. Not all of those findings can be discussed here, but relationships for each domain of well-being will be given.

## 11.2.1   Physical Well-Being

Along with crashes and active travel, transport can affect children's physical well-being in a number of ways. Transport is a means of access to activities outside the home. Active travel was associated with more leisure activities while children's independent mobility (CIM) was associated with more physical activities (Schoeppe et al. 2013). As such, facilitating active and independent travel for children may increase their participation in activities outside the home.

Intrinsic relationships included active travel contributing to overall greater physical activity, though its relationship with obesity is unclear (Schoeppe et al. 2013). A number of other anecdotal (single studies) associations were found for air quality inside school buses (due to exhaust from the bus, but also traffic) (Behrentz et al. 2005) and cars (due to smoking) (Sendzik et al. 2009).

External relationships are significant in that they relate to sickness and death, be it through crashes or air quality. As mentioned, crashes are the primary cause of death for children and youth around the world. Traffic is related to increased blood pressure (Paunovic et al. 2011), childhood asthma (Beatty and Shimshack 2014), and childhood leukemia (Carlos-Wallace et al. 2016). As such, serious consideration must be taken in transport planning to reduce traffic where people live and limit the problem of environmental justice where those who are suffering the problem of traffic are not those creating the traffic.

### 11.2.2   Psychological Well-Being

Psychological impacts of transport may be less obvious and more difficult to measure. Likely as a consequence on that, they are less frequently measured and examined. However, research does exist that relates to this topic. Unlike the physical domain, sufficient research has not been conducted to warrant reviews focused on these different relationships.

As a means of access, transport can improve positive affect (emotions) if it allows the child to access activities that improve or elicit such emotions (Barker 2006). A lack of independent mobility (CIM) was associated with loneliness in children (Pacilli et al. 2013). However, the overall influence of transport on children's life satisfaction is unclear.

A common phrase is "getting there is half the fun" which would mean that the trip itself could have positive psychological impacts. This was born out with studies finding that enjoying the trip was related to walking and positive affect was associated with active modes (Ramanathan et al. 2014). Positive self-esteem was found to be related to children who cycled. However, it was also found that children and adults manage their emotions with respect to mode choices (Jensen et al. 2014). School buses were found to be an emotional battleground (Murray and Mand 2013) and passive modes (here motorized) were more likely to be associated with negative emotions (Ramanathan et al. 2014). Along with increasing stress during trips by passive modes, travel by car and longer trips were associated with negative trip satisfaction (Westman et al. 2017). Thus, positive psychological outcomes were associated mostly with active modes, whereas more negative associations were found for motorized ones.

The majority of external impacts related to crashes, though one traffic noise was consistently found to be an annoyance (Babisch et al. 2012). After suffering a collision, children were found to suffer travel anxiety, travel avoidance, sleep problems or nightmares, their independent mobility was restricted by parents, and finally, children were found to be suffering post-traumatic stress disorder following collisions (Bryant et al. 2004; Ellis et al. 1998).

Although less thoroughly (or repeatedly) studied, transport has the potential to have positive or negative psychological impacts on children's well-being. This is an area of study to develop.

### 11.2.3   Cognitive Well-Being

For cognitive development, access to areas where learning occurs would be one means of measuring this. Transport to school is one obvious measure, but the primary focus of such research is on what mode is used. Some research has examined the different relationships on access to non-local schools as those may provide specializations or better quality. Such relationships often depend on the cultural approach to school facilities such as school siting, financing, and beliefs about what is best for the child. Whether all children can access a range of schools will also depend on the options for independent travel unless a parent has the capacity (time, money) to provide chauffeuring to non-local destinations (Ewing et al. 2004; Torres et al. 2010; Waygood 2010).

For intrinsic impacts, walking was associated with exploring one's environment (Tranter and Pawson 2001) and also positive learning experiences (Kullman 2014), the latter also being associated with CIM (Björklid 2004). Walking alone was also highlighted by some children as a means to think and ponder the world (Romero 2010). Children who came to school by bicycle reported being more alert than those who came by car (Westman et al. 2013). Finally, a number of associations are found between the modes and different measures of mental maps that children have drawn, however there were not consistent findings related to the different modes (Ahmadi and Taniguchi 2007; Joshi et al. 1999).

External impacts on cognitive well-being were limited to negatively affecting reading speed and basic math exercises (Ljung et al. 2009). However, reading comprehension and math reasoning were not found to be affected. It is not clear if this is an understudied relationship or whether studies have been conducted but due to non-significant results were not published. Recently though, research found that smaller cognitive development was associated with higher traffic-related air pollution (Sunyer et al. 2015).

### 11.2.4   Social Well-Being

Children's independent mobility was found to be positively associated with an increase of access to friends (Lim and Barton 2010). Depending on the leisure or physical activity, these could also be considered as means of accessing friends, interacting with members of the public, or cultural learning (which was considered by Pollard and Lee (2003) as a measure of social well-being). Children often want to seek out places where real life is happening, where friends or adults might be

(Banerjee et al. 2014). They do not want to be reliant on parents to facilitate trips to meet friends (Berg and Medrich 1980).

Social interaction with peers was seen as a desirable attribute of travel (Murray and Mand 2013; Romero 2010), and walking was seen by children as an opportunity to socialize with peers (Kirby and Inchley 2013; Zwerts et al. 2010) and this positive association was found in other research. Social capital was found to be developed through CIM (Weller and Bruegel 2009), and community relationships (Panter et al. 2008) and incidental interaction were positively associated to walking (Waygood and Friman 2015; Waygood and Kitamura 2009).

Traffic was found to limit play and social interaction and led to mostly supervised play in low density locations (Berg and Medrich 1980; Holt et al. 2008). Crashes can be considered a negative life event affecting social well-being as children's CIM was found to be limited, which is associated with greater social capital (Bryant et al. 2004; Ellis et al. 1998). Finally, long commute times were not found to reduce time with children, which the authors suggest demonstrates the value of such time for parents (Whitehead-Frei and Kockelman 2010).

### 11.2.5   Economic Well-Being

In Pollard and Lee's (2003) review of child well-being research, they included a domain of economic well-being. For those researchers, this was the amount of financial child support available. In the integrative review of transport and child well-being by Waygood et al. (2017), they considered that CIM was a measure of economic well-being as it reduced the time burden of chauffeuring on parents who are more likely to work to earn income for the household. Mitra (2013) discussed many influences on independent travel to schools. The results included: chauffeuring increased if parents viewed driving as convenient and socially acceptable; and reduced distances to destinations were positively associated with increased CIM. Car-based development was found to increase serve-passenger trips, thus suggesting a greater dependence of children on their parents for transport in such areas (Waygood 2011).

### 11.2.6   Summary

Adults may associate freedom with cars, but for children freedom is active and independent travel (which would include public transport). The research introduced above finds that facilitating active and independent travel could have numerous benefits to children's well-being in all domains. Increased travel by motor vehicles was found to have numerous negative impacts on children's health and well-being. Any development that facilitates increased traffic and speed of private motor vehicles must take this into consideration.

## 11.3   Study Case

Children's travel in Quebec City, Canada will be considered here with respect to different well-being measures. Quebec is the capital city of the province of Quebec in Canada. The City of Quebec had a population of 516,620[2] in 2011 and the metropolitan area in 2014 had a population of 800,900.[3] For the metropolitan area of Quebec City, over 85% of trips to work were by car.[4] In the central part of the city, this is reduced to 27–58%, depending on the neighborhood. The city has a mid-high frequency bus system, Metrobus, with designated lanes in the many parts. However, the city also has a considerable amount of inner-city highways. For utilitarian cycling lanes are being added in the past few years.

In the context of Canada, active travel to elementary schools, based on data from 1996 to 2001, peaked at the age of 10 at under 35% (Pabayo et al. 2011). For the city of London, Ontario (a medium-sized city for Canada with a population of 512,400 in 2016[5]), Ontario 62% of children aged 11–13 used active modes to school, and 72% from school to home (Larsen et al. 2009).

### 11.3.1   Origin-Destination Survey of 2011

General trip data is available from the Origin-Destination Survey (OD Survey) of 2011 for the Quebec metropolitan area.[6] This is a one-day survey in the fall with a sample rate of 7.3% that is conducted by the minister of transport of Quebec (MTQ). The modal share (with population weighting) for the trip to school and for all trips for children aged 6–15 can be seen in Table 11.1. The average walking percentage for 9–11 year olds at 30.5% is lower than the national value found by Pabayo et al. (2011). Once age is taken into consideration, no statistical differences are observed for gender by mode.

The modal share also varies considerably by the built environment. The modal share (with population weighting) for children aged 6–15 by four different built environment types are shown in Fig. 11.1. These built environment types were developed using 17 different measures of the built environment (Ait Soussnae et al. 2015): land-use mix[7]; population density; percentage of roads at less than 50 km/h, at 50 km/h, and above 50 km/h; public parking, density of cycle paths

---

[2]https://www.ville.quebec.qc.ca/apropos/portrait/quelques_chiffres/

[3]http://www.statcan.gc.ca/tables-tableaux/sum-som/l01/cst01/demo05a-eng.htm

[4]http://atlasstat.cmquebec.qc.ca/atlasrecenspub/carto.php

[5]http://www.statcan.gc.ca/tables-tableaux/sum-som/l01/cst01/demo05a-eng.htm

[6]https://www.transports.gouv.qc.ca/fr/salle-de-presse/nouvelles/Pages/enquete-origine-destination.aspx

[7]Entropy measure based on land occupation by five different land uses: residential, civil, industrial, commercial, and recreational.

**Table 11.1** Modal share (%) by age groups for the *trip to school* and *all trips* (2011 Quebec City OD survey)

| Mode | Car | | School bus | | Public transport | | Walking | | Cycling | |
|---|---|---|---|---|---|---|---|---|---|---|
| Age | To school | All trips | To school | All trips | To school | All trips | To school | All trips | To school | All trips |
| 6–15 | 29.3 | 39.5 | 38.2 | 30.2 | 8.7 | 7.8 | 22.6 | 20.8 | 1.0 | .9 |
| 6–8 | 50.1 | 60.2 | 26.7 | 19.4 | .4 | .5 | 22.2 | 19.3 | .7 | .5 |
| 9–11 | 34.5 | 45.2 | 31.9 | 24.6 | 1.3 | 1.3 | 30.5 | 27.3 | 1.7 | 1.4 |
| 12 and 13 | 17.9 | 28.6 | 48.0 | 39.8 | 15.0 | 13.0 | 18.6 | 18.3 | .3 | .4 |
| 14 and 15 | 14.9 | 24.0 | 47.2 | 39.2 | 19.3 | 18.2 | 16.8 | 16.3 | 1.1 | 1.2 |

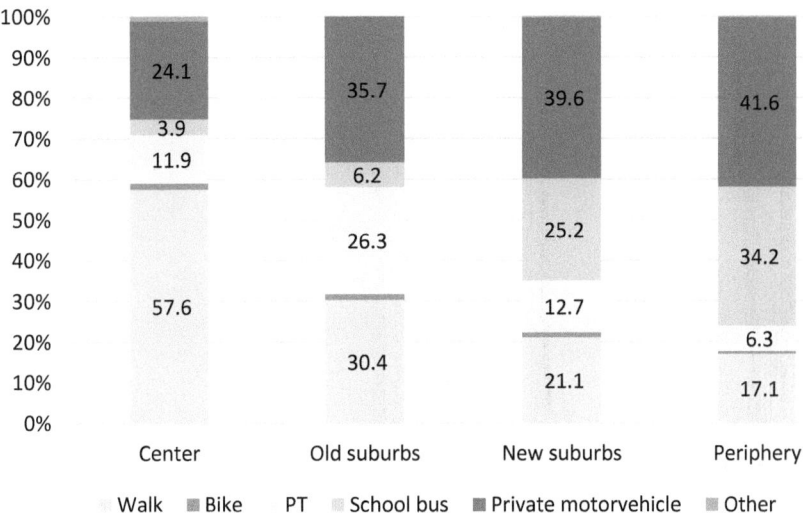

**Fig. 11.1** Modal share for children aged 6–15 across five different built environments

(linear km/km$^2$); ratio of length of sidewalks to road length; intersection density; number of commercial centers by scale (superregional, regional, city, quarter, neighborhood/local); total number of commercial buildings; big-box stores; and small stores. Average values for a sample of those characteristics are given in Table 11.2. Once the built environment is controlled for, the only statistical difference (at a 95% confidence level) by gender is observed for car trips (girls 10% more likely, $p = .032$).

As summarized in the Background, traffic is associated with many negative impacts on children. As such, the amount of traffic created by the different built environments is an important consideration. Previous research (Masters student team research project) (Ait Soussnae et al. 2015) examined the amount of traffic generated using the 2006 Origin-Destination data for Quebec City. Here, traffic is measured as

**Table 11.2** Seven measures of the built environment types used

|  | Mixed land-use | Population density | Intersection density | Sidewalk ratio | 50 km/h | Under 50 km/h | Bicycle path density |
|---|---|---|---|---|---|---|---|
| Center | .37 | 6088 | 101.1 | 1.81 | 88% | 7% | 2.88 |
| Old suburbs | .16 | 3297 | 58.6 | .81 | 85% | 4% | 3.58 |
| New suburbs | .27 | 1732 | 34.6 | .70 | 74% | 12% | 2.16 |
| Periphery | .11 | 1178 | 25.0 | .58 | 68% | 21% | 1.05 |

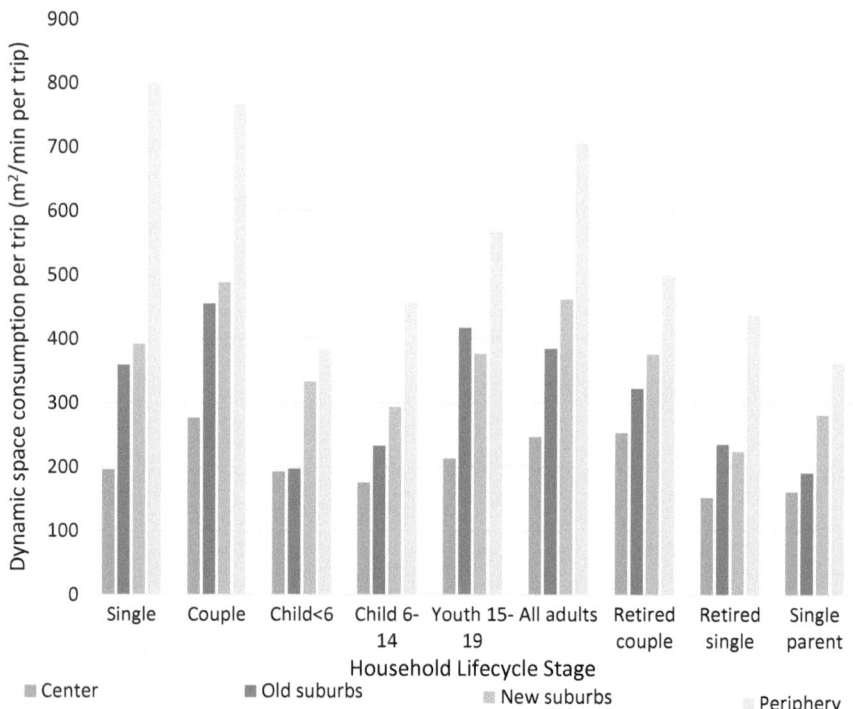

**Fig. 11.2** Dynamic space consumption per trip by household lifecycle stage

dynamic space consumption per trip by household lifecycle stage (Fig. 11.2). The results relate to mode and speed as a vehicle traveling at higher speed "consumes" more space as its stopping distance is larger. This means that no other person or vehicle can occupy that space (safely). For further detail see Héran et Ravalet (2008). In Fig. 11.2, it is clear that for nearly all household types, living in less urban areas is associated with greater traffic production.

In terms of well-being, it is of interest as well to see where children are going; what are children accessing. The percentage of trips for each type and the percentage

**Table 11.3**  Trip purpose by built environment type and by active travel for children aged 6–15

|  | Study | Leisure | Visit | Restaurant/café | Shopping | Serve passenger | Return home | Other |
|---|---|---|---|---|---|---|---|---|
| Centre | 41.4% | 3.7% | 2.1% | .6% | 2.7% | .6% | 45.4% | 3.5% |
| Old suburbs | 39.7% | 4.7% | 1.7% | .2% | 1.9% | 2.1% | 46.1% | 3.5% |
| New suburbs | 41.3% | 2.6% | .4% | .9% | 2.2% | 1.7% | 47.4% | 4.6% |
| Periphery | 40.6% | 3.8% | 1.5% | .4% | 1.8% | 1.7% | 47.2% | 2.9% |
| By active travel | 24.7% | 8.8% | 28.0% | 11.1% | 7.0% | 3.1% | 23.9% | 14.9% |

of those trips by active travel are shown in Table 11.3. Of note is that the children in the center are conducting more "visit" trips, and visit trips have the highest percentage of active travel trips. This is in-line with the relationships mentioned in the literature review. Superfluous traffic (serve passenger trips) is more commonly produced in the areas outside of the center and has the lowest active travel percentage.

## 11.4  Transport and Child Well-Being Survey

The data for this research comes from paper surveys distributed at elementary schools in Quebec, Canada in the fall of 2014 and 2015. In this study schools in all of the built environment types were sought out for participation so as to be able to examine outcomes with respect to that variable. The surveys included a general information section (individual and household characteristics, general travel behavior) and a travel diary for 1 weekday and 1 weekend day. The surveys were conducted at the school with one research assistant for each group of four or five students. In total, 307 students aged 9–12 in grade 5 classes across three different types of built environments completed usable travel diaries. Not all parents returned the consent forms and participation rates ranged from 50% to 100% (the majority of schools had over three quarters participation). The 100% participation rate was achieved by a teacher who introduced the study and requested participation on the meet-the-teacher night at the start of the school year. The 50% participation rate occurred in a class where the regular teacher fell ill and the students were not reminded to bring the consent form by the substitute teacher.

### 11.4.1  General Results

As compared to the OD Survey which included all households with a child aged between 6 and 15 years old, there are differences with the sample. In this sample, the

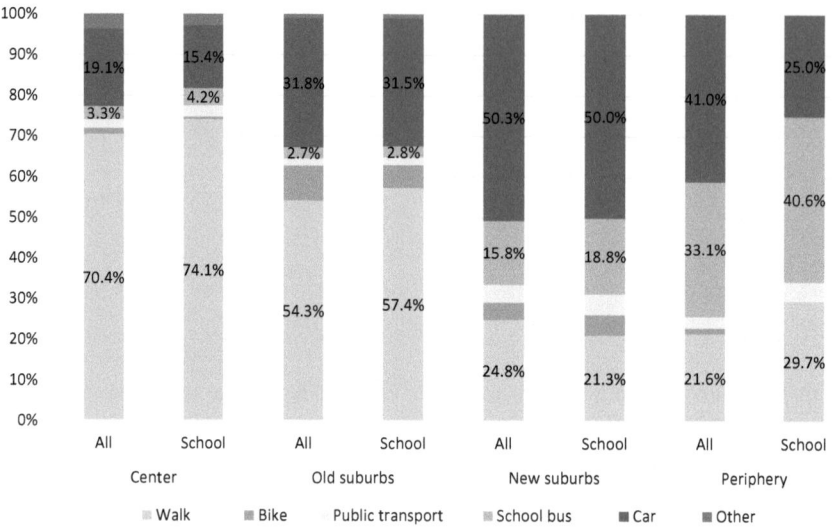

**Fig. 11.3** Modal share for all trips and trips to school for the participants of the study (aged 9–12)

influence of the built environment was a key consideration, which is why there is a more even distribution over the four types. The average Walk Score (walkscore. com) for the schools of each area are: center, 91.6; old suburbs, 58.6; new suburbs, 54.6; periphery, 21.2. The averages for key measures are as follows: female (46.2%), age (10.4 years), household members (4.6), car ownership (0 = 10.4%, 1 = 41.6%, 2 = 41.6%, 3 or more 6.3%). School trips represented 45.9% of all weekday trips.

The results here will be analyzed by mode and by built environment. First, as mentioned, active travel has a number of well-being benefits and the average modal share for all weekday trips can be seen across the four built environments in Fig. 11.3. The modal shares are statistically different for both trip types (i.e. to school, all trips).

As a measure of access, one can look at where children are going by the different modes in Fig. 11.4. For this sample of the population, one can see that active transport is used in most cases, except for access to structured leisure or sport activities. The largest variety in trip destinations was found in the center (14%), and the smallest in the periphery (9%).

Measures of the five domains of well-being are given in Table 11.4. For physical well-being, the number of minutes of active travel gained over the day are given. For social well-being three measures are available: travel with a friend, met a friend at the destination (excluding the trip to school), and saw a known person while travelling (for further details please see Waygood et al. 2017). Psychological well-being is captured by a 5-point measure of whether the trip itself was the worst or best imaginable and a 5-point measure of sad to happy for the activity at the destination. Cognitive well-being, a sub-domain of the psychological domain, is measured by a 5-point scale with the two extremes of bored to alert for activities and trips. The

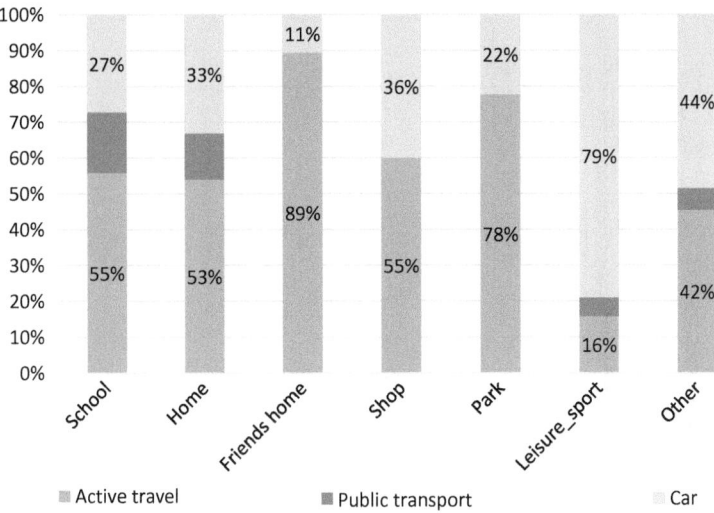

**Fig. 11.4** Mode of transport to different destinations

assumption here is that being more alert relates to a state of a more active brain. Independent travel is a measure of economic well-being as it frees to the parent to do other things. Here, as an additional cost to society, trips by school buses are included as a measure. The differences by mode of travel and built environment are shown in Table. Only significant results are discussed.

## 11.4.2   Physical Well-Being

As a measure of an intrinsic relationship between transport and physical health, the sum of active travel minutes over a day was used. The results find that as the built environment becomes less developed, the children had lower amounts of physical activity through their transport. Assuming that these are representative of normal weekday patterns, this would suggest that over the weekdays, children in the center have 1 h more of physical activity through transport then children in the new suburbs and periphery.

## 11.4.3   Social Well-Being

As a measure of access, the instance of meeting a friend at the destination was analyzed through binary logistic regression, but excluded the trip to school. For mode the results were statistically significant, though the built environment did not have statistically significant differences. For modes, trips by bus were half as likely

**Table 11.4** Differences by mode and built environment for measures of each domain of well-being

| | Physical | Social | | | Psychological | | Cognitive | | Economic | |
|---|---|---|---|---|---|---|---|---|---|---|
| | Active travel[a] (min.) | Travel with friend | Met friend at destination | Saw known person while travelling | Worst (1) to best (5) trip | Destination sad (1) to happy (5) | Bored (1) to Alert (5) | Destination bored (1) to alert (5) | Independent travel (% of all trips) | Trips to/from school by school bus |
| Active travel | – | 26.8% | 36.9% | 38.3% | 4.32 | 4.47 | 4.28 | 4.25 | – | – |
| Public/school bus | – | 42.9% | 22.7% | 40.6% | 3.85 | 3.80 | 3.90 | 3.90 | – | – |
| Car | – | 4.1% | 24.8% | 18.4% | 4.10 | 4.25 | 4.07 | 4.07 | – | – |
| Center | 18.5 | 21.3%[b] | 29.1%[b] | 26.4% | 4.34[b] | 4.43[b] | 4.33[b] | 4.15[b] | 64.3% | 5.6% |
| Old suburbs | 16.1[b] | 20.9%[b] | 34.5%[b] | 42.4% | 4.27[b] | 4.21[b] | 4.26[b] | 4.20[b] | 59.6%[b] | 5.9%[b] |
| New suburbs | 7.1 | 17.4%[b] | 25.7%[b] | 24.7%[b] | 4.24[b] | 4.36[b] | 4.16[b] | 3.98[b] | 38.8% | 22.7% |
| Periphery | 7.3 | 22.7%[b] | 22.2%[b] | 31.8%[b] | 4.12[b] | 4.25[b] | 4.19[b] | 3.76[b] | 22.1% | 26.1% |

[a]All trips by bus counted as 5 min of active travel (to/from stop)
[b]Not statistically different at a 95% confidence level (i.e. p > .05)

to be to a location where the child met a friend, and trips by car were 1.77 times less likely than active travel trips. Thus trips by active travel are much more associated with meeting up with friends.

As a measure of intrinsic relationships, travel with a friend was analyzed for mode of travel and for the built environment. The results for the built environment suggest there are no statistical differences between the areas. For the mode used, trips on public or school buses were twice as likely to be with a friend as active travel trips, while trips by car were 28 times less likely than active travel trips to be with a friend. Thus, it would seem that trips by car are the most isolated from friends. This is in line with comments from children in past research (Barker 2006).

A second measure of intrinsic relationship was included, the children were also asked whether they saw a known person while travelling as a measure related to social capital and community connections (Waygood and Friman 2015; Waygood et al. 2017b). There is an aspect of external relationship here as people need to be out to be seen (e.g. such as out walking). The results show that children going by bus were 1.14 times more likely than those going by active travel to see a known person, while children going by car were 2.76 times less likely than children going by active travel modes. This is in-line with other research from the domain of sociology such as Grannis (2011) where the vast majority of neighborhood connections were related to children's local travel such as walking to school or a bus stop. For the built environment, the analysis found that children in the old suburbs were two times more likely to see a known person than those in the center, but there was no statistical difference for children in the new suburbs and periphery as compared to those in the center.

### 11.4.4 Psychological Well-Being

As a measure of access, the children were asked how their activity at the destination made them feel on a five-point scale from sad to happy. The data were analyzed for mode excluding the trip to school as it is a "forced" destination for all students. Active transport was associated with activities that gave the greatest happiness with the differences between the modes being statistically significant. For the built environment the regression model did not find statistical differences between the types.

As an intrinsic measure, the children were asked to rate the trip as being from worst to best on a five-point scale. This measure from the Satisfaction of Travel Scale (Ettema et al. 2011) captures both affective and cognitive components. The measure was later developed and tested for children (STS-C; Westman et al. 2017). The analysis found statistical differences between active transport and the two other modes. Active travel modes were statistically associated with being better than the two other modes. The built environment did not play a statistically significant role.

## 11.4.5 Cognitive Well-Being

As a measure of access, whether the children rated the activity at the destination as making them bored or alert on a five-point scale was used. Unfortunately, the question was not included in the survey for roughly half of the schools. No statistical significance was found for either mode or the built environment.

As a measure of intrinsic influences, the children were asked the same question for during their trip. The analysis of all trips found that active travel was more associated with trips where the children were alert. The built environment was not found to be significant. Previous research had also found a statistical difference between active and passive modes with bicycling being statistically more associated with being alert than going by car (Westman et al. 2013).

## 11.4.6 Economic Well-Being

As an economic measure, the necessity of chauffeuring children (and thus using the parent's time) is measured through independent trips. The analysis found that children in the center and the old suburbs are not statistically different in their independence, but the children in the new suburbs are 2.84 times less likely to make independent trips of their parents and children in the periphery are 6.34 times less likely than those in the center.

As a measure of a cost to society through additional tax resources required, the percentage of school bus trips is also of interest (one could perhaps argue that trips by car also require more infrastructure than walking and cycling and contribute to congestion, danger, and other health costs, but that will not be directly considered here). Analysis found that children in the center and the old suburbs are not statistically different in their use of public school buses, but the children in the new suburbs are 5.0 times more likely to use a school bus and children in the periphery are 6.0 times more likely than those in the center.

## 11.5 Conclusion

The results of the case study in Quebec City, Canada show a rather consistent story (Table 11.4): active transport is more positively associated with all measures of well-being as compared to travel by car and in comparison to public transport for the psychological and cognitive measures. This continues to support the previous work highlighted in the integrative review by Waygood et al. (2017a) where active and independent travel was positively associated with many measures of well-being.

The built environment was significantly related to differences for a number of the measures. In all but one case, living in the center or older suburbs was associated with more positive outcomes. One distinction between those two built environments was the result where children in the old suburbs were twice as likely as those in center to see someone they know while travelling. This is perhaps in contrast to findings from previous research on this question (Waygood and Friman 2015) where the most urban areas were more associated with seeing a known person while making a trip. In terms of independent trips, most trips by children in the center and old suburbs were independent as opposed to the less urban areas. Few children in those central areas used school buses where as 23–26% of trips to and from school in the outer areas were by this service.

There are a number of ways to improve children's well-being related to transport which involve solutions at various levels and from various sectors. Individual efforts would relate to minimizing car use and using other modes with children to develop their knowledge and skills related to those modes. Walking seems particularly suited to children's curiosity and also to developing neighborhood connections. A change in policy in educational institutes might view the trip to school as part of the school day. The school would, in conjunction with Parent Teacher Associations, organize walking school buses such as the very successful systems developed in Japan which have run for over 50 years (Waygood et al. 2015). For municipalities, reducing speeds would improve safety which, along with reducing the likelihood of severe injury or death, would also be a step in the direction of returning streets to their public social use and not just as a through-put of traffic with the various negative health impacts (Huguenin-Richard 2010). At the planning and policy level, better integration between planning sectors (e.g. transport, land-use, housing) is needed as often important destinations such as sports and recreational facilities, but also child-care and educational facilities are not within walking distances of residences or are not developed at locations easily accessible by modes other than by car. This can lead to problems such as forced car ownership where a low income family may feel they are forced to by a car.

# References

Ahmadi, E., & Taniguchi, G. (2007). Influential factors on children's spatial knowledge and mobility in home-school travel – A case study in the city of Tehran. *Journal of Asian Architecture and Building Engineering, 6*, 275–282.

Ait Soussnae, I., Gagnon, A., & Ouchcham, B. (2015). L'étalement urbain et les transports durables: une contradiction? In Laval, U. (Ed.). Bibliothéque Bonenfant.

Babisch, W., Schulz, C., Seiwert, M., & Conrad, A. (2012). Noise annoyance as reported by 8- to 14-year-old children. *Environment and Behavior, 44*, 68–86.

Banerjee, T., Uhm, J., & Bahl, D. (2014). Walking to school the experience of children in inner city Los Angeles and implications for policy. *Journal of Planning Education and Research, 34*, 123–140.

Barker, J. (2006). *"Are we there yet?": Exploring aspects of automobility in children's lives.* Faculty of Geography and Earth Sciences. Brunel University.

Beatty, T. K., & Shimshack, J. P. (2014). Air pollution and children's respiratory health: A cohort analysis. *Journal of Environmental Economics and Management, 67*, 39–57.

Behrentz, E., Sabin, L. D., Winer, A. M., Fitz, D. R., Pankratz, D. V., Colome, S. D., & Fruin, S. A. (2005). Relative importance of school bus-related microenvironments to children's pollutant exposure. *Journal of the Air & Waste Management Association.* (1995, *55*, 1418–1430.

Berg, M., & Medrich, E. A. (1980). Children in four neighborhoods: The physical environment and its effect on play and play patterns. *Environment and Behavior, 12*, 320–348.

Björklid, P. (2004). Children's independent mobility and relationship with open space: Studies of 12-year-olds' outdoor environment in different residential areas. *Revista Psihologie Aplicta, 3*, 52.

Boothe, V. L., & Shendell, D. (2008). Potential health effects associated with residential proximity to freeways and primary roads: Review of scientific literature, 1999–2006. *Journal of Environmental Health, 70*, 33.

Bryant, B., Mayou, R., Wiggs, L., Ehlers, A., & Stores, G. (2004). Psychological consequences of road traffic accidents for children and their mothers. *Psychological Medicine, 34*, 335–346.

Carlos-Wallace, F. M., Zhang, L., Smith, M. T., Rader, G., & Steinmaus, C. (2016). Parental, in utero, and early-life exposure to benzene and the risk of childhood leukemia: A meta-analysis. *American Journal of Epidemiology, 183*, 1–14.

Davis, A., & Jones, L. J. (1996). Children in the urban environment: An issue for the new public health agenda. *Health & Place, 2*, 107–113.

Dodge, R., Daly, A. P., Huyton, J., & Sanders, L. D. (2012). The challenge of defining wellbeing. *International Journal of Wellbeing, 2*, 222.

Ellis, A., Stores, G., & Mayou, R. (1998). Psychological consequences of road traffic accidents in children. *European Child & Adolescent Psychiatry, 7*, 61–68.

Ettema, D., Gärling, T., Eriksson, L., Friman, M., Olsson, L. E., & Fujii, S. (2011). Satisfaction with travel and subjective well-being: Development and test of a measurement tool. *Transportation Research Part F Traffic Psychology and Behaviour, 14*(3), 167–175.

Ewing, R., Schroeer, W., & Greene, W. (2004). School location and student travel analysis of factors affecting mode choice. *Transportation Research Board Journal of the Transportation Research Board, 1895*, 55–63.

Gilbert, R., & O'Brien, C. (2005). *Child-and youth-friendly land-use and transport planning guidelines.* Winnipeg: Centre for Sustainable Transportation.

Grannis, R. (2011). *From the ground up: Translating geography into community through neighbor networks.* Princeton: Princeton University Press.

Héran, F., & Ravalet, E. P. J. (2008). *La consommation d'espace-temps des divers modes de déplacement en milieu urbain, Application au cas de l'île de France.* PREDIT.

Hillman, M. (1993). *Children, transport and quality of life* (p. 97). London: Policy Studies Institute.

Holt, N. L., Spence, J. C., Sehn, Z. L., & Cutumisu, N. (2008). Neighborhood and developmental differences in children's perceptions of opportunities for play and physical activity. *Health & Place, 14*, 2–14.

Huguenin-Richard, F. (2010). La mobilité des enfants à l'épreuve de la rue: Impacts de l'aménagement de zones 30 sur leurs comportements. *Enfances, Familles, Générations, 12*, 66–87.

Jensen, O. B., Sheller, M., & Wind, S. (2014). Together and apart: Affective ambiences and negotiation in families' everyday life and mobility. *Mobilities Ahead of Print*, 1–20.

Joshi, M. S., Maclean, M., & Carter, W. (1999). Children's journey to school: Spatial skills, knowledge and perceptions of the environment. *British Journal of Developmental Psychology, 17*, 125–139.

Kirby, J., & Inchley, J. (2013). Walking behaviours among adolescent girls in Scotland: A pilot study. *Health Education & Behavior, 113*, 28–51.

Kullman, K. (2014). Children, urban care, and everyday pavements. *Environment and Planning A, 46*, 2864–2880.

Larsen, K., Gilliland, J., Hess, P., Tucker, P., Irwin, J., & He, M. (2009). The influence of the physical environment and sociodemographic characteristics on Children's mode of travel to and from school. *American Journal of Public Health, 99*, 520–526.

Lennard, H. L., & Lennard, S. H. C. (2000). *The forgotten child: Cities for the well-being of children*. Carmel: Gondolier Press.

Lim, M., & Barton, A. C. (2010). Exploring insideness in urban children's sense of place. *Journal of Environmental Psychology, 30*, 328–337.

Ljung, R., Sorqvist, P., & Hygge, S. (2009). Effects of road traffic noise and irrelevant speech on children's reading and mathematical performance. *Noise & Health, 11*, 194–198.

Matthews, H., & Limb, M. (1999). Defining an agenda for the geography of children: Review and prospect. *Progress in Human Geography, 23*(1), 61–90.

Mitra, R. (2013). Independent mobility and mode choice for school transportation: A review and framework for future research. *Transport Reviews, 33*, 21–43.

Murray, L., & Mand, K. (2013). Travelling near and far: Placing children's mobile emotions. *Emotion Space and Society, 9*, 72–79.

Pabayo, R., Gauvin, L., & Barnett, T. A. (2011). Longitudinal changes in active transportation to school in Canadian youth aged 6 through 16 years. *Pediatrics, 128*, E404–E413.

Pacilli, M. G., Giovannelli, I., Prezza, M., & Augimeri, M. L. (2013). Children and the public realm: Antecedents and consequences of independent mobility in a group of 11–13-year-old Italian children. *Children's Geographies, 11*, 377–393.

Panter, J., Jones, A., & van Sluijs, E. (2008). Environmental determinants of active travel in youth: A review and framework for future research. *International Journal of Behavioral Nutrition and Physical Activity, 5*, 34.

Paunovic, K., Stansfeld, S., Clark, C., & Belojevic, G. (2011). Epidemiological studies on noise and blood pressure in children: Observations and suggestions. *Environment International, 37*, 1030–1041.

Pollard, E., & Lee, P. (2003). Child well-being: A systematic review of the literature. *Social Indicators Research, 61*, 59–78.

Ramanathan, S., O'Brien, C., Faulkner, G., & Stone, M. (2014). Happiness in motion: Emotions, well-being, and active school travel. *Journal of School Health, 84*, 516–523.

Romero, V. M. (2010). Children's views of independent mobility during their school travels. *Children Youth and Environments, 20*, 46–66.

Schoeppe, S., Duncan, M. J., Badland, H., Oliver, M., & Curtis, C. (2013). Associations of children's independent mobility and active travel with physical activity, sedentary behaviour and weight status: A systematic review. *Journal of Science and Medicine in Sport, 16*, 312–319.

Sendzik, T., Fong, G. T., Travers, M. J., & Hyland, A. (2009). An experimental investigation of tobacco smoke pollution in cars. *Nicotine & Tobacco Research, 11*, 627.

Sirard, J. R., & Slater, M. E. (2008). Walking and bicycling to school: A review. *American Journal of Lifestyle Medicine, 2*, 372–396.

Sunyer, J., Esnaola, M., Alvarez-Pedrerol, M., Forns, J., Rivas, I., López-Vicente, M., Suades-González, E., Foraster, M., Garcia-Esteban, R., & Basagaña, X. (2015). Association between traffic-related air pollution in schools and cognitive development in primary school children: A prospective cohort study. *PLoS Medicine, 12*, e1001792.

Toroyan, T., & Peden, M. (2007). *Youth and road safety*. Geneva: World Health Organization.

Torres, J., Bussière, Y., & Lewis, P. (2010). Primary schools' territorial policy and active commuting: Institutional influences in Montreal and Trois-Rivières. *Journal of Urban Planning and Development, 136*, 287–293.

Tranter, P., & Pawson, E. (2001). Children's access to local environments: A case-study of Christchurch, New Zealand. *Local Environment, 6*, 27–48.

Waygood, E. O. D. (2010). *How does attending a non-local school affect travel, exercise and community connections? Influences of the built environment, social norms and community isolation*. Transportation Research Board 89th annual meeting, Washington, DC.

Waygood, E. O. D. (2011). *What is the role of mothers in transit-oriented development? The case of Osaka–Kyoto–Kobe, Japan*. Transportation Research Board conference proceedings.

Waygood, E. O. D., & Friman, M. (2015). Children's travel and incidental community connections. *Travel Behaviour and Society, 2*, 174–181.

Waygood, E. O. D., & Kitamura, R. (2009). Children in a rail-based developed area of japan travel patterns, independence, and exercise. *Transportation Research Record, 2125*, 36–43.

Waygood, E. O. D., Taniguchi, A., Craig-St-Louis, C., & Xu, X. (2015). International origins of walking school buses and child fatalities in Japan and Canada. *Traffic Science Japan, 46*, 30–42.

Waygood, E. O. D., Friman, M., Olsson, L. E., & Taniguchi, A. (2017). Transport and child well-being. *Travel Behaviour and Society, 14*, 394.

Weller, S., & Bruegel, I. (2009). Children's place in the development of neighbourhood social capital. *Urban Studies, 46*, 629–643.

Westman, J., Johansson, M., Olsson, L. E., Martensson, F., & Friman, M. (2013). Children's affective experience of every-day travel. *Journal of Transport Geography, 29*, 95–102.

Westman, J., Olsson, L. E., Gärling, T., & Friman, M. (2017). Children's travel to school: Satisfaction, current mood, and cognitive performance. *Transportation, 44*(6), 1365–1382.

Whitehead-Frei, C., & Kockelman, K. M. (2010). Americans' time use a focus on women and child rearing-structural equations modeling. *Transportation Research Record, 2163*, 32–44.

Zwerts, E., Allaert, G., Janssens, D., Wets, G., & Witlox, F. (2010). How children view their travel behaviour: A case study from Flanders (Belgium). *Journal of Transport Geography, 18*, 702–710.

# Chapter 12
# Daily Monitoring of Mobility as an Indicator of Wellbeing Among Individuals with Chronic Disease

**Amit Birenboim, A. Yair Grinberger, Enrico M. Novelli, and Charles R. Jonassaint**

**Abstract** Reduced mobility is associated with decrease in both hedonic and eudemonic aspects of well-being. The current chapter investigates the potential of employing smartphone location tracking to investigate the association between deteriorating mobility and wellbeing among individuals with chronic disease during daily activity. The locations of 36 patients with sickle cell disease, a genetic disorder that affects the production of hemoglobin, were tracked continuously every 2 min using participants' smartphones to allow the calculation of movement parameters such as walking and driving distance and speed. The results of the study were mixed. (1) While smartphone tracking could be performed continuously for long periods of time for some patients (e.g. more than 100 days of tacking), data quality was not consistent for other patients. Twenty-one out the 36 patients enrolled had poor or no spatial information. Based on the results of other studies, we suspect that this is mainly due to motivational factors (e.g. participants did not keep the phone's location services on) and not a fault of the hardware. We conclude that future studies should implement some incentive or feedback mechanism that will enhance motivation of participants. (2) The association between daily mobility parameters and physical and mental wellbeing (i.e. depression, pain level) were in the expected direction, but results were not significant for the most part. While this could be attributed to the small sample of the study, it might also be the case that other indicators which better represent the tempo-spatial context of human behavior should be considered in the future.

A. Birenboim (✉)
Utrecht University, Utrecht, The Netherlands
e-mail: abirenboim@tauex.tau.ac.il

A. Y. Grinberger
Heidelberg University, Heidelberg, Germany
e-mail: yair.grinberger@uni-heidelberg.de

E. M. Novelli · C. R. Jonassaint
University of Pittsburgh, Pittsburgh, PA, USA
e-mail: novellie@upmc.edu; cjonassaint@pitt.edu

© Springer International Publishing AG, part of Springer Nature 2018    219
M. Friman et al. (eds.), *Quality of Life and Daily Travel*, Applying Quality of Life Research, https://doi.org/10.1007/978-3-319-76623-2_12

**Keywords** Sickle-cell disease · Mobility · Smartphone · Wellbeing · Chronic disease

## 12.1   Introduction

As previous chapters in this book suggest, mobility and wellbeing have a reciprocal influence on one another. To date, research in the field has mainly focused on healthy populations and frequently also on older adults who experience decline in their mobility (Nordbakke and Schwanen 2014; Ziegler and Schwanen 2011). One important group which is understudied in the context of wellbeing and mobility is that of non-elderly individuals with chronic conditions. It is often the case that basic daily functioning, including mobility, of individuals with chronic condition is impaired, leading to reduced wellbeing and quality of life (Stewart et al. 1989). Chronic disease is prevalent in the population: 42% of the adult population aged 18–65 in the US is estimated to have at least one chronic condition, and this increases to almost 50% when including older adults (based on data from: Ward et al. 2014). Hence, the investigation of this group is of high social importance.

Sickle cell disease (SCD) is an inherited, chronic disease that affects the production of the oxygen-carrying protein hemoglobin found in red blood cells. It is the most common inherited blood disorder in the United States, affecting approximately 100,000 patients in total (Centers for Disease Control and Prevention 2016).Some of the prominent manifestations of the disease include anemia and acute pain events, both of which are associated with a decrease in physical performance and therefore, often affect mobility of patients. Individuals living with SCD can also experience neuropsychological dysfunction and depression (Jonassaint et al. 2016, 2017; Zempsky et al. 2013). Given the relatively young age and high morbidity of the SCD population, this group serves as a valuable model for examining the link between mobility and wellbeing within the context of severe chronic disease. Data from patients with SCD will inform future studies of other chronic disease groups.

To date, there are limited methods for capturing level of daily functioning and mobility outside of the medical setting beyond self-reported surveys. Methods to objectively monitor daily changes in mobility may provide valuable information for research and intervening on declining health and well-being in SCD and other chronic conditions. Smartphone tracking has been proven a reliable and advantageous method for measuring daily mobility among the general and elderly populations (Birenboim and Shoval 2016; Wan et al. 2013). In this chapter, we test the feasibility of employing this data collection technique among non-elderly adults with chronic disease (i.e. SCD) for daily monitoring of wellbeing in naturally occurring environments. To do that, mobility indicators that were extracted from smartphones' location information were compared with common lab measures of mobility and wellbeing.

Wellbeing is a multifaceted term that is used to refer to the general condition of individuals. The concept has been widely used across disciplines including in healthcare (Stranges et al. 2014), psychology (Diener et al. 1999), mobility and transportation (Ettema et al. 2010) and others, though with somewhat different aims and operationalizations each time. Wellbeing could be measured using several different tools ranging from one item questionnaire (i.e. overall how happy are you in your life) to a more detailed health profile (Guyatt et al. 1993). Given the diverse interpretations of wellbeing, a comprehensive review of the concept and the tools that are used to measure it are beyond the scope of this chapter. It should be noted that the current study adopts a health-related wellbeing or health-related quality of life perspective (Guyatt et al. 1993) which emphasizes aspects of physical and mental health (e.g. pain, depression).

### 12.1.1  The Relation Between Mobility, Chronic Disease and Wellbeing

The simplified model in Fig. 12.1 presents the potential reciprocal effects between chronic disease, mobility, and wellbeing that can be applied to a condition such as SCD. As seen in the model, each of the three elements that comprise the model could affect the other two elements either directly or through the mediation of the third element. Most of the effects that are portrayed in the model are well documented in the literature. Chronic diseases are often associated with deterioration of physical condition that may lead to decrease in mobility levels (arrow a in Fig. 12.1). This includes both reduction in "free-living" daily activity and in physical exercise (Steele et al. 2003). In the other direction (arrow b), reduced mobility may lead to chronic and poor health conditions (Booth et al. 2000). Arguably, the most prevalent examples for this are the negative outcomes of sedentary behavior that increases obesity and the risk of coronary diseases and type 2 diabetes (Ford et al. 2005). Though of less concern to this chapter, chronic conditions may affect wellbeing more directly or through other mediating variables which are not related to mobility

**Fig. 12.1** Potential reciprocal effects between chronic disease, mobility, and wellbeing

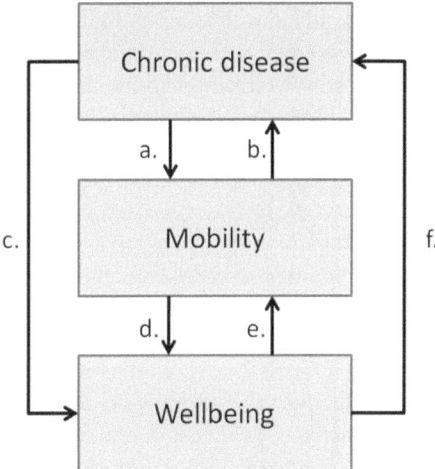

(arrow c). In a large scale study that examined the self-reports of people with chronic condition and their physicians' reports, Stewart et al. (1989) showed that chronic conditions affect various aspects of wellbeing including social functioning, perception of health and others. Additional studies showed that people who suffer from chronic diseases, especially when these involved prolonged pain episodes, were also more inclined to develop depression (see for example: Banks and Kerns 1996).

As other chapters in this book demonstrate, mobility may affect quality of life and wellbeing of individuals directly (arrow d). Mobility plays an essential role in daily life, since most people rely on physical mobility to perform various basic tasks such as commuting, shopping, and socializing. It is important to note that even in our days where information and communication technologies allow us to perform many activities like (e)commerce and (tele)commuting remotely, the ability to be physically mobile is still a crucial competence for most people. In contrast to what some might have predicted in the past, the introduction and advancement of information and communication technologies in the last decades did not reduce the distance that people travel (Aguiléra et al. 2012). Beyond the practical implications of (im)mobility, physical mobility—and especially walking—may support both eudemonic and hedonic aspects of wellbeing (Ettema and Smajic 2015; Olsson et al. 2013). Eudemonically, the ability to move supports a sense of autonomy and mastery (Ziegler and Schwanen 2011). Hedonically, mobility may lead to positive affective experiences (Ettema and Smajic 2015; Mokhtarian and Salomon 2001). Though the effect of wellbeing on mobility (arrow e) has received less attention, a few works strongly support the notion that positive mental wellbeing supports a higher level of mobility and vice versa (see for example: Collins et al. 2008). Though by itself of less interest to our discussion, there is also support that poor mental wellbeing may worsen chronic conditions (arrow f) (Moussavi et al. 2007).

There seems to be substantial evidence to support the effect of mobility on wellbeing and chronic diseases and vice versa. However, it is also important to consider the indirect effects that mobility has on chronic diseases and wellbeing: (1) Mobility acts as a mediating variable between wellbeing and chronic diseases through the chronic disease-mobility-wellbeing axis (connected by the a and d arrows) and the wellbeing-mobility-chronic disease axis (e and b arrows). (2) Mobility may indirectly affect chronic disease and wellbeing. The former is represented by the mobility-wellbeing-chronic disease axis (d–f arrows) the latter by the mobility-chronic disease-wellbeing axis (b and c arrows).

Even when using a very simplified model such as the one in Fig. 12.1, it is clear that the relationship between mobility and wellbeing is multifaceted. The complexity of these relations is emphasized when other mental and/or physical impairments are involved. An important step to a better understanding of the magnitude of the effect of (im)mobility on wellbeing among the general population and among people with chronic disease will include the implementation and development of tools that can measure daily mobility accurately. It is essential that these tools supply valid and reliable information, as well as indicators about the daily mobility of individuals, rather than just the information about mobility potential (e.g. walking competence, car ownership) which is often collected in lab measurements and surveys. Such information could turn out to be highly useful for assessing periodic changes in mobility as a result of changes in the symptoms of a disease. From a clinical perspective, it is also essential that this information be available in near real-time to allow close and efficient monitoring of patients.

## 12.2  Monitoring Physical Mobility of Individuals with Chronic Disease

Even when our discussion about mobility is constrained to deal only with the very basic aspects of physical mobility, we are still left with a very broad spectrum of types of mobility to consider (Stalvey et al. 1999). Mobility may refer to the ability to perform the most basic bodily movements, which may include moving the limbs, standing, and climbing stairs independently (Nitz et al. 2006). But it may also relate to higher level functioning like running, commuting, and performing other activities such as socializing and shopping which are dependent on the ability to move from one place to another by different means of transportation (Vilhelmson 1999).

Many of the tools that were developed to assess mobility functioning are designed to evaluate the elderly population and individuals with physical or mental impairment who suffer from a decline in their mobility (Rossier and Wade 2001; Stalvey et al. 1999). Tools that assess mobility of the general, healthy population are scarcer and will typically focus on higher level mobility aspects, such as assessing the intensity of physical activity (e.g. distance walked in the last week) (Paffenbarger et al. 1993).

People with chronic disease may demonstrate varying quality of physical states and sometimes also mental states which may affect their daily mobility. In some cases, the disease (e.g. SCD, multiple sclerosis) may have a fluctuating pattern of reoccurring attacks which may result in a corresponding, unstable pattern of mobility. Therefore, while some individuals with chronic disease may demonstrate normal mobility levels, others may exhibit lower levels and/or unstable patterns. Given the high prevalence of individuals with chronic disease in the population, it is important that tools that are utilized are general enough to capture varying mobility levels and patterns.

Tools that are currently used to assess mobility can be divided into three broad categories (based on Podsiadlo and Richardson 1991): (1) mobility inventories and scales, (2) lab measurements, and (3) daily mobility information.

### 12.2.1  Mobility Inventories and Scales

This group of instruments includes validated, structured questionnaires, which may take one of three forms: (1) self-reported questionnaire (Paffenbarger et al. 1993), (2) interviewer-administered surveys (Stalvey et al. 1999), and (3) observer-reported questionnaires (Nitz et al. 2006). The main advantages of such surveys are that they are simple to administer and analyze, and they usually score high on reliability tests (Rossier and Wade 2001). On the other hand, these inventories are often too specific (i.e. they address specific mobility deficiencies) and are therefore not always suitable for mobility studies about the general population. Moreover, they are nonpractical for studies that require longitudinal measurements. First, they normally include tens of items, which makes them time consuming. Second, these tools are usually not designed or tested to be administered repeatedly. In addition, due to various biases (e.g. recall bias) the accuracy of the surveys in assessing actual mobility is questionable in many cases (Podsiadlo and Richardson 1991). These make these tools less effective in detecting changes in mobility patterns along time.

## 12.2.2  Lab Measurements

Lab instruments are usually targeted to measure functional mobility and are, therefore, commonly used to assess physical competence among elderly and individuals with some sort of physical impairment (Rossier and Wade 2001; Steffen et al. 2002). Common instruments include measurement of gait speed, balance, and other motor abilities which are essential for daily mobility (Steffen et al. 2002). Tests can be performed using dedicated devices such as treadmills in which gait speed can be measured or in "more natural" settings. In the "timed up & go" test for example, the time it takes an (elderly) individual to rise from an arm chair, walk three meters, turn, walk back, and sit down again is evaluated (Podsiadlo and Richardson 1991).

Lab measurements show high reliability and are considered valid when it comes to assessing basic mobility functioning. However, while easy to administer, some of the tests require special equipment, and they are time consuming and therefore not always practical for implementation (Podsiadlo and Richardson 1991). This is especially true when longitudinal information (i.e. repeat measurements) is desired. It is also not clear how useful lab instruments are in predicting higher level mobility patterns among the general, unimpaired population (e.g. does gait speed predict how often a healthy-individual leaves his house to socialize, or to engage in shopping activities?).

## 12.2.3  Daily Mobility Information

Daily mobility measurements rely on tools that continuously record the location of people. The aim of these tools is to get reliable information about places that individuals visit throughout the day. Up until recently, the recording of the actual daily mobility patterns of people relied on activity diaries that needed to be completed periodically (i.e. once or a few times daily) or on long questionnaires that were administrated at the end of a study period (Birenboim and Shoval 2016). This methodological approach is considered burdensome for both researchers and their study participants. For researchers, the method requires investment in many resources in post-processing of the data, including geo-coding of unstructured addresses and locations (Hicks et al. 2010). For participants, the task of completing a diary is time-consuming and repetitive. Several studies indicated that while the method supplies rich information about their mobility, it is often imperfect due to incomplete or inaccurate information supplied by participants (e.g. participants forget to report, cannot supply accurate position/address) (Birenboim and Shoval 2016).

With the development of advanced tracking technologies since the 2000s, most notably the GPS, researchers have started to develop tools that can accurately and automatically record the locations of people in high tempo-spatial resolutions. This makes it possible not only to record places that participants visit but also to calculate more fine-scale indicators such as walking and driving speed (Barzilay et al. 2011). While early location-tracking studies relied on dedicated devices, such as GPS loggers that participants had to carry with themselves for study purposes (Barzilay et al. 2011), current efforts are invested in utilizing advanced mobile phones (smartphones) for similar purposes (Birenboim and Shoval 2016; Jonassaint et al. 2017; Wan and Lin 2013). The advantage of these devices is that they integrate several location technologies simultaneously, which improves the spatial accuracy of the data. Using smartphones reduces the burden from participants, since these devices are carried by people on a regular basis for personal use. Moreover, since data can be automatically recorded and transferred from the mobile phone to secure servers, researchers can get access to the location information more easily and in real time. Data can also be analyzed in a timely manner using automated scripts (Birenboim and Shoval 2016).

Nevertheless, in contrast to the mobility inventories and lab measurements, daily location tracking might not be sufficient in detecting physical mobility deficiencies and their sources. An occurrence of acute immobility/sedentary behavior, for example, might be interpreted mistakenly as a physical mobility incompetence. This problem can be partly overcome when accelerometers, either smartphone-based or external, are integrated into the data collection procedure (Quigg et al. 2010). In addition, to date, there are no standard mobility indicators that are based on daily location-tracking information which can be used to assess and compare mobility levels of people. Therefore, while smartphones could be useful tools for assessing mobility patterns in the general population, including patterns of individuals with chronic disease, it is important that standard indicators be developed. These indicators should take into account variation between subpopulations (e.g. children, young adults, elderly; males-females).

This chapter examines the feasibility of employing smartphones for basic and clinical research purposes among individuals with chronic disease. While the method could be employed with other populations as well, it has clear advantages when monitoring patients with chronic conditions who may experience unstable physical and mental states for long periods of time (Stewart et al. 1989). It is important that the method not only allow continuous, long-term monitoring, but that it be general enough to permit the evaluation of various mobility aspects.

Inventories and lab measurements are not suitable for this task since they do not allow continuous monitoring of mobility, and they often address a very specific impairment or population.

## 12.3  Method

### 12.3.1  Procedure and Participants

Thirty-six adult patients from the Pittsburgh, US, metropolitan area with a documented SCD diagnosis participated in this study. They were all enrolled in the longitudinal study, Neurovascular Determinants of Cognitive Function in Adults with SCD (PI: Novelli), and were asked by a research assistant whether they would be willing to take part in an ancillary mobility study. Before obtaining informed consent, a research assistant described the purpose of the study and explained to the potential participants that a mobile application tracking their location would be installed on their smartphone if they agreed to participate. It was emphasized that their identifying data would be kept confidential.

As part of the parent study, a battery of tools was employed to assess neuropsychological functioning, depression, pain, hemoglobin level, and more. Mobility was assessed in the lab by a 6-min gait-speed test. Outdoor mobility of participants that took part in the ancillary study was recorded using a dedicated mobile application (SensoMeter) developed by Birenboim and Shoval (see for example: Birenboim 2016, 2017; Shoval et al. 2017). The application was installed on each participant's personal mobile phone; it was configured to record the location of the phone every 2 min based on the phone's GPS and Wi-Fi positioning capabilities, while participants were performing their routine daily activity. The mobile application was available for both iOS and Android devices.

The data that was transmitted automatically to a secured server was exported at the end of the sampling period and was then cleaned and processed using scripts written in Python language that were adjusted to the data structure and sampling interval of every 2 min. In this stage, inaccurate location samples and non-valid days (a day was considered non-valid if it had a gap longer than one hour in the location data) were filtered.

Following strict inclusion criteria, participants were excluded from the final sample as follows:

– Eleven participants were excluded for having less than seven valid days of location-tracking information. A period of 7 days is commonly used as the standard for assessing mobility patterns.
– Six participants had no spatial information at all; this might be a result of a technical problem, and/or a decision of a patient not to share their location (e.g. by uninstalling the mobile application or by turning off location services on their phone).

- Three participants did not have lab information (e.g. no gait-speed measurements).
- Two participants were disabled (i.e. using a wheelchair).
- Four participants had high rates of inaccurate location samples. For example, one participant was tracked for 63 days, but more than 70% of his location samples were considered inaccurate. This raised concerns as to potential bias (e.g. good accuracy only in specific places) that would compromise the integrity of the results.

The final sample included ten participants, all of African-American descent; 40% male; average age 39.5 (std: 9.4, range: 25–58).

### 12.3.2 Data Processing and Analysis

As described above, two types of datasets were collected. The first and more standard one was collected in the clinic as part of the parent study. The second was collected through the mobile application and included location-tracking information. Three lab indicators which are relevant to mobility and wellbeing are reported here. (1) Gait speed as measured during a 6-min-walk lab test. (2) Pain score that was recorded using a 0–10 scale. Based on the pain scale we also extracted a binary variable of pain, where 0 includes patients who reported no pain at all (0 on the 0–10 scale) and 1 stands for all the other scores. (3) The CES-D–Center for Epidemiologic Studies Depression Scale (Radloff 1977). Score for this scale range between 0 and 60, with higher scores indicating the presence of more symptomatology.

The raw data processing of the location tracking information included data cleansing and removal of inaccurate samples and invalid days. At the second stage, location samples were differentiated into walking tracks, driving tracks, and static stays (nodes). Nodes were identified as sequences of subsequent samples, at least 15 min long, in which no point was more than 60 m away from the point starting the sequence, while all other sequences were identified as tracks (except for sequences less than 10-min long starting and ending at the same node, which were merged with the node). Average movement speed was used to identify transport mode, where values of 6 km/h or less were considered to represent walking, 15 km/h or more – driving, and all else – mixed mode or other (e.g. cycling). Several indicators about walking behavior (average and maximum walking speed and average daily walking distance), driving behavior (average daily driving distance), and the number and time spent at various places (daily time spent at home, number of places visited daily), were then calculated for each patient. Due to the scope of the study, analysis was restricted to descriptive and correlative (i.e. Pearson correlation) statistics.

## 12.4   Results and Discussion

Table 12.1 presents descriptive statistics of the mobility and lab indicators that were calculated. The high number of valid days with location information that could be obtained for each participant (62.2 days on average) indicates that smartphones allow tracking of patients for long periods. However, it should be noted that (1) there was a big variation in the tracking periods (standard deviation = 52.03), indicating that only some of the patients were tracked for very long periods of more than 100 days, and (2) many individuals were excluded from the study based on the quality of their data. This puts in question the feasibility of obtaining useful location data using smartphones for long time periods. Nevertheless, we should keep in mind that patients in this study did not receive any incentive for their participation. It is most likely that an incentive or some sort of feedback would dramatically increase the quality of the data.

The average walking speed (1.83 kmph) seems to be underestimated. We suspect that the relatively low location sampling rate (2 min sampling interval) may have caused this, primarily because this sampling resolution cannot differentiate between short stays (e.g. shorter than 4 min) and actual walking activity. In this situation, the (non-detectable) stops would be added to the total time of walking, decreasing speed estimation. In addition, the low sampling rate leads to underestimation of the distance that is walked, especially when there are many curves and turns along the walking route which are not fully captured when the sampling rate is low.

Four out of ten participants scored 15 or more on the CES-D, which is often interpreted as an indication for risk of depression. 70% of the patients reported some pain during the past week.

**Table 12.1** Descriptive statistics of main location and lab indicators

| Type | Indicator | Average | StdDev |
|---|---|---|---|
| Location (mobile) data | Number of valid days sampled | 62.2 | 52.03 |
| | Average walking speed (kmph) | 1.83 | 0.47 |
| | Maximum walking speed (km) | 5.62 | 0.52 |
| | Average daily walking distance (meters) | 989 | 560.2 |
| | Average daily driving distance (meters) | 10,313 | 11838.5 |
| | Daily time spent at home (hrs) | 16.75 | 3.67 |
| | Daily number of places (nodes) visited | 5.55 | 2.53 |
| Lab data | Gait speed (m/s) | 1.11 (4 kmph) | 0.25 |
| | CES-D[a] | 9.60 | 7.09 |
| | Pain (0-10 scale)[b] | 4.43 | 3.69 |
| | Pain (yes/no)[b] | 0.70[c] | |

[a]Score ranges between 0 and 60. Higher score indicates higher depressive symptoms
[b]Based on 7 observations
[c]This means that 70% of the patients reported some pain

To further examine the association between the lab measurements and the daily mobility indicators, a correlation matrix was generated. Since gait speed is a lab instrument that is used to assess mobility, it was implemented in both the rows (mobility indicators) and columns (lab indicators) dimensions of the matrix (Table 12.2).

Surprisingly, average walking speed was negatively and significantly correlated with gait speed. While, as explained above, walking speed is most likely underestimated in our study, this result was still unexpected. While the finding might be explained by technical factors, it is more likely that some other mediating variables led to this result; however, this cannot be supported by the current dataset. In contrast, it seems that gait speed is more similar in its essence to the maximum walking speed parameter. The positive (though not significant) association ($r = 0.381$) between the two is more in line with what one would have expected. Future studies conducted to obtain gait-speed-like information using location data, should examine some variants of the maximum speed rather than the average speed.

The binary variable of pain that was utilized in this analysis (the procedure is known as point-biserial correlation), revealed a strong, negative, and significant association ($r = -0.759$) with average walking speed. This means that as expected, people who reported some pain were more likely to walk more slowly. Giving the negative correlation between walking and gait speed, it is not surprising that gait speed showed an opposite, though not significant pattern. As expected, pain was also negatively correlated with all the other daily mobility parameters though none of these correlations was found significant. This might be attributed to the small sample that was used.

Finally, the correlation between the daily mobility indicators and the depression scale, CES-D, was in most cases in the expected direction but very low and not significant. Average daily driving distance ($r = -0.305$) and gait speed ($r = -0.327$) did show a slightly stronger association.

**Table 12.2** A Pearson correlation coefficient matrix of main location and lab indicators

|  | Pain (yes/no)[c] | CES-D | Gait speed |
|---|---|---|---|
| Avg walking speed[a] | −0.759[b] | 0.191 | −0.651[b] |
| Max walking speed[a] | −0.278 | −0.098 | 0.381 |
| Avg daily walking distance | −0.368 | −0.013 | −0.186 |
| Avg daily driving distance | −0.247 | −0.305 | −0.062 |
| Avg time at home[a] | −0.502 | −0.047 | −0.403 |
| Gait speed[a] | 0.358 | −0.327 | 1.000 |

[a]Based on the entire sample of each individual
[b]p-value < 0.05
[c]Seven observation

## 12.5   Conclusions

The feasibility study reported here was limited in scope, both in terms of sample size and lab instruments that were utilized to assess wellbeing and mobility. While results were statistically not significant for the most part, their general trend was in line with expectations, indicating that increased mobility has a positive impact on the mental and physical wellbeing of individuals with chronic disease. A larger sample and implementation of additional, more specific indicators of mental and physical wellbeing, might result in more significant results and hopefully could also shed light on the underlying mechanisms and relationships between mobility, chronic disease, and wellbeing that were described in the introduction.

It might also be the case that the non-significant results are a consequence of the analytical approach implemented. The relationship between mobility, wellbeing, and chronic condition are mediated by various variables, which do not appear in our model and which were not considered here. The rationale behind the somewhat simplistic approach that was implemented was to identify mobility-related measures of wellbeing that transcend such influences. Our results suggest that this goal cannot be easily obtained. One important element which may thus require attention is the time-space context in which activities are carried, which is known to affect both wellbeing and mobility behaviors (Kwan 2012a, b; Maas et al. 2006; Richardson et al. 2013). While this context remains an elusive element to identify, spatial methods, such as distributional ellipses, may help in exposing it (Kwan 2012a). Consequently, mobility-related indicators of wellbeing must show some consideration of the environment. Indeed, in the case of SCD, it was discovered that the size of the distributional ellipse is correlated with several measures of wellbeing (Jonassaint et al. 2017). Further exploring these relations and relations to other measures may promote the production of measures which do not require complex tempo-spatial analysis, but are still informative regarding the conditions of patients.

The results also show that people could be tracked for long periods of time if needed. Some of the patients in the study were tracked for more than 100 days continuously while supplying good-quality spatial information. However, many of the participants were excluded from the study due to poor data quality or no data. Since previous studies showed that smartphones can generate good spatial information for mobility assessments (Wan et al. 2013), it is likely that the quality of the data is dependent on the motivation of participants (i.e. to keep the phone's location services and the tracking functionality of the application on) more than it is on hardware faults. Therefore, future studies should consider providing incentives for participants that will improve the quality of the spatial data collected. These incentives should not necessarily be monetary; they could, for example, include information and/or feedback for participants about their daily mobility levels.

In order to improve the accuracy of the mobility indicators that are calculated, the sampling rate of the locations should be increased significantly. The current study employed a 2-min sampling rate in order to keep battery drain to a minimum.

However, selective sampling algorithms that increase sampling rate (e.g. 1 Hz) when people are on the move may be employed. Such sampling techniques are already available in some mobile applications (Bhattacharya et al. 2015).

Smartphone location sampling makes a dynamic tool for collecting mobility information that can be used to monitor the status of a chronic disease and the wellbeing of patients. For clinicians, the technology may supply a daily stream of information, which may facilitate a timely response in case undesired mobility patterns are observed. It is important that in future studies researchers also obtain dynamic information about wellbeing and the status of the chronic disease. This could be achieved through repeat mobile surveys that are sent to the mobile phone (Birenboim and Shoval 2016). Once mobility and wellbeing are both monitored continuously, it will be possible to generate more valid insights regarding the relation between the two. This is especially important in cases where the physical and mental states of individuals is less stable as it is with some chronic diseases such as SCD.

Due to the high prevalence of smartphones in the population, it is most likely that practices of smartphone tracking will increase in the near future for both research and clinical purposes (mHealth). Standardization of data collection procedures and indicators is essential in order to allow meaningful and comparable results. Though beyond the scope of this study, it is important to note that smartphone tracking involves many ethical concerns about privacy. Therefore, it is crucial that such ethical issues will be carefully considered and resolved before smartphone tracking is implemented as a common research or clinical procedure.

**Acknowledgements**  This work was supported by the following grants and institutions: The interdisciplinary Healthy Urban Living research program of Utrecht University, NIH grant 1 R01 HL127107-01A1, University of Pittsburgh Vascular Medicine Institute P3HVBI Award and NHLBI K23HL135396-01.

# References

Aguiléra, A., Guillot, C., & Rallet, A. (2012). Mobile ICTs and physical mobility: Review and research agenda. *Transportation Research Part A: Policy and Practice, 46*(4), 664–672. https://doi.org/10.1016/j.tra.2012.01.005.

Banks, S. M., & Kerns, R. D. (1996). Explaining high rates of depression in chronic pain: A diathesis-stress framework. *Psychological Bulletin, 119*(1), 95–110. https://doi.org/10.1037/0033-2909.119.1.95.

Barzilay, Y., Shoval, N., Liebergall, M., Auslander, G., Birenboim, A., Isaacson, M., et al. (2011). Assessing the outcomes of spine surgery using global positioning systems. *SPINE, 36*(4), 263–267. https://doi.org/10.1097/BRS.0b013e3181da3737.

Bhattacharya, S., Blunck, H., Kjargaard, M. B., & Nurmi, P. (2015). Robust and energy-efficient trajectory tracking for mobile devices. *IEEE Transactions on Mobile Computing, 14*(2), 430–443. https://doi.org/10.1109/TMC.2014.2318712.

Birenboim, A. (2016). New approaches to the study of tourist experiences in time and space. *Tourism Geographies, 18*(1), 9–17. https://doi.org/10.1080/14616688.2015.1122078.

Birenboim, A. (2017). The influence of urban environments on our subjective momentary experiences. *Environment and Planning B: Urban Analytics and City Science*. https://doi.org/10.1177/2399808317690149.

Birenboim, A., & Shoval, N. (2016). Mobility research in the age of the smartphone. *Annals of the American Association of Geographers, 106*(2), 283–291.

Booth, F. W., Gordon, S. E., Carlson, C. J., & Hamilton, M. T. (2000). Waging war on modern chronic diseases: Primary prevention through\nexercise biology. *Journal of Applied Physiology, 88*(2), 774–787.

Centers for Disease Control and Prevention. (2016). Sickle cell disease: Data and statistics. Retrieved 31 July 2017, from http://www.cdc.gov/NCBDDD/sicklecell/data.html

Collins, A. L., Goldman, N., & Rodríguez, G. (2008). Is positive well-being protective of mobility limitations among older adults? *The Journals of Gerontology Series B, Psychological Sciences and Social Sciences, 63*(6), 321–327. https://doi.org/63/6/P321 [pii].

Diener, E., Suh, E. M., Lucas, R. E., & Smith, H. L. (1999). Subjective well-being: Three decades of progress. *Psychological Bulletin, 125*(2), 276–302.

Ettema, D., & Smajic, I. (2015). Walking, places and wellbeing. *The Geographical Journal, 181*(2), 102–109.

Ettema, D., Gärling, T., Olsson, L. E., & Friman, M. (2010). Out-of-home activities, daily travel, and subjective well-being. *Transportation Research Part A: Policy and Practice, 44*(9), 723–732.

Ford, E. S., Kohl, H. W., Mokdad, A. H., & Ajani, U. A. (2005). Sedentary behavior, physical activity, and the metabolic syndrome among U.S. adults. *Obesity Research, 13*(3), 608–614. https://doi.org/10.1038/oby.2005.65.

Guyatt, G. H., Feeny, D. H., & Patrick, D. L. (1993). Measuring health-related quality of life. *Annals of Internal Medicine, 118*(8), 622–629. https://doi.org/10.7326/0003-4819-118-8-199304150-00009.

Hicks, J., Ramanathan, N., Kim, D., Monibi, M., Selsky, J., Hansen, M., & Estrin, D. (2010). AndWellness: An open mobile system for activity and experience sampling. In *Wireless health 2010* (WH '10) (pp. 34–43). San Diego.

Jonassaint, C. R., Jones, V. L., Leong, S., & Frierson, G. M. (2016). A systematic review of the association between depression and health care utilization in children and adults with sickle cell disease. *British Journal of Haematology, 174*(1), 136–147. https://doi.org/10.1111/bjh.14023.

Jonassaint, C. R., Birenboim, A., Jorgensen, D. R., Novelli, E. M., & Rosso, A. L. (2017). The association of smartphone-based activity space measures with cognitive functioning and pain sickle cell disease. *British Journal of Haematology*. https://doi.org/10.1111/bjh.14598.

Kwan, M.-P. (2012a). How GIS can help address the uncertain geographic context problem in social science research. *Annals of GIS, 18*(4), 245–255. https://doi.org/10.1080/19475683.2012.727867.

Kwan, M. P. (2012b). The uncertain geographic context problem. *Annals of the Association of American Geographers, 102*(5), 958–968. https://doi.org/10.1080/00045608.2012.687349.

Maas, J., Verheij, R. A., Groenewegen, P. P., de Vries, S., & Spreeuwenberg, P. (2006). Green space, urbanity, and health: How strong is the relation? *Journal of Epidemiology & Community Health, 60*(7), 587–592. https://doi.org/10.1136/jech.2005.043125.

Mokhtarian, P. L., & Salomon, I. (2001). How derived is the demand for travel? Some conceptual and measurement considerations. *Transportation Research Part A: Policy and Practice, 35*(8), 695–719. https://doi.org/10.1016/S0965-8564(00)00013-6.

Moussavi, S., Chatterji, S., Verdes, E., Tandon, A., Patel, V., & Ustun, B. (2007). Depression, chronic diseases, and decrements in health: Results from the World Health Surveys. *The Lancet, 370*(9590), 851–858. https://doi.org/10.1016/S0140-6736(07)61415-9.

Nitz, J. C., Hourigan, S. R., & Brown, A. (2006). Measuring mobility in frail older people: Reliability and validity of the Physical Mobility Scale. *Australasian Journal on Ageing, 25* (1), 31–35. https://doi.org/10.1111/j.1741-6612.2006.00137.x.

Nordbakke, S., & Schwanen, T. (2014). Well-being and mobility: A theoretical framework and literature review focusing on older people. *Mobilities, 9*(1), 104–129.

Olsson, L. E., Gärling, T., Ettema, D., Friman, M., & Fujii, S. (2013). Happiness and satisfaction with work commute. *Social Indicators Research, 111*(1), 255–263. https://doi.org/10.1007/s11205-012-0003-2.

Paffenbarger, R. S., Blair, S. N., Lee, I. M., & Hyde, R. T. (1993). Measurement of physical activity to assess health effects in free-living populations. In *Medicine and science in sports and exercise* (Vol. 25, pp. 60–70). https://doi.org/10.1249/00005768-199301000-00010.

Podsiadlo, D., & Richardson, S. (1991). The timed "up & go": A test of basic functional mobility for frail elderly persons. *Journal of the American Geriatrics Society, 39*(2), 142–148. https://doi.org/10.1111/j.1532-5415.1991.tb01616.x.

Quigg, R., Gray, A., Reeder, A. I., Holt, A., & Waters, D. L. (2010). Using accelerometers and GPS units to identify the proportion of daily physical activity located in parks with playgrounds in New Zealand children. *Preventive Medicine, 50*(5–6), 235–240. https://doi.org/10.1016/j.ypmed.2010.02.002.

Radloff, L. S. (1977). The CES-D scale: A self-report depression scale for research in the general population. *Applied Psychological Measurement, 1*(3), 385–401. https://doi.org/10.1177/014662167700100306.

Richardson, D. B., Volkow, N. D., Kwan, M.-P., Kaplan, R. M., Goodchild, M. F., & Croyle, R. T. (2013). Spatial turn in health research. *Science, 339*(6126), 1390–1392.

Rossier, P., & Wade, D. T. (2001). Validity and reliability comparison of 4 mobility measures in patients presenting with neurologic impairment. *Archives of Physical Medicine and Rehabilitation, 82*(1), 9–13. https://doi.org/10.1053/apmr.2001.9396.

Shoval, N., Schvimer, Y., & Tamir, M. (2017). Real-time measurement of tourists' objective and subjective emotions in time and space. *Journal of Travel Research.* https://doi.org/10.1177/0047287517691155.

Stalvey, B. T., Owsley, C., Sloane, M. E., & Ball, K. (1999). The life space questionnaire: A measure of the extent of mobility of older adults. *Journal of Applied Gerontology, 18*(4), 460–478.

Steele, B. G., Belza, B., Cain, K., Warms, C., Coppersmith, J., & Howard, J. (2003). Bodies in motion: Monitoring daily activity and exercise with motion sensors in people with chronic pulmonary disease. *Journal of Rehabilitation Research & Development, 40*(5), 45–58.

Steffen, T. M., Hacker, T. A., & Mollinger, L. (2002). Age- and gender-related test performance in community-dwelling elderly people: Six-minute walk test, berg balance scale, timed up & Go Test, and gait speeds. *Physical Therapy, 82*(2), 128–137. https://doi.org/10.1093/ptj/82.2.128.

Stewart, A. L., Greenfield, S., Hays, R. D., Wells, K., Rogers, W. H., Berry, S. D., et al. (1989). Functional status and well-being of patients with chronic conditions. *JAMA, 262*(7), 907. https://doi.org/10.1001/jama.1989.03430070055030.

Stranges, S., Samaraweera, P. C., Taggart, F., Kandala, N.-B., & Stewart-Brown, S. (2014). Major health-related behaviours and mental well-being in the general population: The Health Survey for England. *BMJ Open, 4*(9), e005878. https://doi.org/10.1136/bmjopen-2014-005878.

Vilhelmson, B. (1999). Daily mobility and the use of time for different activities. The case of Sweden. *GeoJournal, 48*(3), 177–185. https://doi.org/10.1023/A:1007075524340.

Wan, N., & Lin, G. (2013). Life-space characterization from cellular telephone collected GPS data. *Computers, Environment and Urban Systems, 39*, 63–70.

Wan, N., Qu, W., Whittington, J., Witbrodt, B. C., Henderson, M. P., Goulding, E. H., et al. (2013). Assessing smart phones for generating life-space indicators. *Environment and Planning B: Planning and Design, 40*(2), 350–361. https://doi.org/10.1068/b38200.

Ward, B. W., Schiller, J. S., & Goodman, R. A. (2014). Multiple chronic conditions among US adults: A 2012 update. *Preventing Chronic Disease, 11*, E62. https://doi.org/10.5888/pcd11.130389.

Zempsky, W. T., Palermo, T. M., Corsi, J. M., Lewandowski, A. S., Zhou, C., & Casella, J. F. (2013). Daily changes in pain, mood and physical function in youth hospitalized for sickle cell disease pain. *Pain Research and Management, 18*(1), 33–38.

Ziegler, F., & Schwanen, T. (2011). "I like to go out to be energised by different people": An exploratory analysis of mobility and wellbeing in later life. *Ageing and Society, 31*(5), 758–781.

# Chapter 13
# Mobility in Later Life and Wellbeing

Charles Musselwhite

**Abstract** Transport is more important to older people than ever before. We live in, what is termed by academics in the transport field, as a "hypermobile" society. One where high levels of mobility are needed in order to stay connected to communities, friends and family and to access shops and services. The car has been central to this hyper-connectivity. Being mobile is linked to quality of life. In particular, giving up driving in later life has repeatedly been shown to related to a decrease in wellbeing and an increase in depression and related health problems, including feelings of stress and isolation and also increased mortality. Recent figures from Great Britain suggest around 342,000 over 75 year olds 'feel trapped' in their own homes through lack of suitable transport after giving-up driving. In previous work, myself and my colleague examined why mobility is important to older people. We placed the need for mobility around three main motivational domains, utility (mobility as a need to get from A to B), psychosocial (mobility that effects independence, identity and roles) and aesthetic needs (mobility for its own sake) in a hierarchical manner. This chapter will examine case studies of life beyond the car in three main areas (older people as pedestrians, older people using public transport and older people receiving lifts from friends and family) as well as examining a group of older drivers identifying to what extent the three levels of need, utility, psychosocial and aesthetic are met. Driving a car satisfies all three levels of mobility need. Results suggest that transport provision beyond the car neglects psychosocial needs of mobility and sporadically meets practical and aesthetic needs depending upon the wider social context.

**Keywords** Ageing · Older people · Car driving · Walking · Bus · Motivations · Needs · Passengers · Social support

C. Musselwhite (✉)
Swansea University, Swansea, UK
e-mail: c.b.a.musselwhite@swansea.ac.uk

© Springer International Publishing AG, part of Springer Nature 2018
M. Friman et al. (eds.), *Quality of Life and Daily Travel*, Applying Quality of Life Research, https://doi.org/10.1007/978-3-319-76623-2_13

## 13.1   Introduction

### 13.1.1   Ageing Society

We are living later in life than ever before. Society across the globe is rapidly ageing. In 1950 there were 384million people aged over 60, representing 8.6% of the population (UN 2015). This has risen to almost 900million, 12% of the population, nowadays and is forecast to rise to 2.2 billion, making up 22% of the population, by 2050 (UN 2015). This pattern of ageing is happening across the world, but the rate of increase is faster in high income countries, for example, the United Kingdom (UK) will reach 25% of the population being over 60 by around 2030 (ONS 2013). In the UK, life expectancy is increasing. Females born in 2015 can expect to live 82.8 years from birth, 4 years more than females born in 1991. Males have seen a greater increase in life expectancy of 5.7 years, from 73.4 years for males born in 1991 to 79.1 years for males born in 2015.

### 13.1.2   Increase in Mobility

Being mobile is more important as we age than it has been for previous generations. This is evidenced by the amount of mobility that is occurring among older people and that when mobility is forcibly reduced there is a reduction not only in quality of life, but in general mental health and wellbeing. In the UK, 32.2 million people (70% of the population) currently hold full car driving licences (DfT 2016). For people aged over 70, around 50% hold a driver's licence, which has increased from 32% in 1989 (DfT 2016).

### 13.1.3   Mobility and Quality of Life

The importance of mobility has been linked to life satisfaction and quality of life for older people (Schlag et al. 1996). The need to be mobile and to travel is also related to psychological wellbeing and reduced mobility has been repeatedly shown to be correlated to increases in depression and loneliness (Fonda et al. 2001; Ling and Mannion 1995). This may be due to mediating factors like reduction in out of home activities (Harrison and Ragland 2003; Marottoli et al. 2000; Rosenbloom 2001) and decrease in associated physical and social functioning (Edwards et al. 2009), less frequent health care use for checkups and chronic care (Arcury et al. 2005), reduced social networks (Mezuk and Rebok 2008) and activities (Marottoli et al. 2000) and reduced mobility choices and options (Peel et al. 2002; Taylor and Tripodes 2001). It is also associated with loss of wellbeing due to increased dependency on others (Rosenbloom 2001), norms of using the car (Musselwhite and Haddad 2010; Zieglar and Schwannen 2011), independence (Adler and Rottunda 2006; Davey 2007;

Musselwhite and Haddad 2010; Siren and Hakamies-Blomqvist 2009) and the view of using the car being associated with being young and healthy (Musselwhite and Haddad 2010; Musselwhite and Shergold 2013). Zieglar and Schwannen (2011) conclude that driving cessation constitutes a major life event for older people.

Factors associated with driving cessation include older age (e.g., Anstey et al. 2006; Edwards et al. 2009; McNamara et al. 2013), being female (e.g., Braitman and Williams 2011; Chipman et al. 1998; Dellinger et al. 2004; Gallo et al. 1999; Hakamies-Blomqvist and Wahlström 1998), support of family and friends, both practically and emotionally (Musselwhite and Shergold 2013), lower car use frequency already earlier in life (Hakamies-Blomqvist and Siren 2003; Musselwhite and Haddad 2010; Musselwhite and Shergold 2013; Rabbitt et al. 1996), problems in health and cognitive function (e.g., Anstey et al. 2006; Ball et al. 1998; Brayne et al. 2000; Dellinger et al. 2004; Edwards et al. 2009; Persson 1993; Rabbitt et al. 1996; Sims et al. 2012), and decreased psychological well-being (Anstey et al. 2006). Support of family and friends in terms of practical and psychological support during the process of driving cessation are a vital protective factor in reducing negative affect of giving-up driving. Giving-up driving successfully occurs over time, with long periods of trialling out new modes and destinations (Musselwhite and Shergold 2013).

### 13.1.4  Theoretical Model

Musselwhite and Haddad (2010) propose a three-tier model of needs and motivations for travel in later life (Fig. 13.1). The different levels are hierarchical, grouped together by awareness of that need by participants. Using re-convened focus groups and interviews with drivers and ex-drivers aged over 65, participants discussed the importance of mobility. The hierarchy reflects when such a need was discussed. At the bottom level, utilitarian or practical needs of mobility were almost exclusively talked about first, showing high awareness of such a need. These include the need to get from A to B at quickly, reliably, safely and cheaply as possible. The next level of needs mentioned by participants was grouped together as psychosocial needs. This included for affective or emotional needs that mobility satisfies, including independence, control and the need to be seen as normal in society relating to concepts such as roles, identity, self-esteem and impression management. Finally, the highest level of need, labelled aesthetic needs, articulated later on in discussions was the need to travel for its own sake and just to get out and about, to see nature, a need traditionally termed discretionary. Musselwhite and Haddad (2010) suggest the car satisfies all three levels of need, and there was great concern about such needs being met for those who no longer drive. However, the model has not yet been examined in relation to specific modes of transport being used beyond the car. This chapter aims to explore Musselwhite and Haddad's (2010) model by re-examining data recently collected looking at older people's travel needs in four different contexts, older people as drivers, pedestrians, public transport users and those who frequently get lifts from family or friends.

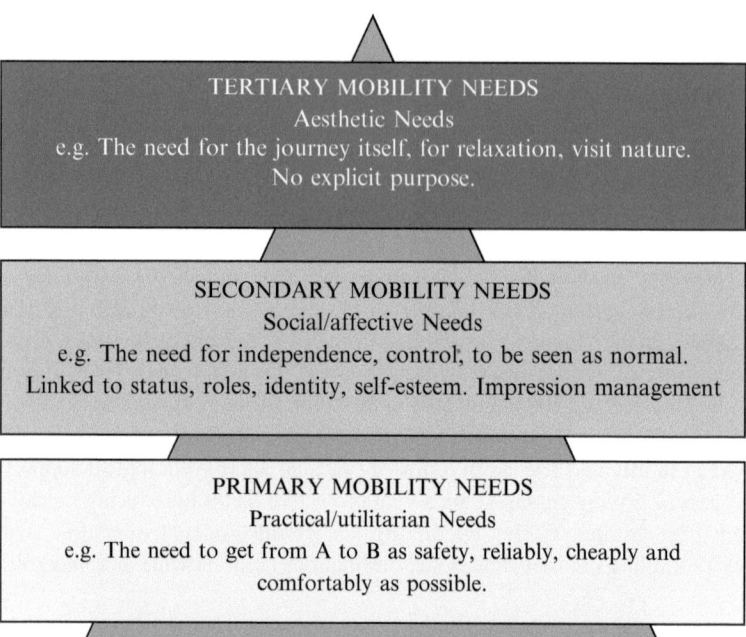

**Fig. 13.1** Hierarchy of travel needs in later life (After Musselwhite and Haddad 2010)

## 13.2 Methods

### 13.2.1 Design

Semi structured interviews were carried out with 48 individuals over the age of 65 years to explore travel and mobility needs and behaviour. The research included three different groups selected on their usual mobility mode: (1) regular drivers; (2) people who usually walk; (3) regular bus users and; (4) non-drivers who regularly rely on friends and family (who don't live with them).

### 13.2.2 Participants

Participants were sought through the research network of older people in South Wales, United Kingdom, answering an advert for people in the four categories. People were placed into each category if they used that mode most often for their journeys. A cut off of 12 people in each category was sought. A total of 48 participants took part (see Table 13.1) with an average age of 74.3 years, 31 were cohabiting with a partner, 11 lived alone and 4 lived in a residential care home (3 in an extra care facility, 1 care home) and 2 lived with their family (both with their

**Table 13.1** Participants in the study

| | n | Age range (average) | Living arrangement | Health (self-score 1 = poor to 9 = good) |
|---|---|---|---|---|
| Context 1: drivers | 12 | 63–87 (73.3) | In couple, = 11 | 6.5 |
| | | | On own = 1 | |
| Context 2: bus users | 12 | 65–88 (72.7) | In couple = 10 | 6.5 |
| | | | On own = 2 | |
| Context 3: lifts from family and friends | 12 | 72–92 (78) | In couple = 4 | 5 |
| | | | On own = 4 | |
| | | | Residential home = 2 | |
| | | | With family = 2 | |
| Context 4: walkers | 12 | 65–85 (71.1) | In couple = 6 | 8 |
| | | | On own = 4 | |
| | | | Residential home = 2 | |
| Total | 48 | 65–92 (74.3) | In couple = 31 | 6 |
| | | | On own = 11 | |
| | | | With family = 2 | |
| | | | Residential home = 4 | |

children). They were asked to self-report their health on a scale from 1 very poor to 9 very good. An average of 6 on the scale was found overall with the highest average, indicating best average health, among the people who walked and lowest among the people getting lifts.

## 13.2.3  Procedure and Tools

Interviews took place in participant's home or at an agreed public location and lasted around 1 h. Participants were free to talk around set themes using apprenticing and abstraction style questions:

Apprenticing (Robertson and Robertson 2013) allowed the participant to describe their everyday experience with mobility, for example the interviewer would ask "take me through a recent trip you went on step by step".

Abstraction (Robertson and Robertson 2013) asks the participant what would happen to their everyday mobility if their experience was different. It involves both counterfactual detail, to ask participants what if they themselves were different (for example if they were older, less mobile or less healthy) and scenario testing (presenting the scenario of the other two contexts, so, for example, for those walking, what would be the difference if they used community transport or drove for that trip).

## 13.2.4  Analysis

A common thematic analysis took place. Data was recorded and then transcribed word for word, and key themes highlighted. Etic (stemming from themes derived from previous theory, models and literature) and emic (stemming from the analysis of the data itself) coding was then employed on the data. Etic codes looked to place the data within categories of practical, psychosocial or aesthetic need based on Mussselwhite and Haddad's (2010) model among the three different groups of participant and additional challenges to the model found through emic style analysis.

## 13.3  Findings

Findings from all four groups of older people are framed here around Musselwhite and Haddad's three tier model (Musselwhite and Haddad 2010). It is clear to see that, as expected, the car easily fulfils all three levels of need among older people, whereas walking, using public transport or getting lifts only partially meets needs, with psychosocial needs especially being neglected.

## 13.3.1  Utilitarian Needs

For all groups the significant importance of the car in meeting utilitarian needs, such as carrying items and the ease of the door-to-door convenience, was frequently mentioned by drivers and missed by non-drivers,

> Bringing stuff back when you've been shopping. I mean I, we struggle to carry it now. (male, driver, aged 76)

How the car keeps people connected to the activities that they see as vital is frequently mentioned throughout the interviews, especially with regards to shopping and meeting appointments,

> We have so many health things going on. We are in and out the hospital for appointments or down the doctors. Doing that now without a car. It's how it takes up a whole day and it's exhausting. (male, bus user, aged 80)

Walking to do shopping or to visit the hospital or doctors was seen as difficult, if not impossible by many due to geographical distance or the physical effort,

> You just can't do it. It mean they expect you'll arrive by car so they schedule it like it. (female, walker, aged 78)

Those that did achieve shopping on foot as a pedestrian, had found ways to overcome the physical burden, either by going regularly or having the shopping delivered,

It's only me, so I don't actually have a great deal to bring back, so all I do is go regularly. I enjoy the walk, so I like to do it daily if I'm feeling up to it and the weather's not too bad. (female, walker, aged 74)

The shop does this wonderful thing where I can shop and they bring it later on in a van! So I can still walk, choose my shopping things and not have to carry it back. If I'm lucky the driver brings it right in to the kitchen too. (Female, walker, aged 79)

Naturally to get shopping or visit services, getting lifts from friends and family was common and satisfied most utilitarian needs,

Having help. I mean we couldn't do it without them. My daughter comes once a week and gets the shopping we need. (Male, friends and family help, aged 81)

Sometimes the help supplemented carrying items for themselves,

I'm lucky to have good neighbours, and they're good friends too. They help me and get stuff in when I need it. The bigger things you know. Or sometimes on offer things, it's the big things on offer I can't carry and I miss out on. Treats like lemonade! (Female, walker, aged 77)

Car drivers become very used to being able to use a car when they want to,

It's just so convenient to go when I want to. To have no timetable. I just can go to the shops anytime and return when I like. (female, driver, aged 77)

However, this is somewhat a perception as is indicated in some conversations about driver's compensating for changes in physiology or health,

I don't drive when it's busy or at night, now. That's a blessing I don't have to. I don't really need to go out at those times anyway and if I do I'll use a taxi or bus. (male, driver, aged 80)

This is somewhat missed for bus users and those getting lifts,

You are reliant on how reliable the bus is. I mean they are every half hour in the day but they don't seem to always run or stick to the timetable. There is, I guess, lots of waiting around for us, that you wouldn't get in a car (female, bus user, aged 80)

I have to wait for Nancy to be ready. She can't do Thursdays or the weekend either. We try to go shopping every Monday but I can't just go when I want then see, like I could when I had a car. (female, lift from friends and family, aged 85)

Where friends and family weren't available these needs were often met with a taxi more often than a bus,

Taxi is expensive but once a week for shopping it's idea. Get a good driver they'll always bring stuff in for you too. (female, walker, aged 78)

People who walk regularly are more able to go when they want but it is dependent on a number of factors,

Walking is quite free, free to use, free to go when you want to, in that sense, you can go when and where you want yes, up to a point. But awful weather or dangerous roads, no pavements and the like stop the routes I walk on. (male, walker, aged 74)

Personal safety was mentioned as being a concern for those walking and for using buses, but never those using cars, either as a driver or getting a lift,

I am worried about being attacked. You hear about it all the time. Old people are always vulnerable and when I'm walking I could be attacked yes I suppose I could. It does play on my mind a little but hey it hasn't happened yet. (male, walker, aged 80)

Concerns about falls are there for those walking and using a bus too, but again not for people using a car. In fact the car was thought to mitigate falls

The driver can be, you know, a bit unkind, can take off with us oldies still finding our seat and you can tumble over. It happened to Mrs Jones up the road. (female, bus user, aged 80)

The pavements can be really bad. I did stumble and have a little fall. Took me a while to get back to it. I don't know if it was because I was old or the pavement was bad. Probably both. (female, walker, aged 78)

It's an advantage of the car isn't it. I'm not stable on my feet nowadays and getting on a bus or walking too far would be difficult for me. I have fallen a couple of times while walking. The car gets me as close as possible <to where I want to go> and that helps. (male, driver, aged 80)

Only walkers mentioned concerns about road safety,

Cars nowadays go so fast, without a concern for us pedestrians. Crossing the road is a particular trouble for me. I don't like walking or crossing near lots of cars. (male, walker, aged 80)

Drivers all stated they wouldn't drive if they felt they were unsafe, even a few admitting they probably weren't as good as they once were,

I would stop immediately I didn't feel safe. I know I'm probably a little slower and slower to react but I am still safe. (male, driver, aged 82)

### 13.3.2  Psychosocial Needs

The independence and perceived freedom that driving gives individuals was frequently discussed and was lamented when people had to give-up driving. Walking places was sometimes mentioned in conjunction with independence, but independence was very much missing from people using buses or getting lifts. Getting lifts was very much seen as reducing independence and the feeling of a sense of being a burden was really felt,

It's the lost independence you know that's the worse, that the car used to give you. I really miss that freedom. (male, bus user, aged 75)

I can get lifts but I feel a burden. They don't make me feel a burden. I just do! I just wish I could still drive myself! (female, lifts from family and friends, aged 83)

Driving and owning a vehicle was related to status,

I drive the car I got when I retired. I worked for that. I'm proud of it. (male, car driver, aged 74)

Using a bus was opposite to gaining status,

> Well I never saw myself using a bus, not when I had a car but now I do, I suppose there is a little embarrassment, people do rib me. But I actually enjoy it. Buses are much better these days. (male, bus user, aged 80)

Walking had some relationship to status as being seen as being fit enough to walk in later life was valued,

> Well I'm proud to be as fit as I am. I'm as fit as someone half my age and fitter than most youngsters these days. (male, walker, aged 80)

The role of the car to help others was often mentioned by drivers but not through walking, using a bus or getting lifts from family and friends,

> I can help look after grandchildren, take and pick up from school, with the car you see and that way I feel I'm a real help, I'm really enjoying being a grandmother. (female, driver, aged, 74)

People talk about the car that they drive in very passionate terms, how it is part of their life. This is not mirrored for those walking, using a bus or getting lifts,

> The car gives you a sense of freedom, of pride, something I connect to. It's mine. I look at it and it's taken me through all good times and bad, to France on holiday, to visit friends and family, to help my wife to and from hospital. I don't want to lose it. (male, driver, aged 80)

## 13.3.3  Aesthetic Needs

Difference between walking and the car is that even in utilitarian or practical trips, enjoyment of walking is mentioned much more frequently. Walking as a source of exercise made the walkers feel good, and gave them a chance to stop and chat. This wasn't mentioned with driving,

> I do really enjoy the walk. I visit more shops than I need to. Stop and natter. Have a look round. (male, walker, aged 76)

> The walking makes me feel better I suppose. I feel less stiff and even though I might feel tired afterwards I feel sort of refreshed. I don't feel that driving, I always got stressed about parking and the traffic and it became such a worry. (female, walker, aged 80)

The car can connect people to aesthetics of the nearby places, with green (countryside, woodlands, parks) and blue (rivers, lakes, seaside) environments being visited, or driven past, mentioned frequently in that sense it can be relaxing,

> Driving past the mountains or through the valleys, open road, all different weathers, all different seasons, it's beautiful. God's own country. (male, driver, aged 70)

There are mixed views over whether driving itself is relaxing,

> Driving isn't what it was. It is so busy now. And much less courtesy on the road. (male, aged 83, driver)

> I find driving is good for me. Helps me relax. I go for a drive when I'm feeling wound up. It's a release. I put the radio on, listen to a good play or book. (male, driver, aged 85)

There are also mixed views on the bus, largely depending upon availability of the services in the area. Those who had frequent bus services tended to see the bus as a third space, as a place for chatting, socialising and visiting places for the sake of the journey. The social situation of the bus also mattered. If it was uncrowded or had people of similar backgrounds and ages then the bus was seen as relaxing and enjoyable, potentially satisfying aesthetic needs. If the bus was infrequent or crowded then it was simply used for utilitarian purposes,

> I love the bus. It's a place I regularly see someone I know to chat to and I often use it to go to places for a cuppa tea and a cake, down to the seaside, nice service that. (female, bus user, aged 79)

> I use the bus to go to my club, have lunch and then come home. I can half a quick half of beer too then. And some more! (male, bus user, aged 80)

> the bus takes so long to get anywhere decent, I'm only using it for the essentials. (male, bus user, aged 84)

Whether aesthetic needs are occasionally met by lifts from family and friends varied depending upon the relationship of the older person and the provider of the lift. More often than not it was felt that going out just to see the world going by was deemed unnecessary and not worthy of taking up the time of someone providing the lift,

> people did offer but I really didn't want to, well it would mean people travelling a long way to come and get me and take me somewhere . . . ... (female, lift from family and friend, aged 89)

> Erm, I hadn't even thought about it really to be honest, er, I probably could have asked two people, erm but I would have felt really cheeky asking. (female, lift from family and friend, aged 80)

## 13.4   Discussion

It is easy to place transport and mobility needs of older people around Musselwhite and Haddad's (2010) three tier model. All three levels of need, practical, psychosocial and aesthetic are discussed in detail by the participants in the interviews. All three levels seem important to older people and their quality of life. This is especially evident when one of the level of needs is not being met by the current transport mode being used. Each level of need is not met in the same way by different modes of transport. Driving your own vehicle meets all three levels of need easily and this can be seen as a major attraction of the car (see Fig. 13.2).

Walking meets psychosocial needs and aesthetic needs well (see Fig. 13.3). However, walking does not satisfy practical needs well. The reason why such needs are not met by walking, however, are largely because of the dominance of a car-based culture, much of which could be changed by good planning and design. For example, the distances and the times of day needed to travel to meet healthcare obligations and appointments at hospitals and doctor surgeries means it is hard to travel to these on foot. Many urban areas across High Income Countries have seen an

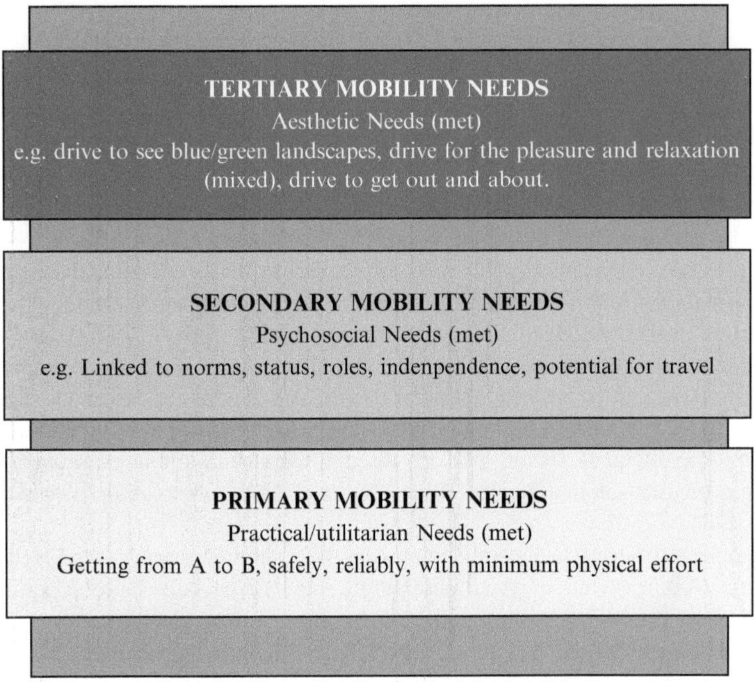

**TERTIARY MOBILITY NEEDS**
Aesthetic Needs (met)
e.g. drive to see blue/green landscapes, drive for the pleasure and relaxation
(mixed), drive to get out and about.

**SECONDARY MOBILITY NEEDS**
Psychosocial Needs (met)
e.g. Linked to norms, status, roles, indenpendence, potential for travel

**PRIMARY MOBILITY NEEDS**
Practical/utilitarian Needs (met)
Getting from A to B, safely, reliably, with minimum physical effort

**Fig. 13.2** The car meets all three levels of Musselwhite and Haddad (2010) older people's mobility needs

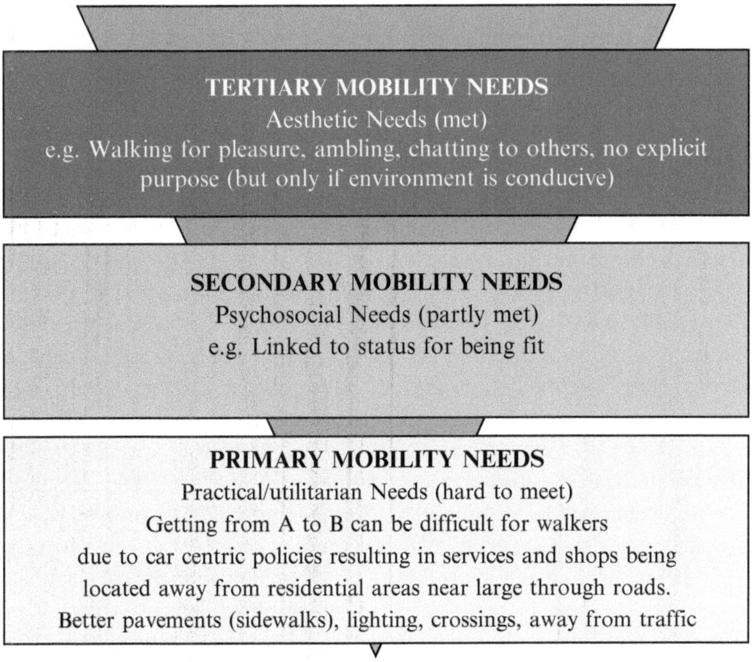

**TERTIARY MOBILITY NEEDS**
Aesthetic Needs (met)
e.g. Walking for pleasure, ambling, chatting to others, no explicit
purpose (but only if environment is conducive)

**SECONDARY MOBILITY NEEDS**
Psychosocial Needs (partly met)
e.g. Linked to status for being fit

**PRIMARY MOBILITY NEEDS**
Practical/utilitarian Needs (hard to meet)
Getting from A to B can be difficult for walkers
due to car centric policies resulting in services and shops being
located away from residential areas near large through roads.
Better pavements (sidewalks), lighting, crossings, away from traffic

**Fig. 13.3** Walking meets aesthetic needs, some psychosocial needs but few mobility needs

agglomeration of healthcare at the fringes of the central districts, built on cheap land, placing staff and facilities together, passing on the cost of transport and mobility to staff and patients. The easiest way to attend such healthcare is by car or possibly in some cases by bus. Older people have more healthcare appointments than other age groups and hence spend more time at such locations. Solutions include better planning to ensure healthcare is provided within walking distances of major conurbations. Planning, needs to value transport and accessibility and in particular placing accessibility on foot high up on the benefits when making decisions about agglomeration of healthcare. Healthcare appointments need to be made taking into account older people's travel needs. They need to be allowed to make them at times of day when walking can occur, keeping older people from having to walk in the dark or in poor weather, for example. There also needs to be a re-focus on reducing the necessity to attend in person, perhaps through tele-health and tele-care facilities or having smaller satellite health clinics in local places for routine appointments (Musselwhite et al. in press).

People also struggle to walk to satisfy their shopping needs. Again, in High Income Countries out of town shopping centres, especially large supermarkets, based on accessibility by car and bulk buying are inaccessible on foot. Out of town shopping centres and large supermarkets have a knock-on effect on local shops, reducing the number of smaller supermarkets and convenience shops in neighbourhoods that are walkable too. This is, of course, circular in nature, so with fewer local shops, the less likely people are to walk, the fewer walking, the less likely shops are needed in the local area. Again, planning could change this, helping local shops to stay open with reduced rents or taxes, building in shops to planning conditions, as well as reducing the ease and the amount of out of town shops allowed. There were also some good examples given, where shops will deliver the shopping for people, reducing the need to carry heavy items. Encouraging use of shopping online can also help. People who walk cannot always visit family and friends easily.

Accessibility for walking also needs to be improved at the microscopic level. There needs to be well kept pavements, free from clutter and away from busy traffic. These need to be maintained and gritted in poor weather. They need to be well-lit, and have benches, for resting, and trees, for shelter from sun or rain, along them.

Many people nowadays have friends and family dispersed around the country and without using motorised transport and staying connected with such people is hard. Older people are more likely than any other age group to say they would like to visit friends and family more often but mobility stops them doing so. Telephone and video calls (such as skype and similar) help people stay connected but generally raising awareness of the importance of family or friend visits and keeping people from being isolated and lonely is vital. Services provided to support people from being isolated and lonely need to take into account mobility and accessibility.

Using the bus with heavy items can be problematic and there are safety concerns about sharing with other passengers and most notably the bus driver driving the bus off before the person has sat down. There are examples of bus companies training their drivers to be age aware and to consider the needs of older passengers more.

Gilhooly et al. (2002) found the highest barrier to public transport use amongst older people was personal security in the evening and at night, followed by transport running late and having to wait. A report using accompanied journeys in London has highlighted similar problems for older people including crowds at the bus stop or on the bus, not being able to sit on buses, fear of falling getting on and off buses and fear of falling over when the bus moves off (TfL 2009). Broome et al. (2010) in an Australian study found that driver friendliness, ease of entry/exit and information usability were prioritised barriers and facilitators for older people on buses.

The psychosocial element tends to be absent once driving has ceased especially for public transport users and people who get lifts from family and friends. The independence and freedom is not only absent from people who mainly gets lifts, but there is an additional sense of being a burden on other people. This can be mitigated through reciprocation, the offer to cook or buy a meal or to offer payment for petrol or parking, for example, but this does not come close to the freedom associated with driving oneself. The ability to drive when and where you please is also lost in other forms of transport, even when people do not do that. This is termed the potential for travel (Metz 2000) and no other transport quite affords such luxury. However, there is somewhat of a disconnect between perception of freedom that car offers and the reality which is often constrained. For example, older people talked about deliberately restricting their driving to times and roads they felt comfortable on, avoiding busy traffic, poor visibility, difficult turns or merges reducing the freedom of the car. Walking also offers similar perception of freedom to travel when people want but again restrictions on walking in poor weather or in the dark occur. Also, walking is restricted by how far physically the person can walk.

The dominance of the car as a desirable vehicle that satisfied human psychological needs is hardly matched by other modes. People are sold freedom, independence, esteem and identity through advertising and marketing by the car, that other modes just don't match. Car companies spend huge resources on getting the aesthetics right targeting both psychosocial and aesthetic travel needs, making the car a desirable space to be in. Bus companies are beginning to do so, offering better quality interior, leather seating, air conditioning, climate control, large windows, ambient lighting, wifi, but more still needs to be done to get close to cars.

Aesthetic needs are best met by the car. People can travel to see the world going by, to see nature, to just get "out and about". This is especially the case for people who drive themselves, but can occur with lifts from friends and family. There is anxiety about asking for lifts, viewing such travel as unnecessary and burdensome. Recognition that such "discretionary" travel is in fact important for health and wellbeing needs further emphasis (Musselwhite 2017). Travel does not always have to have an explicit purpose for it to be worthwhile and valuable. The bus can serve this need and can be seen as a "third space", a space for "people watching", for watching the world go-by, for interacting with other passengers. However, the bus must be (perceived as) comfortable and accessible before this can happen. Aesthetic needs can be met by walking, if the public realm is well designed to allow it to happen. There must be space for people to walk, to sit and watch. Places need to be desirable to facilitate walking, as much as they are accessible (Musselwhite in press). They must have character and identity, reflecting local culture and history to give people a sense of place and legitimacy to be there. There should be continuity to facilitate walking yet some mystery and intrigue to entice people in, to make people want to dwell.

## 13.5   Conclusion

Overall, it can be seen that driving satisfies all three levels of needs better than other modes do. Figures 13.2, 13.3, 13.4, and 13.5 show how far each need is met by each form of transport. Psychosocial needs are only met by driving and by walking. There is potential for aesthetic needs to be met by all modes of transport dependent on other factors. For walkers, this is getting an attractive and desirable public realm to walk in. For people getting lifts, this is making the people provide lifts understand how important a journey itself is or a journey to visit countryside or the seaside is. For those using buses, it is dependent upon having good quality bus services that serve

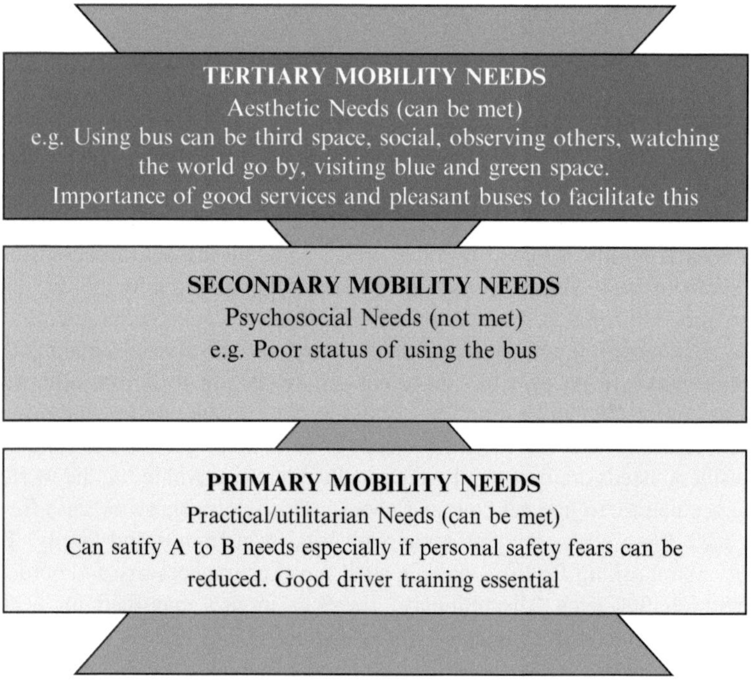

**TERTIARY MOBILITY NEEDS**
Aesthetic Needs (can be met)
e.g. Using bus can be third space, social, observing others, watching the world go by, visiting blue and green space.
Importance of good services and pleasant buses to facilitate this

**SECONDARY MOBILITY NEEDS**
Psychosocial Needs (not met)
e.g. Poor status of using the bus

**PRIMARY MOBILITY NEEDS**
Practical/utilitarian Needs (can be met)
Can satify A to B needs especially if personal safety fears can be reduced. Good driver training essential

**Fig. 13.4** Using the bus can meet practical and aesthetic mobility needs but not psychosocial mobility needs of older people

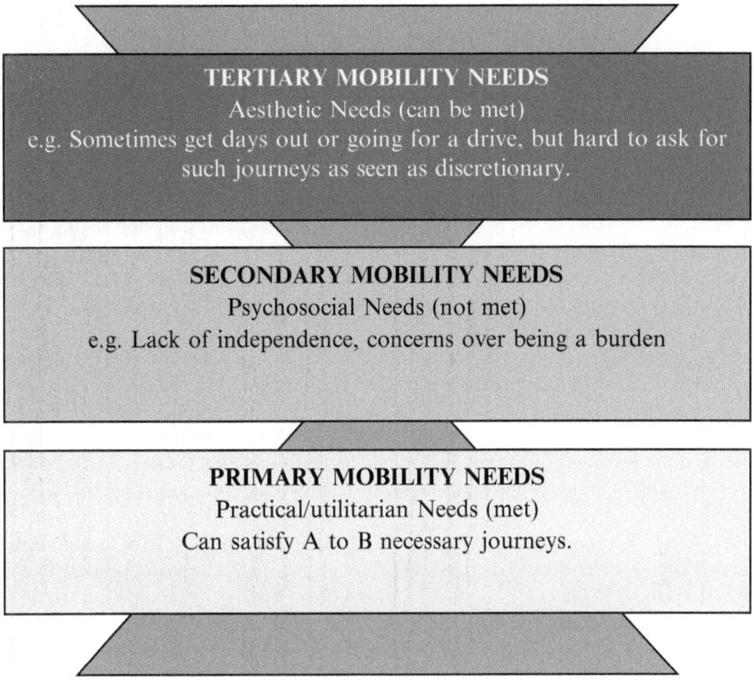

**TERTIARY MOBILITY NEEDS**
Aesthetic Needs (can be met)
e.g. Sometimes get days out or going for a drive, but hard to ask for
such journeys as seen as discretionary.

**SECONDARY MOBILITY NEEDS**
Psychosocial Needs (not met)
e.g. Lack of independence, concerns over being a burden

**PRIMARY MOBILITY NEEDS**
Practical/utilitarian Needs (met)
Can satisfy A to B necessary journeys.

**Fig. 13.5** Getting a lift can meet practical mobility needs and sometimes can be aesthetic mobility needs but does not meet psychosocial mobility needs of older people

attractive areas. Practical mobility needs can be met across all modes of transport, though there is greatest difficulty in doing this through walking, especially through modern day car-centric planning, followed by using the bus because of difficulty in carrying items and concerns over personal safety. In understanding services beyond the car, there is a need to address all three levels of need, most notably a need to address psychosocial needs that are limited in other modes of transport and ensuring aesthetic and practical needs can be met. Practical support is found quite widely, but without understanding the affective elements of car use will not fulfil older people's needs and as a result will not necessarily help reduce negative health associated with giving-up driving. More of this support is needed as society becomes ever more geared around the car and future generations of older people will have used a car almost all of their adult life and geared their life around the car, making the move to alternative ways of travelling even more difficult.

# References

Adler, G., & Rottunda, S. (2006). Older adults' perspectives on driving cessation. *Journal of Aging Studies, 20*(3), 227–235.

Anstey, K. J., Windsor, T. D., Luszcz, M. A., & Andrews, G. R. (2006). Predicting driving cessation over 5 years in older adults: Psychological well-being and cognitive competence are stronger predictors than physical health. *Journal of the American Geriatrics Society, 54*, 121–126.

Arcury, T. A., Gesler, W. M., Preisser, J. S., Sherman, J., Spencer, J., & Perin, J. (2005). The effects of geography and spatial behavior on health care utilization among the residents of a rural region. *Health Services Research, 40*, 135–156.

Ball, K., Owsley, C., Stalvey, B., Roenker, D. L., Sloane, M. E., & Graves, M. (1998). Driving avoidance and functional impairment in older drivers. *Accident Analysis & Prevention, 30*, 313–323.

Braitman, K. A., & Williams, A. F. (2011). Changes in self-regulatory driving among older drivers over time. *Traffic Injury Prevention, 12*, 568–575.

Brayne, C., Dufouil, C., Ahmed, A., Dening, T. R., Chi, L. Y., McGee, M., & Huppert, F. A. (2000). Very old drivers: Findings from a population cohort of people aged 84 and over. *International Journal of Epidemiology, 29*, 704–707.

Broome, K., Nalder, E., Worrall, L., & Boldy, D. (2010). Age-friendly buses? A comparison of reported barriers and facilitators to bus use for younger and older adults. *Australasian Journal on Ageing, 29*(1), 33–38.

Chipman, M., Payne, J., & McDonough, P. (1998). To drive or not to drive: The influence of social factors on the decisions of elderly drivers. *Accident Analysis & Prevention, 30*, 299–304.

Davey, J. A. (2007). Older people and transport: Coping without a car. *Ageing and Society, 27*, 49–65.

Dellinger, A. M., Kresnow, M. J., White, D. D., & Sehgal, M. (2004). Risk to self versus risk to others: How do older drivers compare to others on the road? *American Journal of Preventive Medicine, 26*(3), 217–221.

DfT (Department for Transport, UK). (2016). *Transport Statistics Great Britain: 2016*. London: DfT. Available at: https://www.gov.uk/government/statistics/transport-statistics-great-britain-2016. Accessed 15 Sept 2017.

Edwards, J. D., Perkins, M., Ross, L. A., & Reynolds, S. L. (2009). Driving status and three-year mortality among community-dwelling older adults. *Journal of Gerontology Series A: Biological Sciences and Medical Sciences, 64*, 300–305.

Fonda, S. J., Wallace, R. B., & Herzog, A. R. (2001). Changes in driving patterns and worsening depressive symptoms among older adults. *The Journal of Gerontology, Series B: Psychological Sciences and Social Sciences, 56*(6), 343–351.

Gallo, J. J., Rebok, G. W., & Lesikar, S. E. (1999). The driving habits of adults aged 60 years and older. *Journal of American Geriatrics Society, 47*, 335–341.

Gilhooly, M.L.M., Hamilton, K., O'Neill, M., Gow, J., Webster, N., Pike, F., & Bainbridge, C. (2002). *Transport and ageing: Extending quality of life via public and private transport.* ESCR Report L48025025, Brunel University Research Archive.

Hakamies-Blomqvist, L., & Siren, A. (2003). Deconstructing a gender difference: Driving cessation and personal driving history of older women. *Journal of Safety Research, 34*, 383–388.

Hakamies-Blomqvist, L., & Wahlström, B. (1998). Why do older drivers give up driving? *Accident; Analysis and Prevention, 30*, 305–312.

Harrison, A., & Ragland, D. R. (2003). Consequences of driving reduction or cessation for older adults. *Transportation Research Record, 1843*, 96–104.

Ling, D. J., & Mannion, R. (1995). Enhanced mobility and quality of life of older people: Assessment of economic and social benefits of dial-a-ride services. In *Proceedings of the Seventh International Conference on Transport and Mobility for Older and Disabled People* (Vol. 1). London: DETR.

Marottoli, R. A., Mendes de Leon, C. F., Glass, T. A., Williams, C. S., Cooney, L. M., & Berkman, L. F. (2000). Consequences of driving cessation: Decreased out-of-home activity levels. *Journals of Gerontology: Series B, Psychological Sciences and Social Sciences, 55B*(6), 334–340.

McNamara, A., Chen, G., George, S., Walker, R., & Ratcliffe, J. (2013). What factors influence older people in the decision to relinquish their driver's licence? A discrete choice experiment. *Accident Analysis & Prevention, 55*, 178–184.

Metz, D. (2000). Mobility of older people and their quality of life. *Transport Policy, 7*, 149–152.

Mezuk, B., & Rebok, G. W. (2008). Social integration and social support among older adults following driving cessation. *Journal of Gerontolology Social Science, 63B*, 298–303.

Musselwhite, C. B. A. (2017). Exploring the importance of discretionary mobility in later life. *Working with Older People, 21*(1), 49–58.

Musselwhite, C. (in press). Creating a convivial public realm for an ageing population. Being a pedestrian and the built environment In C. Musselwhite (Ed.), *Transport, travel and later life*. Emerald Publishing.

Musselwhite, C. B. A., & Haddad, H. (2010). Mobility, accessibility and quality of later life. *Quality in Ageing and Older Adults, 11*(1), 25–37.

Musselwhite, C. B. A., & Shergold, I. (2013). Examining the process of driving cessation in later life. *European Journal of Ageing, 10*(2), 89–100.

Musselwhite, C., Freeman, S., & Marston, H. R. (in press). An introduction to the potential for the mobile eHealth revolution to impact on hard to reach, marginalised and excluded groups. In H. Marston, S. Freeman, & C. Musselwhite (Eds.), *Mobile e-Health*, Human–Computer Interaction Series, Springer. https://doi.org/10.1007/978-3-319-60672-9_1.

Office for National Statistics. (2013) *National population projections*, 2012-based. Available at: http://www.ons.gov.uk/ons/dcp171778_334975.pdf. Accessed 15 Sept 2017.

Peel, N., Westmoreland, J., & Steinberg, M. (2002). Transport safety for older people: A study of their experiences, perceptions and management needs. *Injury Control & Safety Promotion, 9*, 19–24.

Persson, D. (1993). The elderly driver: Deciding when to stop. *Gerontologist, 33*, 88–91.

Rabbitt, P., Carmichael, A., Jones, S., & Holland, C. (1996). *When and why older drivers give up driving*. Basingstoke: AA Foundation for Road Safety Research.

Robertson, S., & Robertson, J. (2013). *Mastering the requirements process, third edition: Getting requirements right*. New York: Addison-Wiley.

Rosenbloom, S. (2001). Sustainability and automobility among elderly: An international assessment. *Transportation, 28*, 375–408.

Schlag, B., Schwenkhagen, U., & Trankle, U. (1996). Transportation for the elderly: Towards a user- friendly combination of private and public transport. *IATSS Research, 20*(1).

Sims, J., Rouse-Watson, S., Schattner, P., Beveridge, A., & Jones, K. M. (2012). To drive or not to drive: Assessment dilemmas for GPs. *International Journal of Family Medicine, 2012*, 417512.

Siren, A., & Hakamies-Blomqvist, L. (2009). Mobility and well-being in old age. *Topics in Geriatric Rehabilitation, 25*, 3–11.

Taylor, B. D., & Tripodes, S. (2001). The effects of driving cessation on the elderly with dementia and their caregivers. *Accident Analysis and Prevention, 33*, 519–528.

TfL. (2009). *Older people's experience of travel in London*. London: Transport for London. Available at: http://www.tfl.gov.uk/cdn/static/cms/documents/older-peoples-transport-experiences-report.pdf. Accessed 15 Sept 2017.

United Nations (UN). (2015). *World population ageing*. New York: United Nations. Available at http://www.un.org/en/development/desa/population/publications/pdf/ageing/WPA2015_Report.pdf. Last accessed 15 Sept 2017.

Zieglar, F., & Schwannen, T. (2011). I like to go out to be energised by different people: An exploratory analysis of mobility and wellbeing in later life. *Ageing and Society, 31*(5), 758–781.

# Part IV
# The Future

# Chapter 14
# Travel and Wellbeing: Future Prospects

**Margareta Friman, Dick Ettema, and Lars E. Olsson**

**Abstract** In this chapter, ideas and directions for future research are presented. Various interventions, as a means of counteracting mispredictions by the individual traveler and breaking travel habits, are discussed and illustrated. We elaborate upon what is known about individuals' predictions and their accompanying thoughts about possible consequences regarding wellbeing when performing a travel mode change. It is argued that one overall goal of every transport policy should be providing sustainable travel, accompanied by sustained or increased wellbeing. The authors conclude that, while there is a vast amount of research on judgment and decision making, there is still a need for knowledge of how to aid people's judgments as regards switching to sustainable alternatives. Specifically, researchers are urged to unveil how to prevent a loss of, or support a gain in, wellbeing when switching to sustainable travel.

**Keywords** Daily travel · Sustainable travel · Travel behaviour change · Travel · Wellbeing · Interventions · Wellbeing consequences · Decision making

## 14.1 Introduction

This book presents an interdisciplinary perspective on travel and wellbeing. It is a multifaceted subject that has so far received only modest attention in the academic transport community, and in the public and private transport sector. This lack of attention is somewhat surprising considering that travel involves issues of human, social, economic, and political importance. This book proposes a cross-disciplinary

M. Friman (✉) · L. E. Olsson
CTF Service Research Center, Department of Social and Psychological Studies, Karlstad University, Karlstad, Sweden
e-mail: Margareta.friman@kau.se; lars.e.olsson@kau.se

D. Ettema
Department of Human Geography and Spatial Planning, Utrecht University, Utrecht, The Netherlands
e-mail: D.F.Ettema@uu.nl

© Springer International Publishing AG, part of Springer Nature 2018     255
M. Friman et al. (eds.), *Quality of Life and Daily Travel*, Applying Quality of Life Research, https://doi.org/10.1007/978-3-319-76623-2_14

focus by bringing together a series of works by authors from a variety of disciplinary orientations (e.g., transport geography, psychology, engineering, and public health). We hope that this breadth and diversity will convey an inclusive view of the complex nature of people's travel and quality of life. This chapter provides a brief overview and summarizes some important evidence in this field. We point to gaps in knowledge and diagnose difficulties that will provide a roadmap for future research. The issues considered here are also debated in other chapters of this book, albeit from different perspectives.

Chapters of this book show how travel can influence quality of life (e.g., Lancée, Burger, Veenhoven, Chap. 2), and there is growing recognition that the daily commute can be both unpleasant and fatiguing (Gärling, Chap. 6), as well as positive and favorable as an experience (Mokhtarian, Chap. 4). In the US, the Office for National Statistics (2014) presents evidence that people who regularly travel to work are, on average, less satisfied with their lives than those who work from home as their main job. By comparing international data on travel mode choice and quality of life, in a number of high-income cities, Buehler et al. (2017) show that, even though Vienna, Austria has implemented transport policies that restrict car use and promote public transport, cycling, and walking, it has improved its ranking on a number of quality of life indicators (2005–2015). Vienna is now ranked as one of the top five cities when it comes to quality of life, even though this city has reduced its car mode share more than other comparable cities. Air pollution is a well-known problem and a severe one in cities like Mexico City, Kabul, New Delhi, Beijing and Paris, but also in cities like Oslo, where restrictions on diesel cars have now been implemented. Traffic noise has well-documented effects on cardiovascular, respiratory, and metabolic health and studies have reported long-term associations between urban noise and premature death (Recio et al. 2016). Shifting to electrical vehicles is likely to improve traffic noise levels (Walker et al. 2016), as well as pollutant concentrations (Ferrero et al. 2016). One alternative is a sustainable transport system that relies on active travel modes. Several studies can confirm that active travel is beneficial for quality of life in that people who choose an active commute mode (walking and cycling) evaluate their lives as more satisfactory than those who choose to travel by car (e.g. Buehler et al. 2017; Gatersleben and Uzzell 2007; Rissel, Crane, Petrunoff, Chap. 14). A longitudinal study (Martin et al. 2014) conducted in the UK showed greater life satisfaction among public transport users than among car users over time. One explanation for this is that public transport use includes active elements, for instance walking back and forth to bus stops. Travelers using public transport generally walk two to three times further than car drivers (Besser and Dannenberg 2005; Litman 2015); changing from the car to public transport leads to a reduced body mass index (BMI) (Flint et al. 2016). Other explanations that have been put forward to explain the link between travel and wellbeing include the time people spend on travel. People with long commutes to and from work (totaling between 60 and 90 min) are systematically worse off and report significantly less life satisfaction than people with short commutes (Stutzer and Frey 2008; Hansson et al. 2011). On the other hand, travel time can be filled with meaningful activities or involve social interactions which provide psychological stimulation and positive emotions, such as feelings of excitement, fun, and pleasure. Activities on the move may also counteract boredom (Ettema et al. 2012; Mokhtarian 2005), making travelers less dissatisfied with their journeys. Other components of the transport system that influence quality of life include accessibility (Currie and Delbosc, Chap. 5). Not being able to travel to attractive places leads to a sense of alienation that has been found to negatively affect life satisfaction (Lucas 2012; Stanley et al. 2011). In particular, for older people (aged 75 and older), a positive relationship has been observed between leisure travel and life satisfaction (Nawijn and Veenhoven 2011; Musselwhite, Chap. 9).

In conclusion, scientific evidence for the link between travel and wellbeing has been presented, showing that human wellbeing and quality of life are affected by external influences on traffic (e.g., air pollution, noise, accidents), the length of the trip, the transport mode, activities done during travel, accessibility, and individual characteristics. Much of this book has been devoted to case-study applications that illustrate the relationship between travel and longer-term wellbeing, such as life satisfaction. Researchers have devoted time and resources to studying this relationship among different groups of travelers, by different modes, and for travel for different purposes, much needed and valuable knowledge. However, far fewer researchers have begun to apply their findings on travel and wellbeing to understanding voluntarily travel behavior change or to designing intervention programs with positive links to wellbeing outcomes. This issue is relevant since many policies are nowadays being implemented worldwide in order to persuade or force individuals to change their car use.

The following section focuses on travel behavior change and wellbeing consequences. In this section, we discuss what happens *before* travel behavior change, the focus being on individual predictions and on thoughts of possible consequences regarding wellbeing. It turns out that people may not always make the most optimum travel mode choices in relation to their long-term wellbeing. The third section of this chapter focuses on interventions as a means of counteracting possible negative wellbeing consequences and of breaking travel habits. In the final conclusions section, we discuss important avenues for future research.

## 14.2 Travel Behavior Change and Wellbeing Consequences

It is well known that alternatives to the car may reduce personal utility when essential sacrifices are included (Wall et al. 2007), such as giving up flexibility or having freedom in life. It is also known that choices are based on the feelings that people anticipate will arise from these choices (Mellers et al. 1999; Shiv and Huber 2000). Research on affective forecasting (Wilson and Gilbert 2005) has shown that people mispredict how much pleasure or displeasure future events will bring. As a result, people sometimes make choices that do not maximize their happiness. Car users might predict that public transport will bring them stress and worries because they expect crowded buses with no possibilities of getting a seat, instead of a comfortable trip where they can relax or prepare for work. Fortunately, travelers are reasonably capable of predicting the valence (i.e., good or bad) of future travel experiences; however, they are much less capable of forecasting its intensity and duration. Studies focusing on the wellbeing consequences experienced by car users undergoing a travel behavior change suggest that outcomes are not always as negative as the car users themselves predict (Pedersen et al. 2011a). Consequently, when predicting satisfaction with public transport, car users foresee being less satisfied (which they also correctly are); however, they tend to predict that they will feel much worse than they actually report feeling, during a free trial. This is defined as forecasting bias (Wilson et al. 2003), which explains how similar and intense experiences are more likely to be stored in memory. One example of this is frequently-experienced negative critical incidents while using public transport, such as a lack of time-keeping, which makes people eventually assess the service as unreliable (e.g., Friman et al. 2001). When people generate predictions based on such "peak" incidents, they tend to overestimate the intensity (e.g., the degree of stress or anger) of their future emotional reactions (Pedersen et al. 2011b).

People are also frequently poor predictors of how their affective experiences evolve over time (i.e., duration), and their possibility of adapting to different circumstances (Wilson and Gilbert 2003). When people decide where to work and live, they must consider how far they are prepared to commute. When making trade-offs between different options, people mispredict their ability to adapt, something which has consequences for their long-term wellbeing (Frey and Stutzer 2014). For instance, a high salary and an upmarket residence are often preferable to a short commute.

For many people, a travel behavior change is a major shift in life. From mainly taking the car to combining walking and public transport, for example. Adapting one's life to departure and arrival times, choosing one's clothes depending on the weather, and route planning can all induce stress that brings dissatisfaction with life in general. However, most people will return, after some time, to a relatively stable level of wellbeing or happiness under the hedonic treadmill effect (Loewenstein and Ubel 2008). This phenomenon is explained by people's tendency to adjust to changes in their circumstances; for instance, people adjust their desires as regards what to attain using a certain travel mode. When going by car, people can get to all of their activities at any given time during the day. Switching to public transport entails being restricted to scheduled routes and timetables. Adjusting to the current situation lessens the gap between people's expectations and the delivery of the service, making people more satisfied (or less dissatisfied).

The hedonic treadmill effect may depend on specific circumstances (Diener et al. 2006), suggesting that people do not always revert to a base level. Whether or not people revert to a base level in wellbeing after switching their travel behavior is unclear. A related mechanism is adaptation (Ubel et al. 2005), which means that, by looking for other sources of pleasure, individuals actively seek to improve a setting that invokes negative responses. Bringing along devices for relaxation (e.g., music players) or work (e.g., books, laptops) is a strategy people use to reduce the impact of an otherwise unstimulating environment (Ettema et al. 2012), however, there might also be other strategies that could be encouraged. In a study by Frey and Stutzer

(2014), individuals' commuting decisions were analyzed using data on subjective wellbeing. The results showed that people who spend more time commuting report less life satisfaction and it is concluded that commuters are not fully compensated for the burden of commuting by a higher salary, a better living environment, or a lower rent. Frey and Stutzer (2014) conclude that people do not adapt very well to commuting and even seem to become more sensitive to the burden of commuting over time.

Schwarz and Xu (2011) describe how the expected positive affect of driving a luxury car was evaluated significantly higher than the anticipated positive affect of driving a budget car. However, when asking drivers of luxury and budget cars to report their wellbeing during their last commute, no differences are observed in their travel experiences. Attention paid to the driving characteristics (e.g., comfort, design of the vehicle, speed) is likely to be much less pronounced than the attention paid to daily hassles and the tasks of the working day to come.

The focusing illusion suggested by Schkade and Kahneman (1998) is another important psychological process influencing people's travel mode changes. When people are induced to believe that they must travel by car (such as when living in car-friendly cities), they greatly exaggerate the difference that the alternatives would have on their longer-term wellbeing, such as life satisfaction. An illusion arises when people focus on a limited set of factors relating to travel, factors which then bias their expectations positively or negatively. Initially, car users can harbor a negative attitude toward cycling as they tend to focus too much on the annoying and stressful factors, such as the right clothing for the weather or on helmet use. By focusing on the negative factors, they tend to overlook the other more enjoyable factors, such as having the opportunity to enjoy the scenery or to interact with people. A gap in our knowledge concerns how to get car users to pay attention to the things in life that will be the same no matter whether they travel by car or by alternative travel modes.

Research shows how satisfaction with everyday travel affects our emotional wellbeing, in turn bringing implications for our longer-term wellbeing (Friman et al. 2017). However, few studies have examined, in real life, how long-term wellbeing is influenced by travel mode change. A related study by Abou-Zeid et al. (2012) shows that, before a change in travel mode (a 1-week trial), car commuters had rated their satisfaction with public transport lower than commuting by car; however, during the first few days after changing, many had increased their level of satisfaction with commuting by car. Surprisingly, changing had made them focus more on the positive aspects of life with car travel. After the 1-week trial, some had rated the service as satisfactory and these people were also more likely later on to occasionally use public transport. This study was replicated (Abou-Zeid and Ben-Akiva 2012), with the results showing again that a change leading to a lower level of satisfaction with travel made the car users return to their cars. Those more satisfied initially with the service kept on commuting by public transport after the study had ended. Interestingly, the satisfaction gap between those remaining with the service and those returning to their cars increased after the trial. Testing public transport had apparently served to strengthen the participants' initial attitude toward this travel mode. In yet another study focusing on travel behavior change, Pedersen et al. (2011b) found that car users reported greater satisfaction with public transport during a trial compared to their initial expectations regarding the service. Two years after the trial, their memory of using public transport had returned to, and was even slightly lower than, the expected level of satisfaction. It was concluded that car users' perceptions of alternatives may be biased even after they have used the alternative with a positive outcome. Martin et al. (2014) analyzed longitudinal data with the aim of investigating how travel behavior changes correlate with changes in longer-term wellbeing, something which is naturally influenced by many more factors than travel. The findings showed that a travel behavior change, from car or public transport to walking or cycling, is associated with greater long-term wellbeing. Possible explanations for this include the intrinsic enjoyment of physical activity and its positive effects on physical health.

In summary, studies show that people misjudge their long-term wellbeing as regards different travel modes and different time commutes. This seems especially pronounced when making trade-offs between different options that are difficult to evaluate beforehand. However, research indicates that both travel decisions and travel behavior changes have implications for long-term wellbeing, such as life satisfaction. There may thus be a need for guidelines or interventions aimed at correcting or reducing the effect of mispredictions. More knowledge is needed of how to aid car users' evaluations of alternative travel modes. Furthermore, there may also be a need for interventions aimed at self-management in order to support and aid the prevention of travel change related problems and to contribute to the (pro)active creation and maintenance of wellbeing.

## 14.3   Interventions as a Means of Counteracting Negative Wellbeing and Breaking Habits

Most people value 'instant utility' (Kahneman 1999). Future oriented behavior will be easier to conduct when it yields positive feelings in the present. For instance, cycling for good health in the future will be easier if the infrastructure and milieu are of high quality. When people make behavioral changes, they take the predicted emotional consequences into account. However, as has been discussed in the previous section, such predictions tend to be biased. The first part of this section focuses on how to reduce impact bias using a variety of interventions or defocusing techniques. The second part focuses on how travel behavior interventions can break travel habits when the intervention is related to people's stage or motivation of change.

Pedersen et al. (2012) tested two defocusing techniques on car users: a generic technique (low personal relevance and involvement) and a self-relevant technique (high personal relevance and involvement). The results showed that car users' predictions about their future wellbeing, when travelling by public transport, were notably higher when they were subjected to a self-relevant defocusing technique (in which participants listed their daily activities and indicated how much time they spend on these daily activities). Using a self-relevant defocusing technique, car users may be inclined to think about how their commute might not negatively impact on other life domains, or life in general, even if they were to commute by public transport. Comerford (2011) used a defocusing technique on bus travelers called Affective Averaging. The purpose of this technique was to construct a representation of the average commuting experience and to thus counteract forecasting errors. Bus travelers were approached on-board buses and invited to rate how much they were enjoying "the time spent traveling to work or university today". People not travelling by bus were asked to predict the average enjoyment rating given by the bus travelers. A random sample of people, not traveling by bus either, were likewise asked to predict the average enjoyment rating given by the bus travelers. Before the random sample of people gave their predictions, they were presented with the Affective Averaging procedure. Comparing the ratings given by the three groups showed no difference between bus travelers giving online ratings, and guided by the Affective Average technique, and the predictions given by people in the Affective Averaging condition. Thus, Affective Averaging successfully attenuated the bias and caused the respondent to form a representation of the average travel experience of a commute. Information on average commute experiences may be difficult to access spontaneously, but seems to be important when people are making predictions about their future wellbeing.

Biased predictions can also be attenuated by means of personal experiences when trying out new behaviors. One popular policy measure is a free travel card for public transport during a prespecified time period (1-month, 2 weeks, or even 1-day) (Thøgersen 2009). Previous research shows that having car-using students try out public transport services gives them information about bus systems (e.g., schedules, routes, stops), increasing their knowledge and perceived behavioral control (Gärling et al. 2017). The fact that the students also reassessed the cost of public transport travel can be taken as evidence that actual experiences lead to better, or more correct, judgments. When experiencing a service (e.g., public transport, car pool), it may turn out to be the case that many more aspects than were expected influence satisfaction, thus possibly dampening a negative pre-attitude.

In order to change a behavior, one needs to be ready to make a change; the biggest barrier to change is often in people's minds. One approach to changing travel behavior is to use a stage or processual model (Friman et al. 2017). The transtheoretical model of change (Prochaska and DiClemente 1984) suggests that behavior change is a sequence of the stages through which individuals progress toward a desired kind of behavior. The TTM consists of five major stages, as previously described in transport studies (Diniz et al. 2015; Redding et al. 2015; Crawford et al. 2001). During the first stage (precontemplation), the individual has no intention of changing his/her behavior and is unaware of the negative consequences of his/her current behavior, or believes that these consequences are insignificant. During the next stage (contemplation) the individual is starting to think about changing his/her behavior within the next 6 months. However, while contemplating, he/she overestimates the cost of change and thus remains undecided regarding the benefits. During the ensuing preparation stage, the individual is planning to make a change within a month, and has begun taking small steps toward changing. When people reach the action stage, they have recently changed their behavior and are actively trying to modify this (problem) behavior, and to acquire new behaviors. Finally, individuals transition to the maintenance stage once they have been able to maintain a change for more than 6 months, and are actively trying to prevent a relapse. Relapsing means regressing by one or more stages, something which may occur at any stage (Bamberg 2007). A recent review (Friman et al. 2017) shows that transport interventions for behavioral change greatly support processes such as consciousness raising, self-efficacy, social support, and skill improvement. Furthermore, travel-based interventions have most frequently been implemented during the contemplation stage, followed by the preparation stage. The selected studies included in the review by Friman et al. (2017) confirm that interventions supporting the various processes defined in the TTM successfully trigger a change in travel behavior. Positive changes concern a reduction in car travel (number of trips) and an increase in trips using active modes (e.g., public transport, bicycle rides, and walking). Additionally, carpooling increases as regards the number of trips made. Changes in willingness to use a specific mode, actual main mode use, and trip distance in meters per day all followed the same pattern.

In summary, it has become important to explore why people are slow to adopt alternatives to the private car. Explanatory factors include freedom of choice (Steg et al. 2001), resistance to changes of habit (Verplanken et al. 1994), affective attachment (Mann and Abraham 2006), and the pleasure of driving (Gatersleben 2007; Steg 2005). Bias as regards predicting future wellbeing is an additional major factor. Biases and misprediction may result in negative pretravel attitudes to alternative travel modes. Different interventions can be implemented, however, in order to successfully counteract such biases. Self-relevance and average commute experiences are two techniques that have been applied successfully. Another technique is giving car users the opportunity to try out a new behavior by providing free travel cards for public transport. More techniques and their effect on predictions should be explored in order to use this knowledge when designing future interventions.

Changing travel behavior is easier said than done. Many people attempt to change their travel behavior without succeeding in the long run. This failure can be simply explained by people not knowing how to change. A recent review (Friman et al. 2017) indicates that future interventions need to take a process perspective into account in order to help people to assess their readiness to change, and to improve their wellbeing. In future studies, more knowledge is needed of the effects of different interventions aimed at changing people's travel behavior. More specifically, we need a better understanding of how, and in what way, interventions impact upon people's wellbeing and quality of life.

## 14.4 Conclusion

This chapter sought to achieve two things. The first was to discuss what is known about individuals' predictions and accompanying thoughts about possible consequences regarding wellbeing when performing a travel mode change. The second was to discuss and illustrate various interventions as a means of counteracting mispredictions and breaking travel habits. The overall aim of this chapter has been to provide ideas and directions for future research. In light of this discussion, we have come to the conclusion that the need exists for knowledge of how to aid people's judgments as regards switching to sustainable alternatives. There is also a need for research into how to prevent a loss of, or to support a gain in, wellbeing when traveling sustainably. The overall goal of every transport policy should be to provide sustainable travel accompanied by sustained or increased wellbeing.

**Acknowledgements** Financial support provided to Margareta Friman and Lars E Olsson for their work on this chapter was obtained through grant #2014-05335 from the Swedish Governmental Agency for Innovation Systems.

## References

Abou-Zeid, M., & Ben-Akiva, M. (2012). Well-being and activity-based models. *Transportation, 39*(6), 1189–1207.

Abou-Zeid, M., Witter, R., Bierlaire, M., Kaufmann, V., & Ben-Akiva, M. (2012). Happiness and travel mode switching: Findings from a Swiss public transportation experiment. *Transport Policy, 19*(1), 93–104.

Bamberg, S. (2007). Is a stage model a useful approach to explain car drivers' willingness to use public transportation? *Journal of Applied Social Psychology, 37*, 1757–1783.

Besser, L. M., & Dannenberg, A. L. (2005). Walking to public transit: Steps to help meet physical activity recommendations. *American Journal of Preventive Medicine, 29*(4), 273–280.

Buehler, R., Pucher, J., & Altshuler, A. (2017). Vienna's path to sustainable transport. *International Journal of Sustainable Transportation, 11*(4), 257–271.

Comerford, D. A. (2011). Attenuating focalism in affective forecasts of the commuting experience: Implications for economic decisions and policy making. *Journal of Economic Psychology, 32* (5), 691–699.

Crawford, F., Mutrie, N., & Hanlon, P. (2001). Employee attitudes towards active commuting. *International Journal of Health Promotion and Education, 39*(1), 14–20.

Diener, E., Lucas, R. E., & Scollon, C. N. (2006). Beyond the hedonic treadmill: Revising the adaptation theory of well-being. *American Psychologist, 61*(4), 305.

Diniz, I. M., Duarte, M. D. F. S., Peres, K. G., de Oliveira, E. S., & Berndt, A. (2015). Active commuting by bicycle: Results of an educational intervention study. *Journal of Physical Activity and Health, 12*(6), 801–807.

Ettema, D., Friman, M., Gärling, T., Olsson, L. E., & Fujii, S. (2012). How in-vehicle activities affect work commuters' satisfaction with public transport. *Journal of Transport Geography, 24*, 215–222.

Ferrero, E., Alessandrini, S., & Balanzino, A. (2016). Impact of the electric vehicles on the air pollution from a highway. *Applied Energy, 169*, 450–459.

Flint, E., Webb, E., & Cummins, S. (2016). Change in commute mode and body-mass index: Prospective, longitudinal evidence from UK Biobank. *The Lancet Public Health, 1*(2), 46–55.

Frey, B. S., & Stutzer, A. (2014). Economic consequences of mispredicting utility. *Journal of Happiness Studies, 15*(4), 937–956.

Friman, M., Edvardsson, B., & Gärling, T. (2001). Frequency of negative critical incidents and satisfaction with public transport services. I. *Journal of Retailing and Consumer Services, 8*(2), 95–104.

Friman, M., Huck, J., & Olsson, L. E. (2017). Transtheoretical model of change during travel behavior interventions: An integrative review. *International journal of environmental research and public health, 14*(6), 581.

Gärling, T., Bamberg, S., & Friman, M. (2017). The role of attitude in choice of travel, satisfaction with travel, and change to sustainable travel. In D. Albarracin & B. T. Johnson (Eds.), *Handbook of attitudes: Applications*. London: Routledge.

Gatersleben, B. (2007). Affective and symbolic aspects of car use. In *Threats from car traffic to the quality of urban life: Problems, causes and solutions* (pp. 219–233). Emerald Group Publishing Limited.

Gatersleben, B., & Uzzell, D. (2007). Affective appraisals of the daily commute: Comparing perceptions of drivers, cyclists, walkers, and users of public transport. *Environment and Behavior, 39*(3), 416–431.

Hansson, E., Mattisson, K., Björk, J., Östergren, P. O., & Jakobsson, K. (2011). Relationship between commuting and health outcomes in a cross-sectional population survey in southern Sweden. *BMC Public Health, 11*(1), 834.

Litman, T. (2015). *Evaluating public transit benefits and costs*. Victoria Transport Policy Institute.

Loewenstein, G., & Ubel, P. A. (2008). Hedonic adaptation and the role of decision and experience utility in public policy. *Journal of Public Economics, 92*(8), 1795–1810.

Lucas, K. (2012). Transport and social exclusion: Where are we now? *Transport Policy, 20*, 105–113.

Mann, E., & Abraham, C. (2006). The role of affect in UK commuters' travel mode choices: An interpretative phenomenological analysis. *British Journal of Psychology, 97*(2), 155–176.

Martin, A., Goryakin, Y., & Suhrcke, M. (2014). Does active commuting improve psychological wellbeing? Longitudinal evidence from eighteen waves of the British Household Panel Survey. *Preventive Medicine, 69*, 296–303.

Mellers, B., Schwartz, A., & Ritov, I. (1999). Emotion-based choice. *Journal of Experimental Psychology: General, 128*(3), 332.

Mokhtarian, P. L. (2005). Travel as a desired end, not just a means. *Transportation Research Part A: Policy and Practice, 39*(2–3), 93–96.

Nawijn, J., & Veenhoven, R. (2011). The effect of leisure activities on life satisfaction: The importance of holiday trips. In *The human pursuit of well-being* (pp. 39–53). Springer Netherlands.

Office for National Statistics. (2014). *Commuting and personal well-being*. Washington, DC: Office for National Statistics.

Pedersen, T., Friman, M., & Kristensson, P. (2011a). Affective forecasting: Predicting and experiencing satisfaction with public transportation. *Journal of Applied Social Psychology, 41*(8), 1926–1946.

Pedersen, T., Friman, M., & Kristensson, P. (2011b). The role of predicted, on-line experienced and remembered satisfaction in current choice to use public transport Services. *Journal of Retailing and Consumer Services, 18*, 471–475.

Pedersen, T., Kristensson, P., & Friman, M. (2012). Counteracting the focusing illusion: Effects of defocusing on car users' predicted satisfaction with public transport. *Journal of Environmental Psychology, 32*(1), 30–36.

Prochaska, J. O., & DiClemente, C. C. (1984). Self change processes, self efficacy and decisional balance across five stages of smoking cessation. *Progress in Clinical and Biological Research, 156*, 131.

Recio, A., Linares, C., Banegas, J. R., & Díaz, J. (2016). The short-term association of road traffic noise with cardiovascular, respiratory, and diabetes-related mortality. *Environmental Research, 150*, 383–390.

Redding, C. A., Mundorf, N., Kobayashi, H., Brick, L., Horiuchi, S., Paiva, A. L., & Prochaska, J. O. (2015). Sustainable transportation stage of change, decisional balance, and self-efficacy scale development and validation in two university samples. *International Journal of Environmental Health Research, 25*(3), 241–253.

Schkade, D. A., & Kahneman, D. (1998). Does living in California make people happy? A focusing illusion in judgments of life satisfaction. *Psychological Science, 9*(5), 340–346.

Shiv, B., & Huber, J. (2000). The impact of anticipating satisfaction on consumer choice. *Journal of Consumer Research, 27*(2), 202–216.

Stanley, J. K., Hensher, D. A., Stanley, J. R., & Vella-Brodrick, D. (2011). Mobility, social exclusion and well-being: Exploring the links. *Transportation Research Part A: Policy and Practice, 45*(8), 789–801.

Steg, L. (2005). Car use: Lust and must. Instrumental, symbolic and affective motives for car use. *Transportation Research Part A: Policy and Practice, 39*(2), 147–162.

Steg, L., Vlek, C., & Slotegraaf, G. (2001). Instrumental-reasoned and symbolic-affective motives for using a motor car. *Transportation Research Part F: Traffic Psychology and Behaviour, 4*(3), 151–169.

Stutzer, A., & Frey, B. S. (2008). Stress that doesn't pay: The commuting paradox. *The Scandinavian Journal of Economics, 110*(2), 339–366.

Thøgersen, J. (2009). Promoting public transport as a subscription service: Effects of a free month travel card. *Transport Policy, 16*(6), 335–343.

Ubel, P. A., Loewenstein, G., & Jepson, C. (2005). Disability and sunshine: Can hedonic predictions be improved by drawing attention to focusing illusions or emotional adaptation? *Journal of Experimental Psychology: Applied, 11*(2), 111.

Verplanken, B., Aarts, H., van Knippenberg, A., & van Knippenberg, C. (1994). Attitude versus general habit: Antecedents of travel mode choice. *Journal of Applied Social Psychology, 24*, 285–300.

Walker, I., Kennedy, J., Martin, S., & Rice, H. (2016). How might people near national roads be affected by traffic noise as electric vehicles increase in number? A laboratory study of subjective evaluations of environmental noise. *PloS one, 11*(3), e0150516.

Wall, R., Devine-Wright, P., & Mill, G. A. (2007). Comparing and combining theories to explain proenvironmental intentions: The case of commuting-mode choice. *Environment and Behavior, 39*(6), 731–753.

Wilson, T. D., & Gilbert, D. T. (2005). Affective forecasting knowing what to want. *Current Directions in Psychological Science, 14*(3), 131–134.

Wilson, T. D., Meyers, J., & Gilbert, D. T. (2003). "How happy was I, anyway?" A retrospective impact bias. *Social Cognition, 21*(6), 421–446.